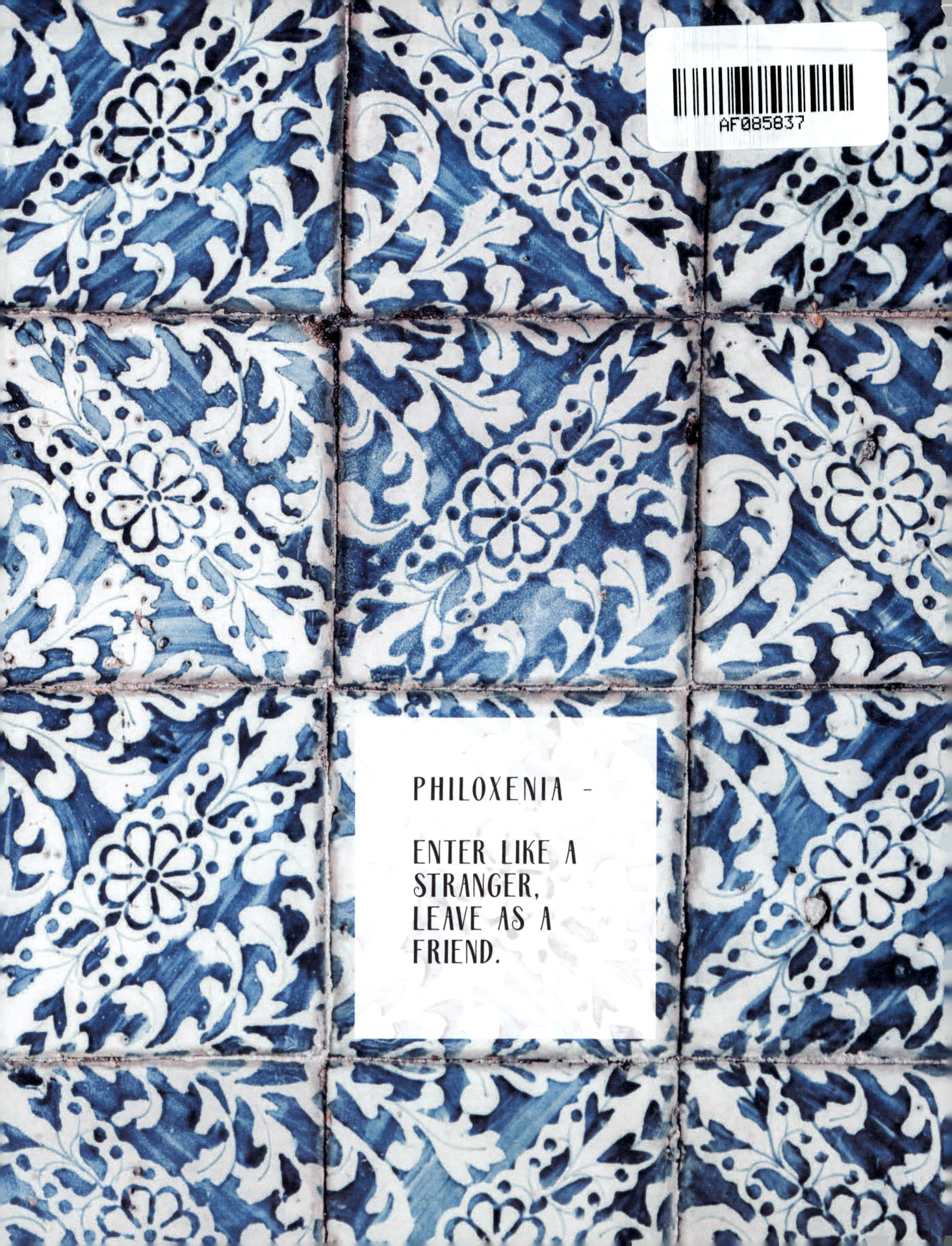

PHILOXENIA –

ENTER LIKE A STRANGER, LEAVE AS A FRIEND.

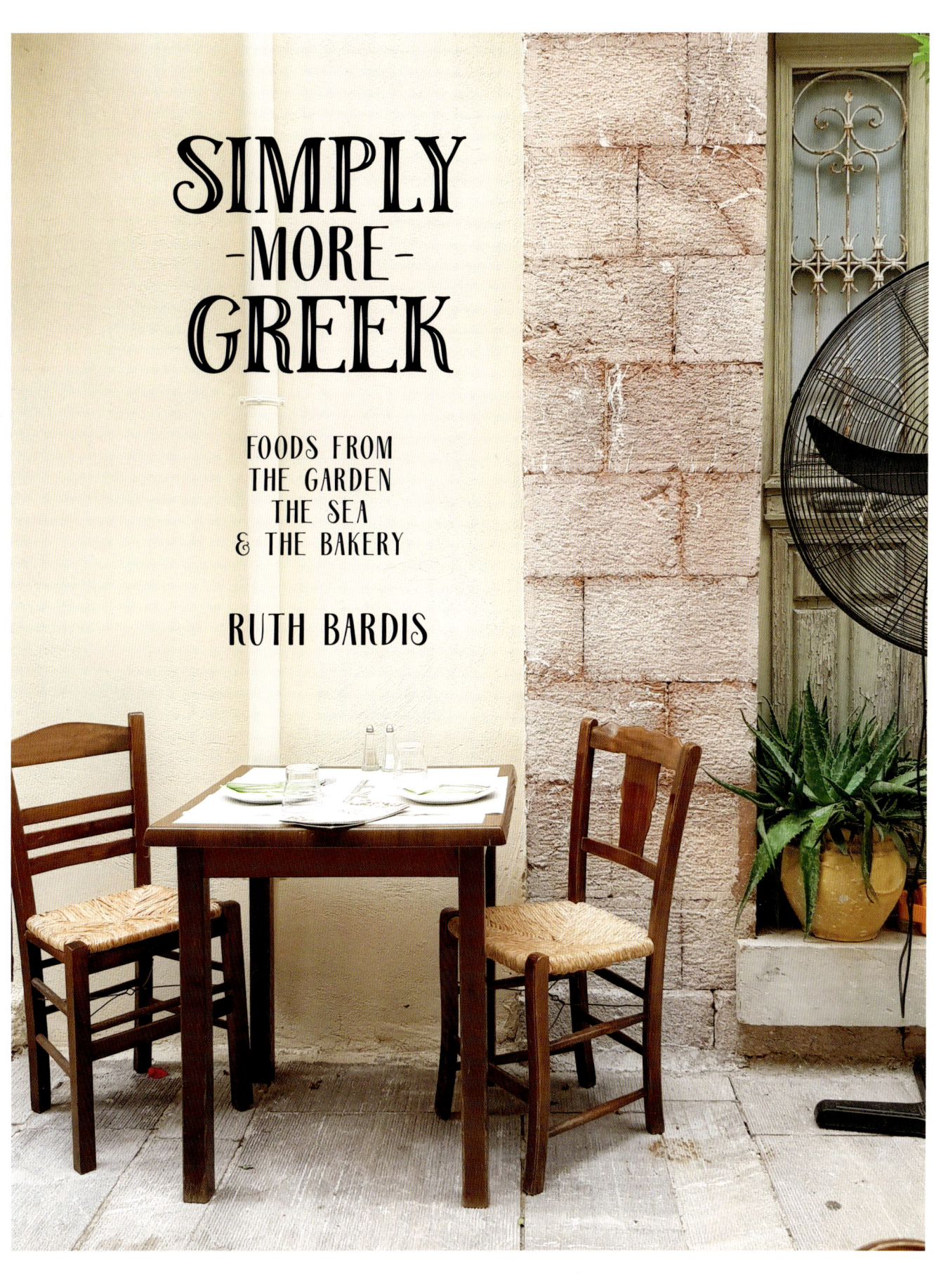

SIMPLY -MORE- GREEK

FOODS FROM THE GARDEN THE SEA & THE BAKERY

RUTH BARDIS

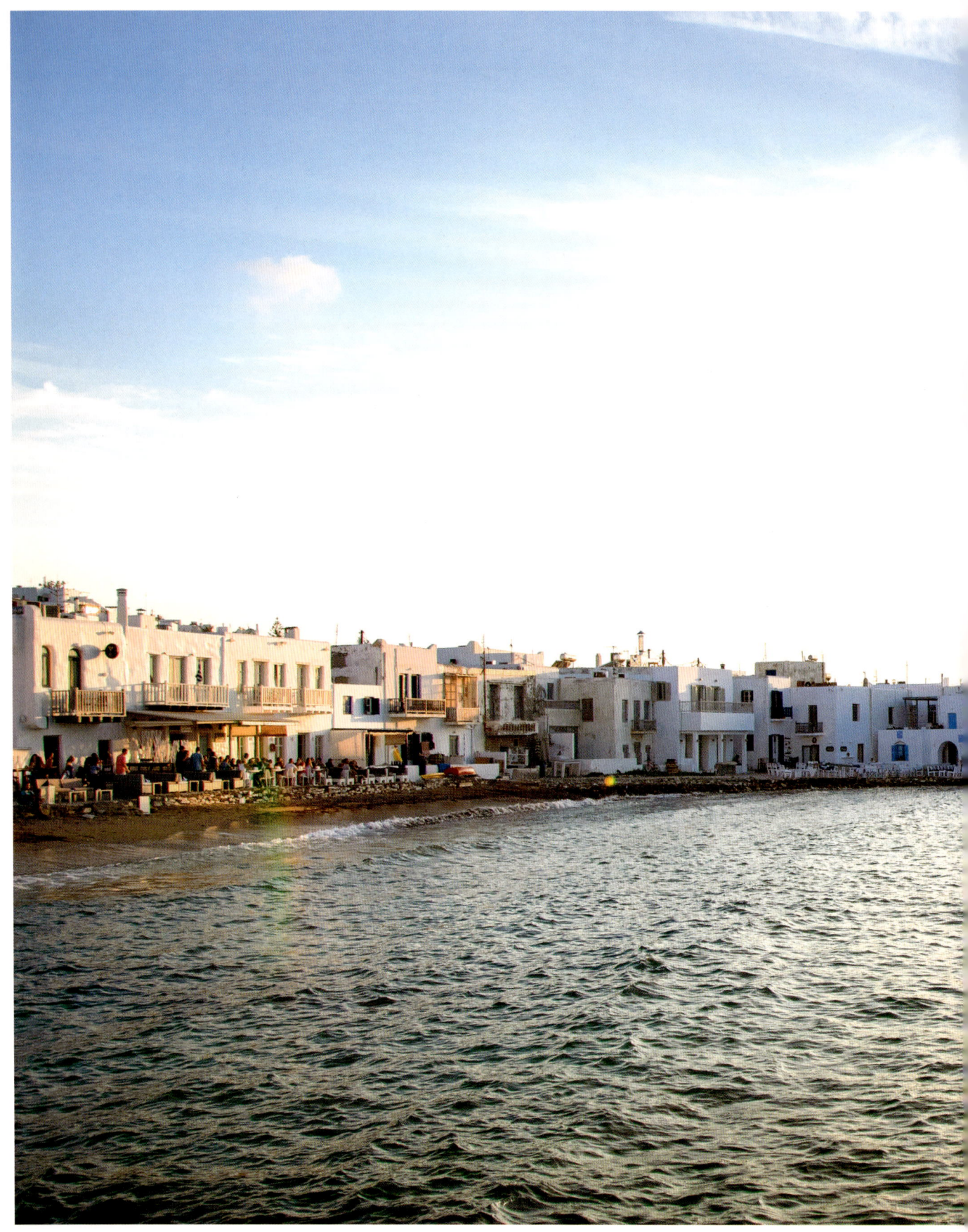

ATHANASIOS,

I was able because you gave me wings to fly.
Of course, book three is for you!

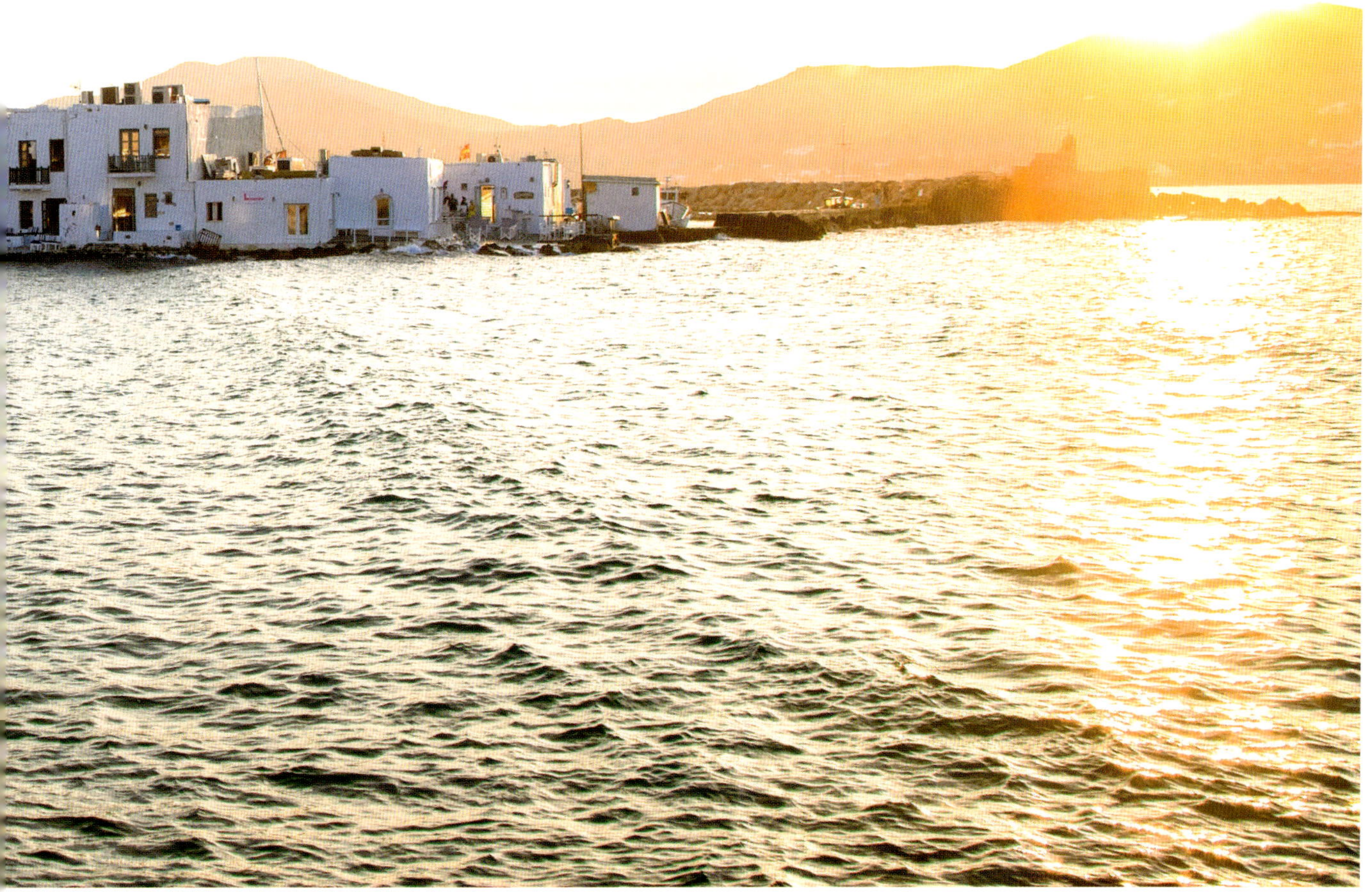

ΕΠΙΣΤΡΕΦΩ
RETURNING

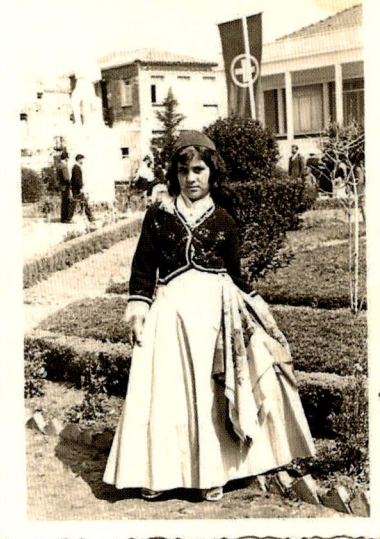

I have just arrived at my mother's birthplace, Gargaliani, Greece, two hours from the regional capital, Kalamata. It is a place that remains empty most of the year except through the summer when the extended family use it as a holiday hub to enjoy the Greek summer. There is a sense of serenity, a powerful feeling of connection to this place. I enter via a metal gate that has recently been added to prevent any foreigners or trespassers to enter. Up and around the stairs I go, feeling a million emotions run through my head as I think of my mother's childhood. I pass by overgrown weeds that have yet to be trimmed by whichever family member resides there next. There is a long concrete fence surrounding the property on the roadside and a large water tank to the other side. There are but a few windows and a newly restored ceramic tile roof on a small stone home. I sit on a concrete bench and look toward the house. I allow my mind to journey. *No need for haste*, I tell myself. I do not want to miss anything. I want to take it all in, the smell of the air, the warmth of the sun, and the sound of birdsong. I can think slowly in this place. I must. I do. I want to be thankful for this part of my history. I feel captivated and so nostalgic. This is part of my story, my Greek narrative, my culinary journey engraved in me, which starts right here. A part of me feels as though it is returning home. It starts with my mother, and therefore, I write my third Greek cookbook. She was poor; they were poor. They had a garden, they had the sea nearby, and they baked in wood-fired clay ovens.

My beginnings are half in this place as they are also on the island of Kefalonia, the hometown of my father. I need to savor this time; I ought to contemplate, imagine the true experiences, the ones lived by my mother, and enjoy the smells, the air of the place that once was her home.

I travel in my mind to the 1950s. I know the countless childhood stories my mother has communicated with me. I glance around and picture my mother as a child, especially in the summer. Her olive skin is now tanned from the sun. She has curly black hair, no shoes on her feet, and wears rags for clothes. She secretly departs and goes to neighboring houses to pluck fruit from trees or steal vegetables from other gardens and eggs from chicken barns to eat. Food was scarce for her. She was the second youngest child, so food was not always a priority for her among her many siblings. If she were caught stealing, she would get a good spanking, and therefore she would be mischievous and think of creative ways to provide extra food for herself. She would hide any extra food she found and place it between rocks and bricks to have on days when they had no food to eat.

I am here now. The daughter of this young girl who grew up in this home. The young girl who had many dreams. Dreams she once had of feasting and eating like some of her richer neighboring friends, wearing shoes that had no holes and clothes that were not ripped. She dreamed of wearing dresses that would be bright, beautiful, elegant, and becoming. She looked down at her fingers and dreamed of a gold band and diamond ring that would be given to her by a man who would promise to love and be hers forever. *Someday*, she dreamed, *he will take me away, and together we will have children, many children, and a family full of joy and laughter*. She dreamed of a house decked out in simple but beautiful things. She dreamed of little heads, all crowding around her to hear stories, be hugged, and be loved by her, their mother.

Maybe one day, she dreamed. *Maybe one day*.

And now I, the daughter of this young girl in my forties, am standing in this place. My mother's dreams came alive in ways she never really thought would come to pass.

I have not had to experience the difficulties my mother endured, nor have I had to dream those types of dreams. Yet as I sit here, I want to put myself in the shoes of my mother as a young girl uncertain of what her future would hold.

I see a water tank. I walk toward it and place my hands on this large tank now painted white.

Here I am thankful.

Here I pray and thank God for protecting my mother. Just shy of her eighth birthday, she accidently fell into this water-filled tank. She recalls swallowing water at a rate that was choking her, and she was unable to float. She was rescued. She survived.

To my left there is a vine, overgrown and much in need of pruning. The leaves are bright green, and the dark red grapes are draping. I gather some grapes. I do not even bother to wash them. There is no need. There have been no pesticides or sprays on this vine. They are organic, just the way they should be. I place a few in my mouth. They are flavorful and juicy. I am unsure how many of these my mother was able to consume as she was not permitted to help herself because of the scarcity of food.

Poverty was hard.

I stop and think of my grandfather. I picture him seated on a wooden and woven chair on this front porch, gently moving the beads of his *komboloi* (worry beads) and slurping a strong, unsweetened Greek coffee. His mind travels, wondering if these days of hardship will ever end. He was strong and tall, close to seven feet. A white-haired man, twenty-five years older than my grandmother. He was a hardworking family man who, just short of becoming a centenarian, died of tuberculosis.

I head to the kitchen. There is not much here. A few pots and pans.

I gaze outside the tiny kitchen window above the sink and think of my grandmother. She stood here over this exact sink. A short lady with her hair tied back and covered with a headscarf and an apron around her waist. Her hands are strong from the work in the field, though they are now starting to wrinkle. She has pigmentation and dark spots from the sun. The dark circles around her blue eyes are becoming more prominent. She is weary, she is fragile, and yet she finds the strength and resilience to endure.

Endure for survival, she must be telling herself.

What she has is not fancy, what she cooks is not abundant, nor is it many of the days sufficient for all her family. However, it is simple. It is hearty. It is derived from hands that planted a garden, harvested at the right time, and gathered from the ground or caught from the sea.

I look back at the vine. This vine, I tell myself, has yielded many leaves for many a *dolmadakia* rolled by my grandmother. The grapes were picked and pressed for juice to be turned to wine and used as a sweetener for desserts. What beauty and fruitfulness comes from the garden!

My grandmother toiled land for barley and harvested olives from their olive groves.

She had olive oil, she had flour. She had skilled hands. So she kneaded. She baked.

She provided food simply from the garden and the sea.

I must leave.

I descend the stairs and lock the metal gate. My history lies behind this gate. I shed a tear and take a few last pictures. I treasure this time, these glimpses, the experiences, the stories. I take with me the love and memories and bring it to my world—and predominantly to my food world—today. I am not in a village nor even in Greece. My life is far from here, and though I have abundance in comparison to my mother, I cannot help but remember these humble beginnings. No matter where my world is, where I go, or where I end up, these beginnings will always come with me. They are what brought me to the now, these many years later.

I do not want to lose the lessons learned, the skills acquired for resilience, and how it all started for that young girl, my mother back in the '50s. It proved to be healthy, it proved to sustain, and it proved we do not need much.

I want to cook just like them. Just like her. Just like a Greek of old.

From the garden, the sea, and the bakery

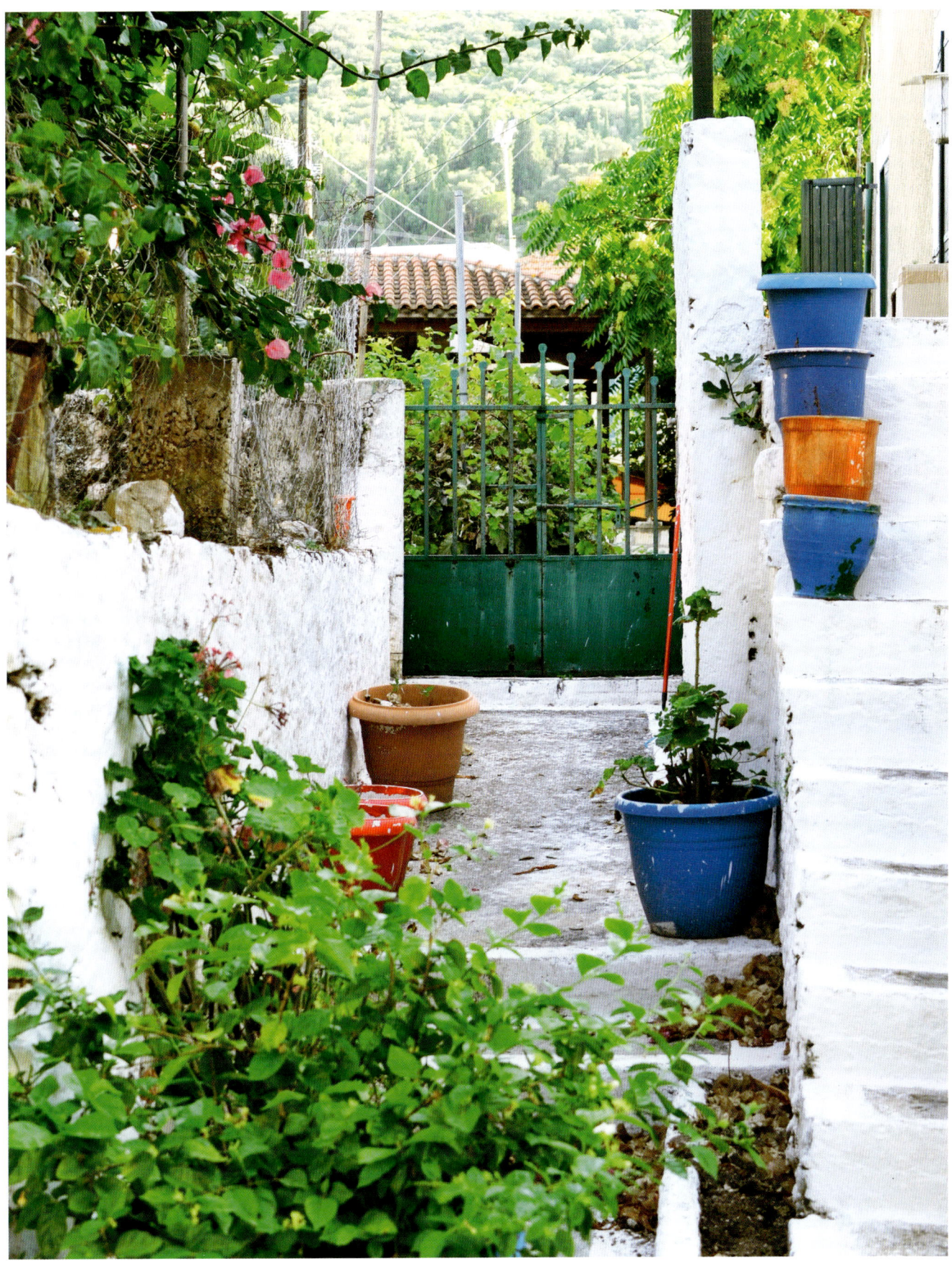

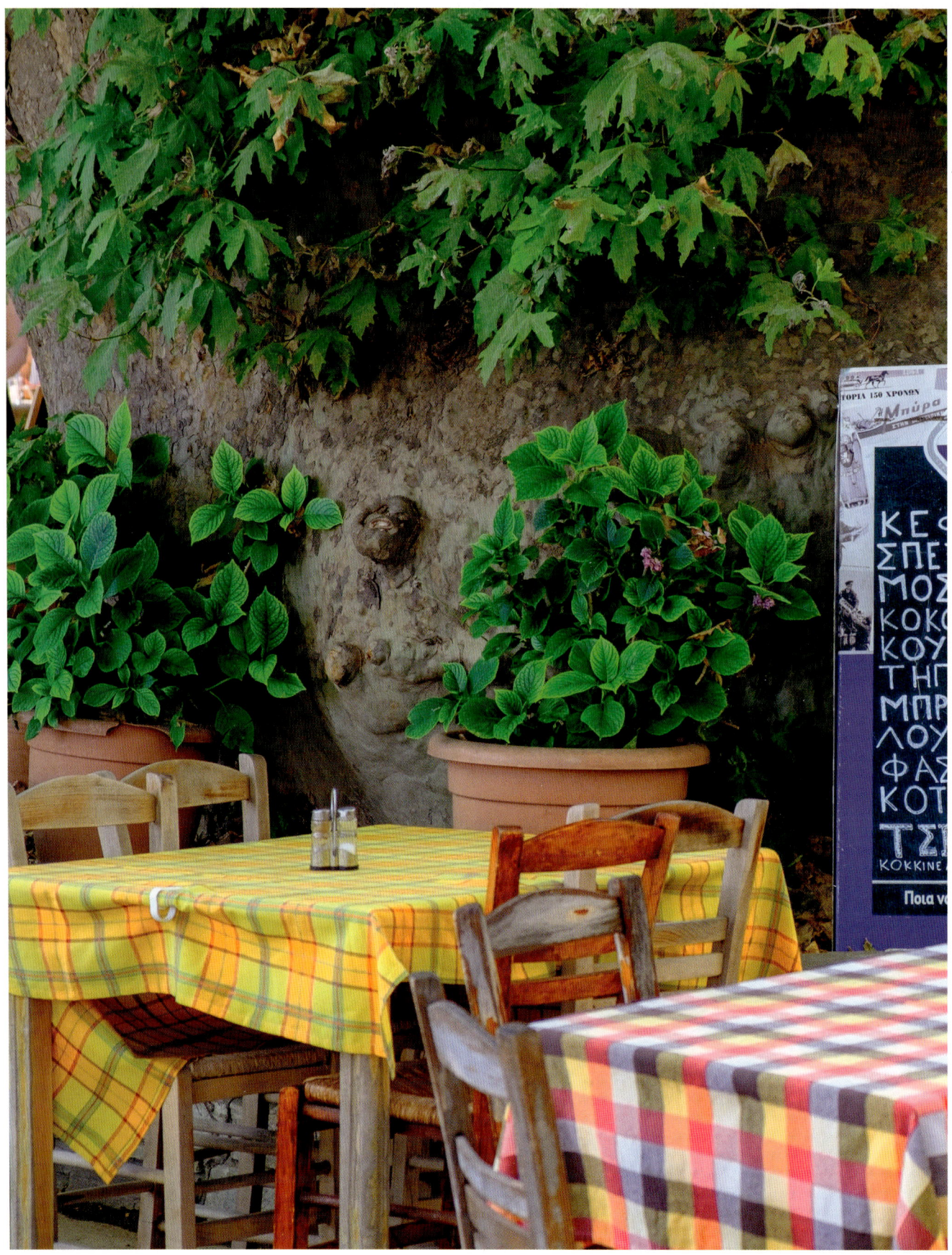

CONTENTS

14	Preface
15	Simply More Greek
16	Greece and Vegetarianism
20	Greek Folk Medicine ΕΛΛΗΝΙΚΑ ΓΙΑΤΡΟΣΟΦΙΑ
25	The Garden Ο ΚΗΠΟΣ
29	Α Light ΕΛΑΦΡΙΑ
43	Β Cooked ΜΑΓΕΙΡΕΜΕΝΑ
73	Γ Accompaniments ΣΥΝΟΔΕΥΜΑ
97	The Richness of the Sea Ο ΘΑΛΑΣΣΙΟΣ ΠΛΟΥΤΟΣ
131	The Baker Ο ΦΟΥΡΝΑΡΗΣ
135	Α The Savory Baker ΠΙΤΕΣ ΚΑΙ ΨΩΜΙΑ
175	Β The Sweet Baker ΤΗΣ ΓΛΥΚΑΣ ΤΑ ΚΑΜΩΜΑΤΑ
202	The Garden and Its Nutrients ΤΑ ΘΡΕΠΤΙΚΑ ΣΥΣΤΑΤΙΚΑ ΤΟΥ ΚΗΠΟΥ
222	Index
231	Cook's Notes
232	Acknowledgments

PREFACE

The best meals I have eaten have been in Greece, and maybe the things I have best learned about Greece have been around the table. Though I was born outside of Greece, my Greek heritage on both my mother's and father's side grow stronger in me as each day goes by. My husband, born and raised in Greece, is the one who continues to stir my hunger to know even more about Greece and its food. He regularly shares stories evoking memories of his life back in Greece, which awaken in me a deeper love and desire to want to taste for myself some more of the inexhaustible, exquisite meals Greece has to offer. Greece has exceptional food and is widely known for produce such as olives, bread, wine, honey, yogurt, beans, greens, and the like. The traditional way of eating and cooking are slowly dissipating as each generation passes. The market is being flooded with quick fast-food options, there is less quality time in the kitchen, and meals are eaten with a phone in hand.

This does not need to be so!

Greece, abundant in history, theories, passions, architecture, and so on, has also a beauty found in the "Greek way," and that is simplicity in enjoying a meal together. Something is to be said about dining around a table, uncomplicated as the food may be, and conversing, sharing, and eating. We are losing simple gestures such as the physical touch of being greeted with a kiss on both cheeks (as Greeks do) and enjoying company in an unhurried manner. This is part of the Greek way. I understand we are not all privileged to live among the pine, oak, and olive groves, nor even along a coastline of blue waters, fetching the catch of the day, undistractedly listening to the cicadas that fill the air, and drinking ouzo while the sun sets. However, we can still retain the tradition and continue to cook, serve, and eat like Greeks on the motherland. What we eat, how we eat, and why we eat the way we do, inclusive with the richness of the Greek culture regarding hospitality, are traditions we would do well to preserve.

I would suggest that, before you cook from this book, make yourself a cup of Greek coffee and take your time reading and familiarizing yourself with *Simply More Greek*. As Patience Gray in her classic book, *Honey from a Weed*, rightly says, "A book about food can be as fatiguing as sitting through a six-course dinner." I hope this book becomes more to you than that.

The aim of this book is to add "simply more Greek food" primarily from the garden, the sea, and the bakery to your repertoire of meals.

SIMPLY MORE GREEK

Over the course of history, the Greeks have created a gastronomy of delicious, healthy, and plentiful dishes. They have incorporated simple yet pleasurable flavors to tantalize the taste buds, marrying together proteins with fruits, simmering stews of vegetables in mountains of herbs and copious amounts of olive oil. There are endless dishes of freshly caught fish from the sea, rice-stuffed vegetables with raisins and spices, lentil soups, pulses, and fresh crispy salads for every season. They add nuts and fruit into layers of thin dough and bathe pastries in sweet syrups of honey and citrus rinds. No wonder Greek gastronomy has long had a reputation of promoting good health. Food is based primarily on fresh ingredients such as vegetables, fruit, and fish, and the cooking oil of choice is the venerated extra-virgin olive oil.

In this book, I lay out "simply more" Greek dishes that can be found for those desiring to cook beyond their usual repertoire. Maybe for some these dishes are unchartered territory, unknown and unsung outside their place of origin. My previous publications, *Hellenic Kanella: Memories Made in a Greek Kitchen* and *Beyond the Greek Salad: Regional Foods From All Around Greece* compile over 180 recipes of traditional foods and include meat dishes. However, in this book, there are no meat dishes but exclusively other traditional recipes that highlight dishes made with vegetables (produce from the garden), seafood (produce from the sea), and the bakery (both savory and sweet). They are recipes I have compiled from my extensive reading and research on Greek gastronomy. They are recipes that have come from Greece and recipes that look familiar but are made with other produce depending on the region in Greece. I know there are plenty of dishes that most are familiar with when they think of Greek food, but I have stepped out to showcase other amazing dishes that may sound similar but are vastly different in ingredients and taste. Even for Greeks, local specialties remain local, and therefore one would need to travel to specific regions to try these recipes unless they are recreated in their home. This is my purpose for this book. These recipes come from a mixture of local regional recipes and monasteries around Greece. They capture the essence of eating seasonally and without any meat. You will discover a plethora of delicious foods such as *pastitsio* and *stifado* made with mushrooms, sardines wrapped in vine leaves, silver beet rolls stuffed with rice and herbs, stuffed onions with spices and pine nuts. There are legumes with greens, seafood with raisins, octopus with honey, fresh salads and various dips. There is a whole chapter on traditional baked recipes such as feta cheese and fennel bread rings, greens, cheese and other variety of pies and different ways to make pastry. To end there is a chapter on desserts with recipes such as rice pudding cake, apple cake with whiskey, pastry parcels with nuts, yogurt jelly cake, and plenty more. As true as I can be to classical recipes, I have attempted to keep the recipes as authentic as possible. However, in some instances I have intensified the flavors to enhance the overall dishes yet retain their traditional character. The desire with all my books is that recipes are cooked with the same ingredients and methods as they would be in a home kitchen in the villages and cities of Greece. As always, there will be a variance in cooking style from region to region. So let us explore together and see a greater assortment of Greek vegetables, seafood, and pastry dishes.

Greece & Vegetarianism

I need to parenthetically say that the philosophical information I relay below is purely a view and not the one that I personally hold to. Eating meat, in my opinion, does not harm our soul, nor have I written this book to highlight the religious view of the Greeks, but rather I wish to expand a little on how far back we can trace vegetarian eating in Greece. The Bible says, "It is not what goes into the mouth that defiles a person, but what comes out of the mouth; this defiles a person" (Matthew 15:11, ESV).

Pythagoras, the Greek philosopher and mathematician (570 BCE–495 BCE), first adopted the concept of vegetarianism in ancient Greece. He intricately connected religion and philosophy, believing that asceticism and the absence of certain foods—withdrawing from certain pleasures—would allow a person to reach a more purposeful life. There was also a mystical conception that the soul would pass through the body of several living things after death. He thought that animals should be treated with respect and that slaughtering animals brutalized the human soul. Simultaneously, he also saw the benefits of a meat-free diet regarding its health advantages. Other Neoplatonic philosophers also wrote about strict eating such as Plutarch (c. 46 CE), whose sixteen-volume work *Moralia* includes the essay "On the Eating of Flesh," Porphyry (c. 232 CE), who wrote "On Abstinence From Animal Food," and Apollonius, who was also vegetarian. There was a link between them all, and that link was a belief that eating the vegetarian way was medicinal and aided in better health.

Whatever the case, history has proven and medical science confirmed that eating the Mediterranean way (not necessarily strictly vegetarian) aids in better health, prolongs life, and decreases ailments. Today in Greece, meat is eaten in moderation, but for this book, I will share a plethora of vegetarian meals, seafood dishes, breads, and pastries. I will briefly note some main components and benefits from eating vegetarian Greek food. No doubt the strictness and selection of foods have changed slightly with the easing of certain absences over the centuries. Most Greeks today eat a balanced diet of all things, though vegetables stand as the main ingredients from day to day.

The word "vegetarian" for some can immediately be off-putting and yet for others relatively exciting. I trust that if you have picked up this book, it will be the latter. Vegetarian meals, if executed well, are substantially fulfilling, pleasing to the eyes, tasteful, and nutritious all in one. A vegetarian-based lifestyle is one that Greeks have adopted for centuries. As you read this, you may be thinking, *Really, Greek food is largely vegetarian?* How about the famous Greek souvlaki slathered with tzatziki sauce, the luscious meat-based moussaka, or the famous Greek roast lamb? Yes, no doubt these constitute part of a Greek's repertoire of food, but they are not the primary meals eaten daily. A few generations ago, meat was eaten on special occasions, during festivities, or to break the Lenten fast, and it was also mostly eaten by the wealthy as it was considered an extravagance. It wasn't until meat became more widely available that it was served more readily.

A Greek's plant-based diet consists of a high consumption of olive oil (high level of antioxidants), fish (omega-3 fatty acids), vegetables and fruits (dietary fiber), legumes and nuts (key sources of protein), seeds, dairy (bone and digestive health), and wine (antioxidants and anti-inflammatory properties). Saturated fats are minimal. This way of life is constituted of a set of skills and knowledge in what is eaten, as well as social interaction. Communal meals have been proven to aid in longevity.

Known as the gold standard of healthy eating, there is substantial research confirming that eating the Mediterranean way is one of the best in the world and has numerous health benefits. I will not give substantial scientific evidence here as there is plenty of that written by health professionals and that information is accessible in other books and resources. Here is a synopsis. It is said that diet is the main factor contributing to cardiovascular health. Therefore, the Mediterranean diet, being rich in minimally processed plant-based foods, abundant in monounsaturated fat from extra-virgin olive oil, and low in saturated fat, meats, and dairy products, seems the ideal nutritional model for cardiovascular health and blood sugar control. In addition, this affects weight loss and weight management. Nutrient-rich foods are key, along with minimally processed foods and added sugars, which are high in calories. Bone and brain health are also linked to eating this way. Obviously, diet is a big part of the package of health behaviors, together with regular exercise and other things which form a healthier lifestyle. We must start somewhere.

My intention for this book is to tantalize your taste buds to see the beauty and benefits of eating more seafood and vegetarian Greek food. My selection of recipes is specifically chosen as to not double up from recipes in my other two cookbooks. There are an insurmountable number of recipes around Greece showcasing healthy dishes. This collection is just a sample!

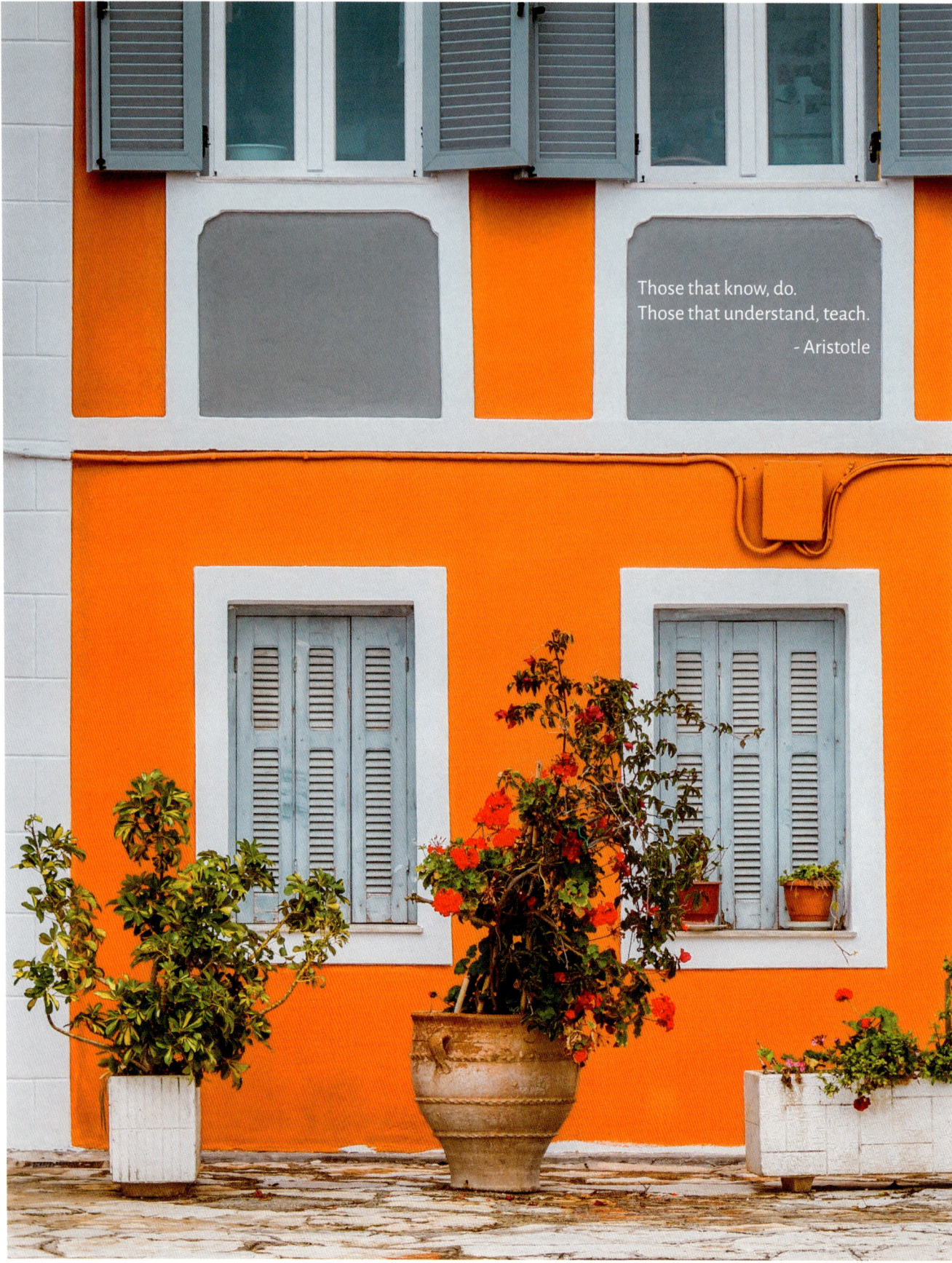

Those that know, do.
Those that understand, teach.
- Aristotle

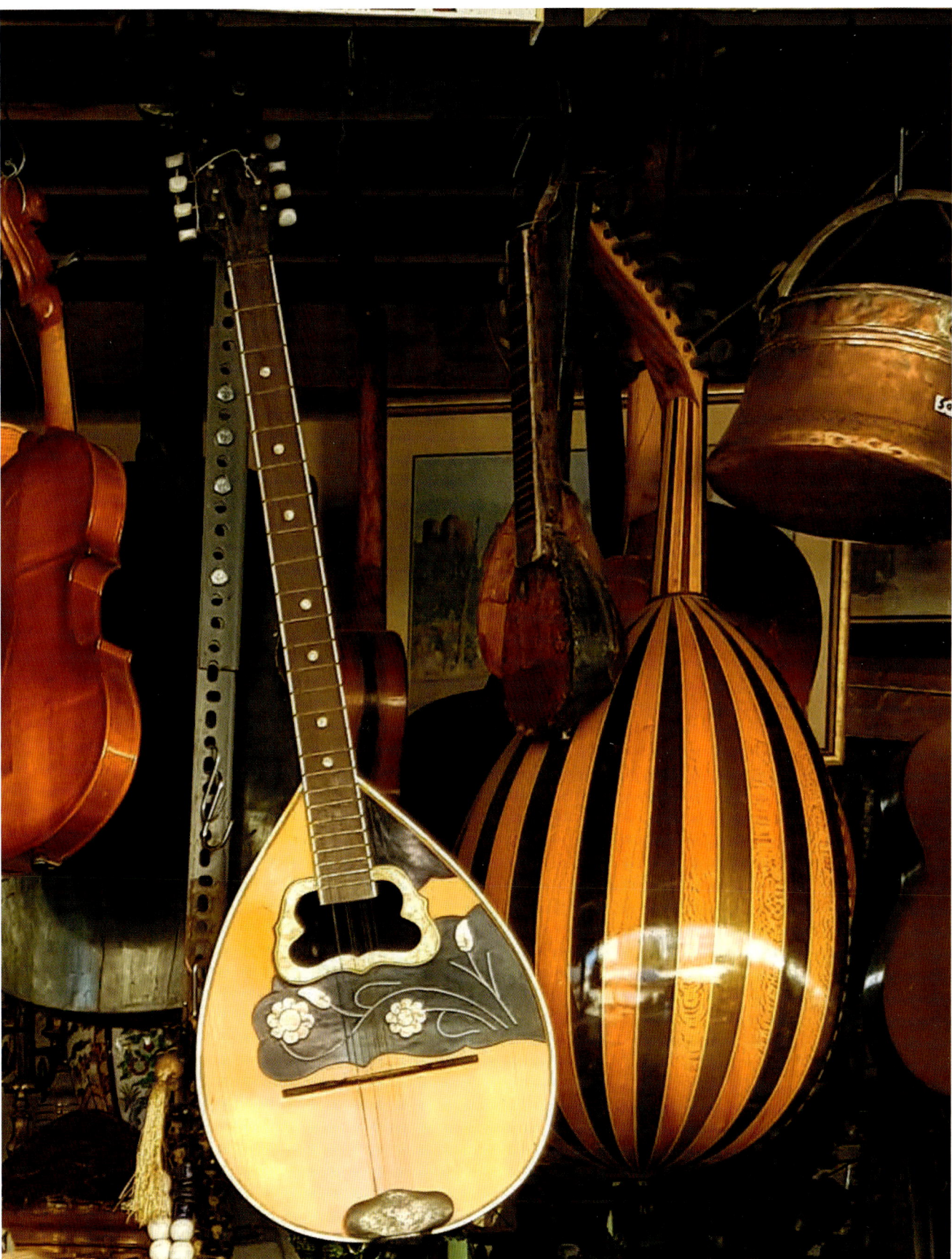

ΕΛΛΗΝΙΚΑ ΓΙΑΤΡΟΣΟΦΙΑ
GREEK FOLK MEDICINE

> Foolish the doctor who despises knowledge acquired by the ancients.
> — HIPPOCRATES

Please note: I am not a health professional. Consult your physician for any further clarification. See your doctor before implementing any of the ancient remedies below.

A specific number of herbs are a fundamental basis for many Greek meals and herbal remedies used from ancient times. The ancient Greeks were thirsty for knowledge and no doubt paved the way for philosophy, math, and science. The Greeks sought good health for military activity and sports in order to prevent injury and promote fitness. Various techniques were used like using olive oil to raise body temperature and warming up before events to prevent injuries. Greeks in ancient times associated disease with displeasing the gods and punishment for things they did or did not do. This belief continued until Hippocrates, the classical Greek physician known as the father of medicine, shifted ancient Greek medicine views from spirituality to using logic and pointing out the correlation of sicknesses affecting the body primarily, not superstitions. Hippocrates stated, "Let your food be your medicine, and your medicine be your food." He was pro-medicine but recognized the more pure, whole, and unrefined a substance is, the higher its nutritional value and the better it is assimilated and metabolized by the body.

I, too, am not substituting medicine by any means. What I write is just informative as to how the Greek culture over centuries has adapted, changed, and addressed food, both for consumption and for medicinal purposes. I find it quite humorous at times to see how herbs and ingredients were (and sometimes even now) used to aid different symptoms, some with value, some maybe not so much.

The facts below are known as λαϊκή ιατρική (layfolk medicine), or also known as old wives' tales. Take it as you will, fact or fiction, but ancient Greeks kept to many of these practices. Medicine was not as it is today, and so foods and produce were used to aid in many practical ways in the home and to the benefit of one's health. Unless you have an aging relative, you will not know many of these tips and tricks. They are slowly dissipating as each generation passes and as pharmacies fill the shelves with products for every ailment. My grandparents and parents (even still) would extensively use herbs and natural remedies to aid in sicknesses. If we had a sore throat, my father would bring out Greek honey on a teaspoon and insist we swallow it slowly. A day later, if that was not enough, ouzo liquor would be boiled with honey and lemon juice, and down you drank it, underage or not. If we had a sore tummy, chamomile would be brewed from fresh chamomile flowers to ease our pain. If we were burning with fever, a wet face towel was draped over our foreheads to cool us down. Any pain in the ears would be treated with a drop of lukewarm olive oil in the ear. My favorite was the remedy used for the common cold or chronic pain called cupping (βεντούζες) done on one's back. One would lie flat on their stomach. A small amount of oil is rubbed onto the skin on one's back to reduce any irritation. A cotton ball is soaked in alcohol, lit on fire, and then placed in a cup, which is then turned onto the skin or treatment area to create suction. This suction stimulates the pores and creates blood flow.

So who would have known matches, alcohol, and a cup could be used as treatment!

These things are usually passed down from generation to generation. Here are just some for your perusal and amusement.

WINE
ΚΡΑΣΙ

DISINFECTANT:
Wine was used to disinfect wounds.

CHAMOMILE
ΧΑΜΟΜΗΛΙ

HAIR TREATMENT:
To enhance blond hair, do a final rinse with chamomile tea when shampooing.

MINT
ΔΥΟΣΜΟΣ

DIGESTIVE AID:
Chew on mint sprigs to settle stomach after overeating.

MOSQUITO REPELLENT:
To repel mosquitos, rub mint leaves on your skin.

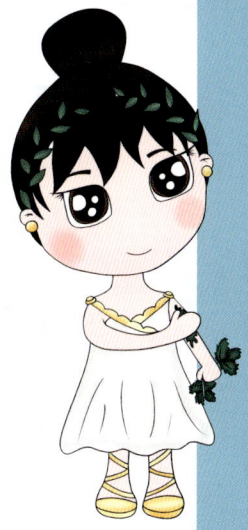

MOUNTAIN TEA
ΦΑΣΚΟΜΗΛΟ

STOMACH RELIEF:
A cup of brewed mountain tea alleviates stomach reflux.

DILL
ΑΝΗΘΟΣ

SLEEP AID:
Place dill over the eyes before going to bed. Said to promote sleep.

PARSLEY
ΜΑΪΝΤΑΝΟΣ

FOR BRUISES:
Chop 40g parsley and boil in 40ml vinegar. Then rub onto the bruise.

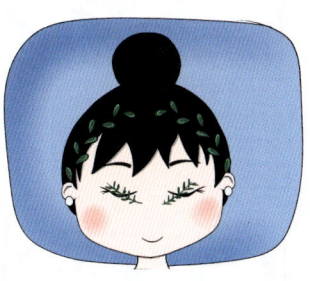

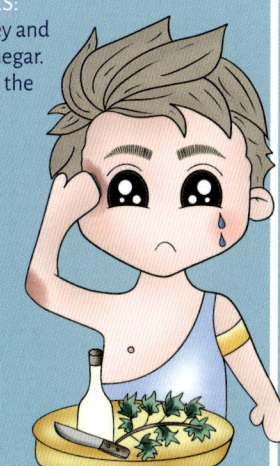

OLIVE LEAF AND OIL
ΕΛΙΑ ΚΑΙ ΕΛΑΙΟΛΑΔΟ

FOR DIABETICS:
To help combat diabetes, boil 30g olive leaf in one liter water until approximately one cup water remains. Strain and drink in the morning.

FOR ACID REFLUX OR ULCERS:
Two spoonfuls of olive oil in the morning and evening.

FOR CONSTIPATION:
For relief, drink a spoonful of olive oil morning and evening.

CUMIN
ΚΥΜΙΝΟ

FOR FLATULENCE:
Chew on cumin seeds to help counteract any flatulence after eating bean dishes. In ancient times, cumin seeds were regarded as one of most effective digestive aids.

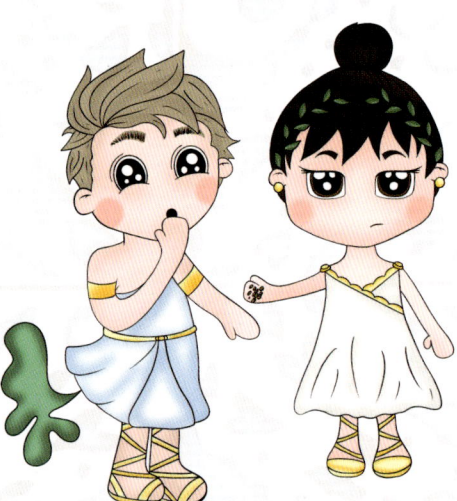

OUZO LIQUOR
ΟΥΖΟ ΛΙΚΕΡ

FOR A SORE THROAT:
Boil ouzo liquor together with some honey and lemon juice and consume hot. Be careful you don't get burned.

LEMON
ΛΕΜΟΝΙ

FOR VOMITING OR DIARRHEA:
A cup of Greek coffee with 3–4 drops of lemon juice aids to stopping vomiting and diarrhea.

DIGESTIVE AID:
Drink warmed lemon juice with a pinch of baking soda to help digestion.

PAIN RELIEF:
Fill a cup with water, add the squeezed juice of one lemon, add one teaspoon honey, and drink to relieve headaches.

ROSEMARY
ΔΕΝΤΡΟΛΙΒΑΝΟ

TO BOOST MEMORY:
Ancient Greek students wore wreaths of rosemary to aid memory.

MILK
ΓΑΛΑ

NATURAL FACE MASK:
Soak bread in milk, squeeze out excess milk, and place the bread over face for thirty minutes while lying down. Rinse well. Use once a month. Milk is associated with promoting a youthful complexion, hence why Cleopatra would bath in milk on a regular basis.

GARLIC
ΣΚΟΡΔΟ

FOR WOUNDS AND MOSQUITO BITES:
Crush garlic (a natural antiseptic) and rub on wounds and mosquito bites.

FOR HIGH BLOOD PRESSURE:
Eat one whole clove daily to reduce blood pressure.

HONEY
ΜΕΛΙ

COLD AND FLU RELIEF:
Brew 2–3 herbal teas in a day and add a spoonful of Greek honey.

FOR DIARRHEA:
Combine grated apple a spoonful of honey with some olive oil and consume.

THYME
ΘΥΜΑΡΙ

RELIEF FOR STIFF MUSCLES:
Steep thyme leaves in white wine and then massage your neck using the liquid.

MOUTHWASH:
Oil of thyme is used as an antiseptic mouthwash.

FOR COUGH AND BRONCHITIS RELIEF:
Drinking thyme tea relieves cough and helps in healing bronchitis.

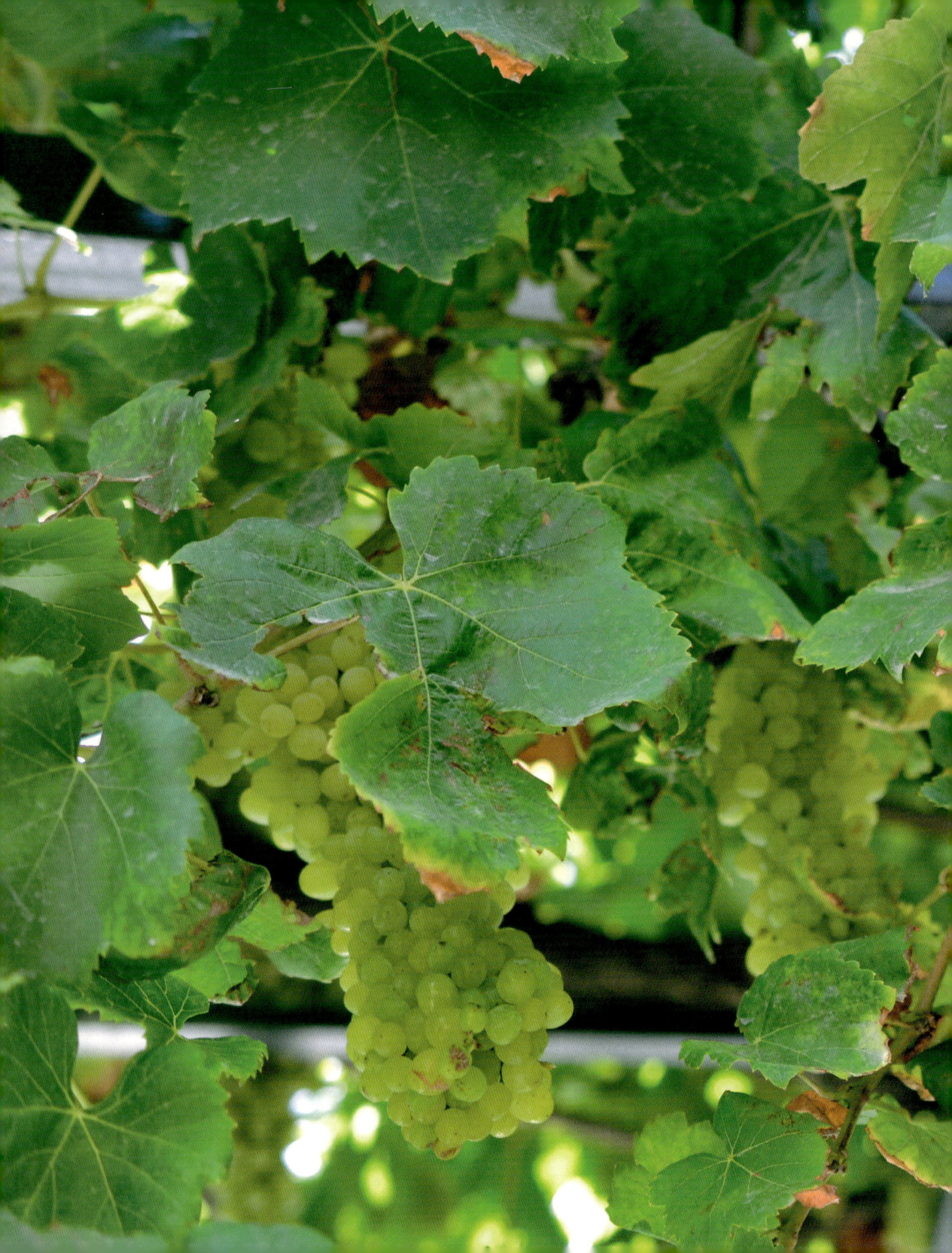

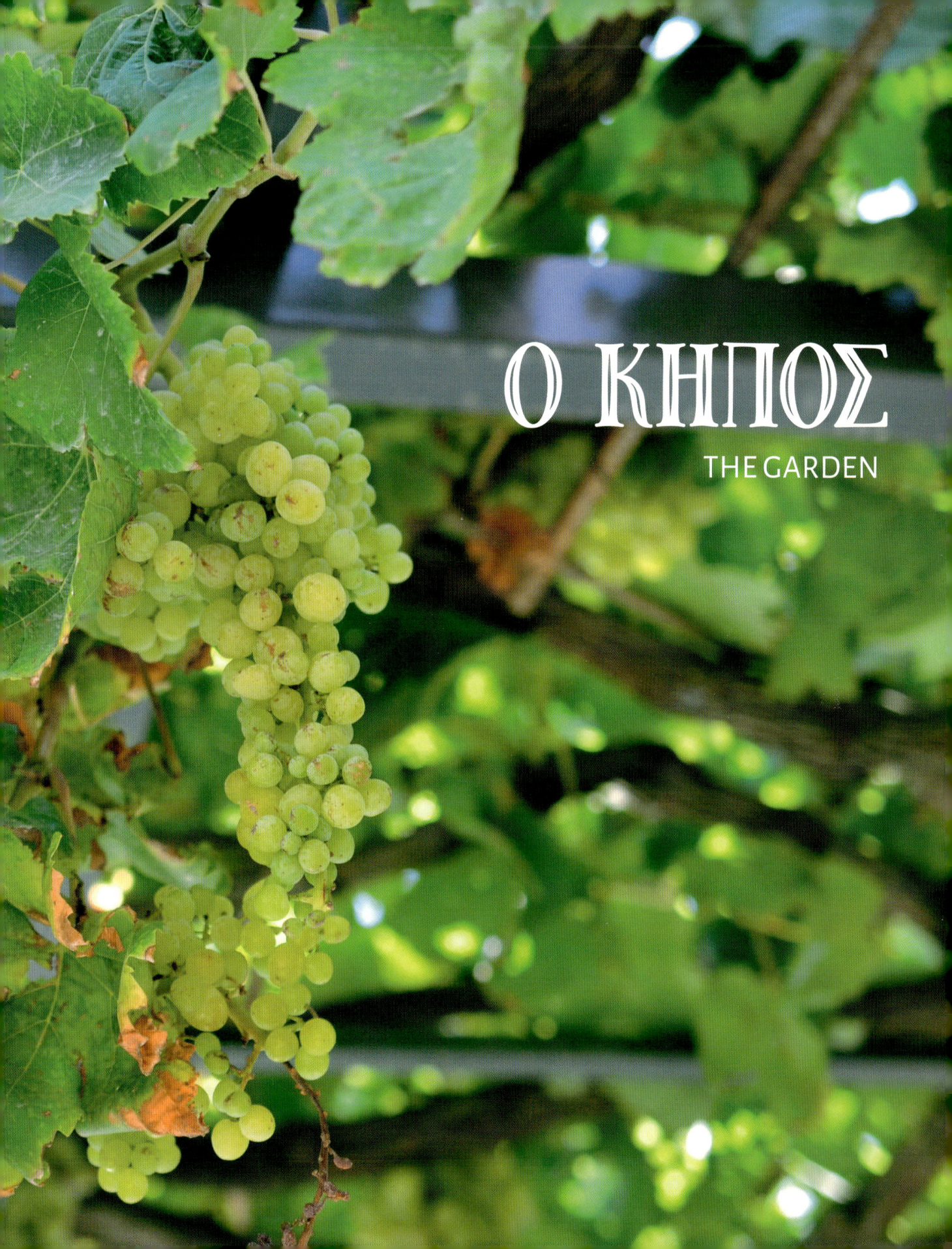

Ο ΚΗΠΟΣ
THE GARDEN

Ο ΚΗΠΟΣ

Ο ΚΗΠΟΣ
THE GARDEN

If anyone knows much about Greeks, they will most probably know that they have a love of eating produce derived from their gardens. Greeks have always cultivated, enjoyed, and harvested organic produce in every inch of space given on their land, in additional pots, and in empty drums of olive oil and the like. A focus on food traditions and not just the nutrients is utterly important. There is a diverse cultural heritage of traditional foods and methods when growing one's own produce and then cooking from the garden. In classical Greek texts such as Plato's *Republic*, Plato lists vegetables both fresh and seasonal as a critical component of one's diet. Fresh herbs and spices are also an integral part of Greek cooking.

Most Greek children have held the hands of their grandparents and parents as they browse the garden, cutting off ripened tomatoes and fresh greens. Most balconies or outdoor areas have a vine draped over them, creating shade and a welcoming space to talk loudly, eat homemade food over long periods, share stories, and make memories with the next generation. One of my fondest memories as a child was picking lemons and figs from homegrown plants. Even as we walked the streets or drove by in our car, if fruit trees or edible greens were on the side of the road, my parents would stop and ensure we ate or collected some to cook at home. My parents instilled in me the importance, the benefits, and the pleasure of cultivating and eating from the garden. They bought a farm when I was incredibly young. My father started to work the soil and planted dozens of fruit trees. We would watch the process, help in watering and watching the plants grow, and ultimately see the fruit and enjoy the produce. It was thrilling as a young girl to see what could happen when seeds were planted and, together with some love and care, be involved in the process. As I grew, I was educated by my parents and via my own research to understand that the richness of antioxidants is increased when produce ripens on the vine or tree in comparison to temperature-controlled produce. We would do well to attempt to eat from our land and learn from our ancestors!

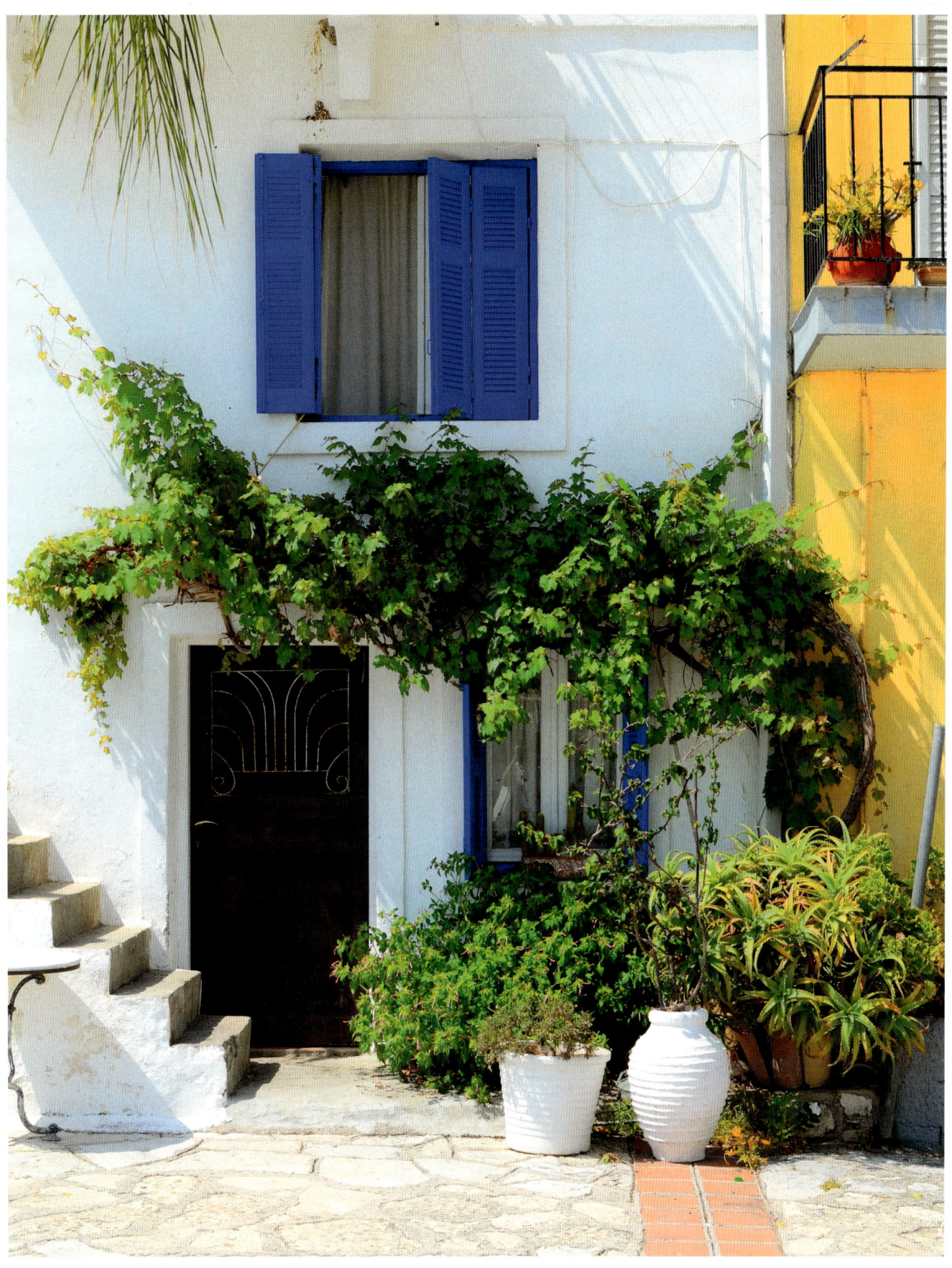

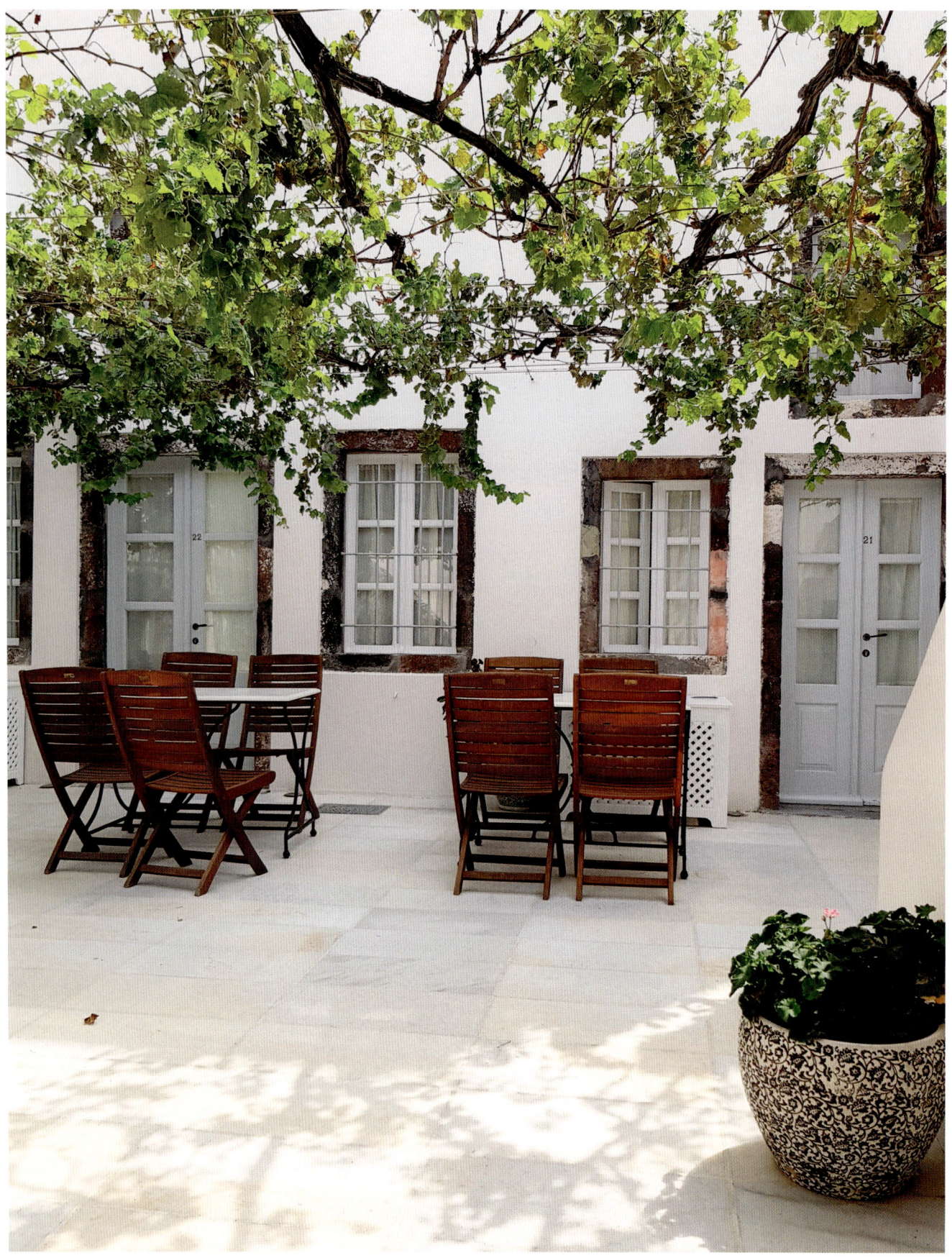

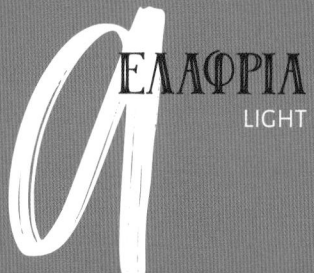
ΕΛΑΦΡΙΑ
LIGHT

ΡΕΒΙΘΟΣΑΛΑΤΑ ΜΕ ΠΙΠΕΡΙΕΣ ΚΑΙ ΛΙΑΣΤΗ ΝΤΟΜΑΤΑ
31 CHICKPEA SALAD WITH MARINATED CAPSICUM AND SUN-DRIED TOMATO (GF)

ΡΟΒΙΤΣΑ ΣΑΛΑΤΑ ΜΕ ΑΝΗΘΟ
32 MUNG BEAN AND DILL SALAD (GF)

ΑΘΗΝΑΪΚΗ ΡΟΚΑ ΣΑΛΑΤΑ ΜΕ ΝΤΟΜΑΤΑ, ΛΕΜΟΝΙ ΚΑΙ ΧΟΝΤΡΟ ΑΛΑΤΙ
33 ATHENIAN ROCKET SALAD WITH TOMATO, LEMON JUICE, AND ROCK SALT (GF)

ΠΡΑΣΙΝΗ ΣΑΛΑΤΑ ΜΕ ΦΡΑΟΥΛΕΣ ΚΑΙ ΣΑΛΤΣΑ ΜΕΛΙΟΥ
35 GREEN SALAD WITH STRAWBERRIES AND HONEY DRESSING (GF)

ΣΑΛΑΤΑ ΜΕ ΜΑΥΡΟΜΑΤΙΚΑ ΦΑΣΟΛΙΑ
37 BLACK-EYED BEAN SALAD (GF)

ΣΑΛΑΤΑ ΜΕ ΨΗΤΑ ΠΑΝΤΖΑΡΙΑ, ΜΑΪΝΤΑΝΟ ΚΑΙ ΜΕΛΙ
39 ROAST BEETROOT AND PARSLEY SALAD WITH HONEY DRESSING (GF)

ΧΩΡΙΑΤΙΚΗ ΣΑΛΑΤΑ
40 GREEK SALAD (GF)

GF DENOTES GLUTEN-FREE RECIPES

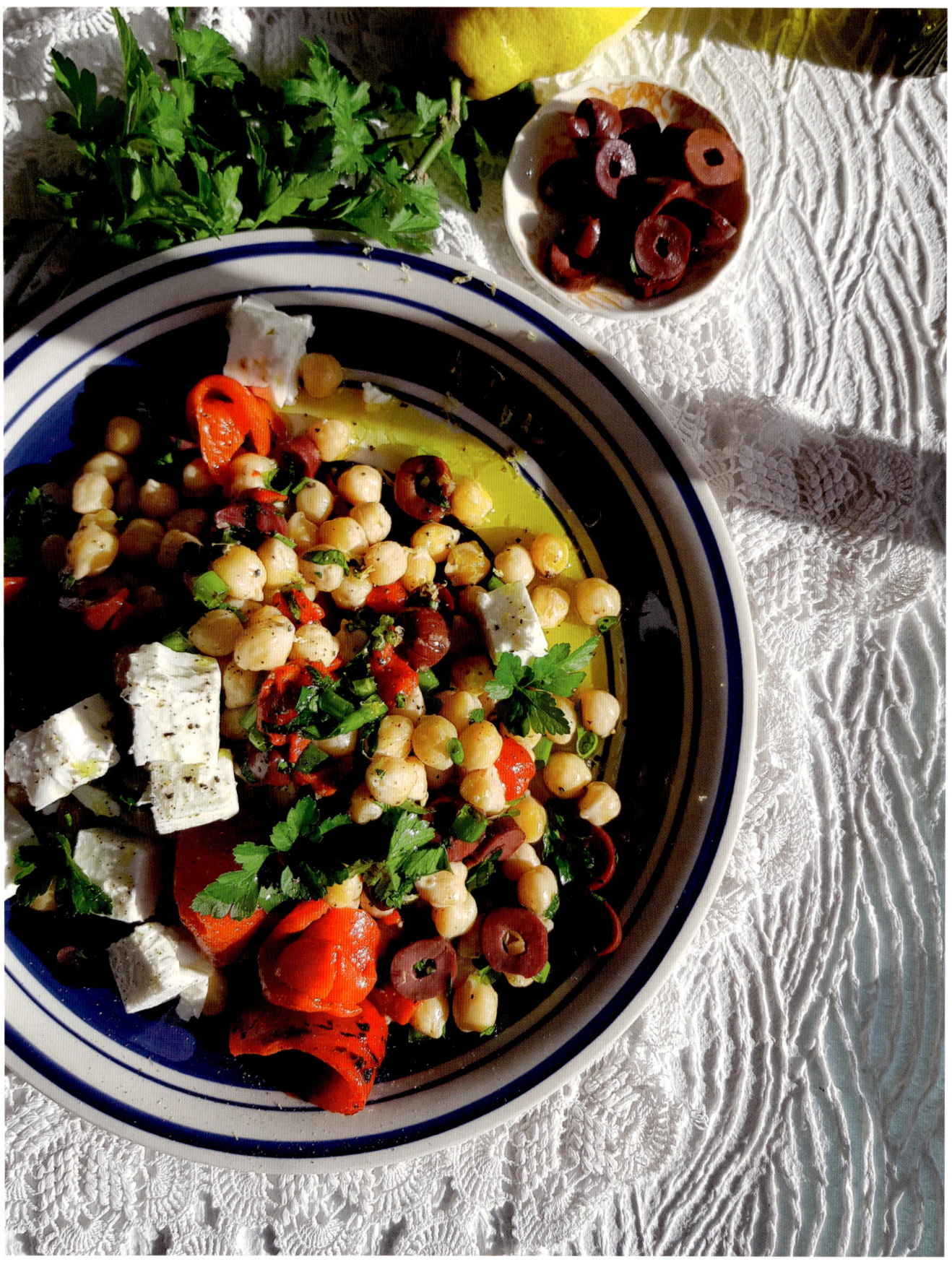

Chickpeas are part of the legume family. They are grown in northern and central Greece. Used in stews, soups, and dips, chickpeas are also eaten in salads. This salad can be made and stored in the fridge for up to 3 days. The flavors permeate and taste better by the day. The lemon juice in the dressing can be substituted with vinegar if preferred. I use dried chickpeas, which I soak overnight then boil till soft. You can use canned chickpeas if you prefer, omitting the cooking step below. Best served a few hours after it has been made.

Serves: 4 · 1 hour (plus overnight soaking) · GLUTEN FREE

Place dried chickpeas in a bowl and cover with fresh water. Allow to soak a minimum 10 hours or overnight.

Drain and add to a pot covered with fresh water and the halved onion. Bring to a boil, and then simmer on low heat for 30–50 minutes or until chickpeas are cooked through but not falling apart.

Place the dressing ingredients into a jar and shake to combine well. Taste and adjust seasoning if needed. It should be a little salty and sour. Set aside.

Drain chickpeas, discard onion, and place into a bowl. While the mixture is still warm, pour half the dressing over it and mix through. Now add the remaining ½ onion, olives, sun-dried tomatoes, capsicums, spring onion, parsley, mint, and half the feta cheese. Toss to combine.

Just before serving, pour the remaining dressing over the salad. Taste again and adjust seasoning if needed. Sprinkle over the remaining feta cheese and serve as a side.

Ρεβιθοσαλάτα με πιπεριές και λιαστή ντομάτα

- CHICKPEA SALAD WITH MARINATED CAPSICUM AND SUN-DRIED TOMATO -

1 cup dried chickpeas

1 small onion, halved and peeled

DRESSING

1–2 lemons, juiced, to taste

1 lemon, zested

½ cup olive oil

Salt and pepper, to taste

1 small chili pepper sliced (optional)

½ cup Kalamata olives, chopped

½ cup sun-dried tomatoes, chopped

½ cup marinated (or fresh) capsicums, chopped

½ cup spring onion, chopped

¼ cup parsley, chopped

¼ cup mint, chopped

1 cup feta cheese, crumbled

Ροβίτσα σαλάτα με άνηθο
- MUNG BEAN AND DILL SALAD -

Mung beans, also known as small green beans, are quite common in the Peloponnese. They are typically eaten as a soup or salad. This tiny bean has so many nutrients; it is a good source of folate, dietary fiber, protein, phosphorus, iron, copper, magnesium, manganese, potassium, and vitamin K. This salad is quick and easy to prepare. It can also be made a day in advance, refrigerated, and served with a fresh squeeze of lemon juice. It is a great accompaniment to fish.

Serves: 4 · 1 hour · GLUTEN FREE

½ cup mung beans, dried

2 medium tomatoes, diced

¼ cup parsley, chopped

¼ cup dill, chopped

¼ cup mint, chopped

1 small onion, diced

DRESSING

1–2 lemons, juiced, to taste

½ teaspoon cumin powder

Salt and pepper, to taste

¼ cup olive oil

Place the mung beans in a pot covered with water. Bring to a boil, and then simmer on low for 45 minutes or until mung beans are soft but not mushy. Drain and allow to cool.

Place the tomatoes, parsley, dill, mint, and onion into a bowl. Add the cooled mung beans together with the dressing ingredients. Toss to combine.

Refrigerate for a minimum one hour, and then spoon onto a serving platter and serve with additional chopped dill and a splash of olive oil.

Can be refrigerated up to 2 days. Tastes even better the next day.

I first tried this salad in a taverna in Athens only because I was intrigued at how simple it was and that it was the only other salad (other than the traditional Greek salad) on the menu. I looked around and found every table served had a bowl of it, front and center. *Why was such a simple salad so popular?* After having tried it, I still crave it from this taverna, and I always ensure it is my first stop when visiting Athens. It is one of those salads where the quality of the tomatoes is most essential. They need to be ripe and in season. It is so simple and yet so refreshing. The pepperiness of the rocket leaves tastes wonderful with the sweet juicy tomatoes, lemon juice, and rock salt!

Serves: 4 · 10 minutes · GLUTEN FREE

In a small bowl, whisk the salt, olive oil, lemon juice, and black pepper. Set aside.

Place rocket and tomatoes in a salad bowl. Pour over the dressing. Taste and adjust seasoning.

Add olives if preferred. Serve immediately as a side.

*If you prefer, you could slice tomatoes and grill on a hot plate together with some olive oil and salt until they are charred. Then add to the salad.

Αθηναϊκή ρόκα σαλάτα με ντομάτα, λεμόνι και χοντρό αλάτι

- ATHENIAN ROCKET SALAD WITH TOMATO, LEMON, AND ROCK SALT -

DRESSING

¾ **teaspoon rock salt**

¼ **cup olive oil**

1–2 lemons, juiced, to taste

Pepper, to taste

150 g (5.3 oz.) rocket, washed

6 large vine tomatoes, cut into eighths*

10–12 Kalamata olives (optional)

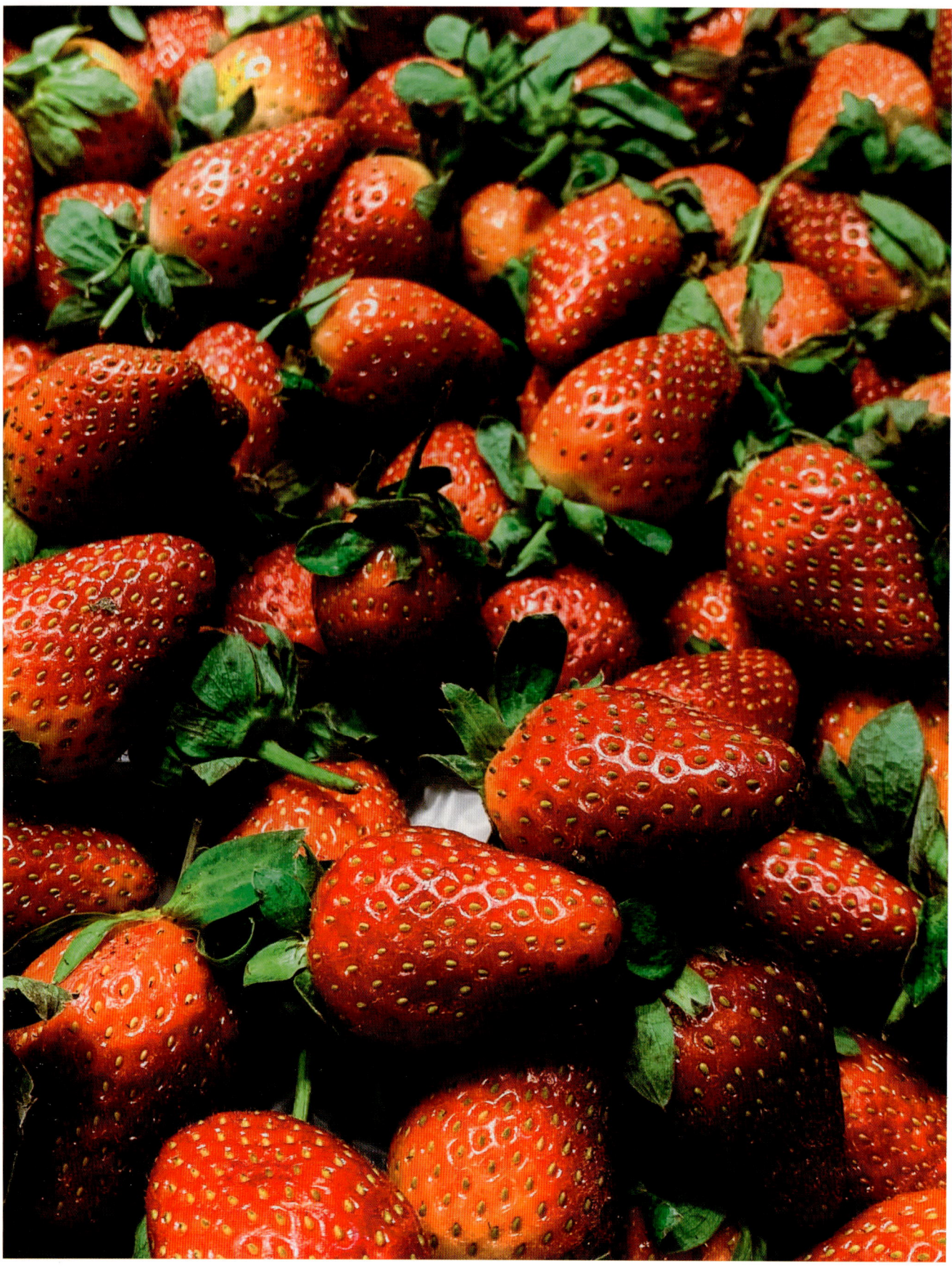

I am a huge fan of crispy and crunchy salads that have both fresh fruits and vegetables. Greek foods have long included both, though more predominately in stews. The combination of the sweetness of strawberries together with the mild and somewhat bitter greens and sweet honey dressing are delicious. Ensure you have a good quality honey and use only the best extra-virgin olive oil you can find. This salad is best made when strawberries are in season. Always taste and adjust dressing before adding to the salad and always add dressing just before serving. You can add more strawberries and almonds if desired.

Serves: 4–6 · 10 minutes · GLUTEN FREE

Place the dressing ingredients into a glass jar. Close and shake well to incorporate. Taste and adjust seasoning if needed. Dressing should be sweet and slightly tart from the vinegar. Set aside.

Place all the salad ingredients into a large bowl. Pour the dressing over the salad greens and gently toss to coat. Place the salad onto a serving dish.

Scatter the feta cheese and almonds over the top. Serve immediately.

Πράσινη σαλάτα με φράουλες και σάλτσα μελιού

- GREEN SALAD WITH STRAWBERRIES AND HONEY DRESSING -

DRESSING

¼ cup olive oil

1 tablespoon whole grain mustard (optional)

3–4 tablespoons balsamic vinegar, or to taste

2–3 tablespoons runny honey

180 g (6.35 oz.) combination of mixed greens (rocket, Italian lettuce, baby spinach)

1 tablespoon parsley, chopped

8 mint leaves, chopped

¼ cup spring onion, chopped

300 g (10.5 oz.) strawberries, sliced

TO SERVE

½ cup feta cheese, crumbled

3–4 tablespoons almonds, sliced and roasted

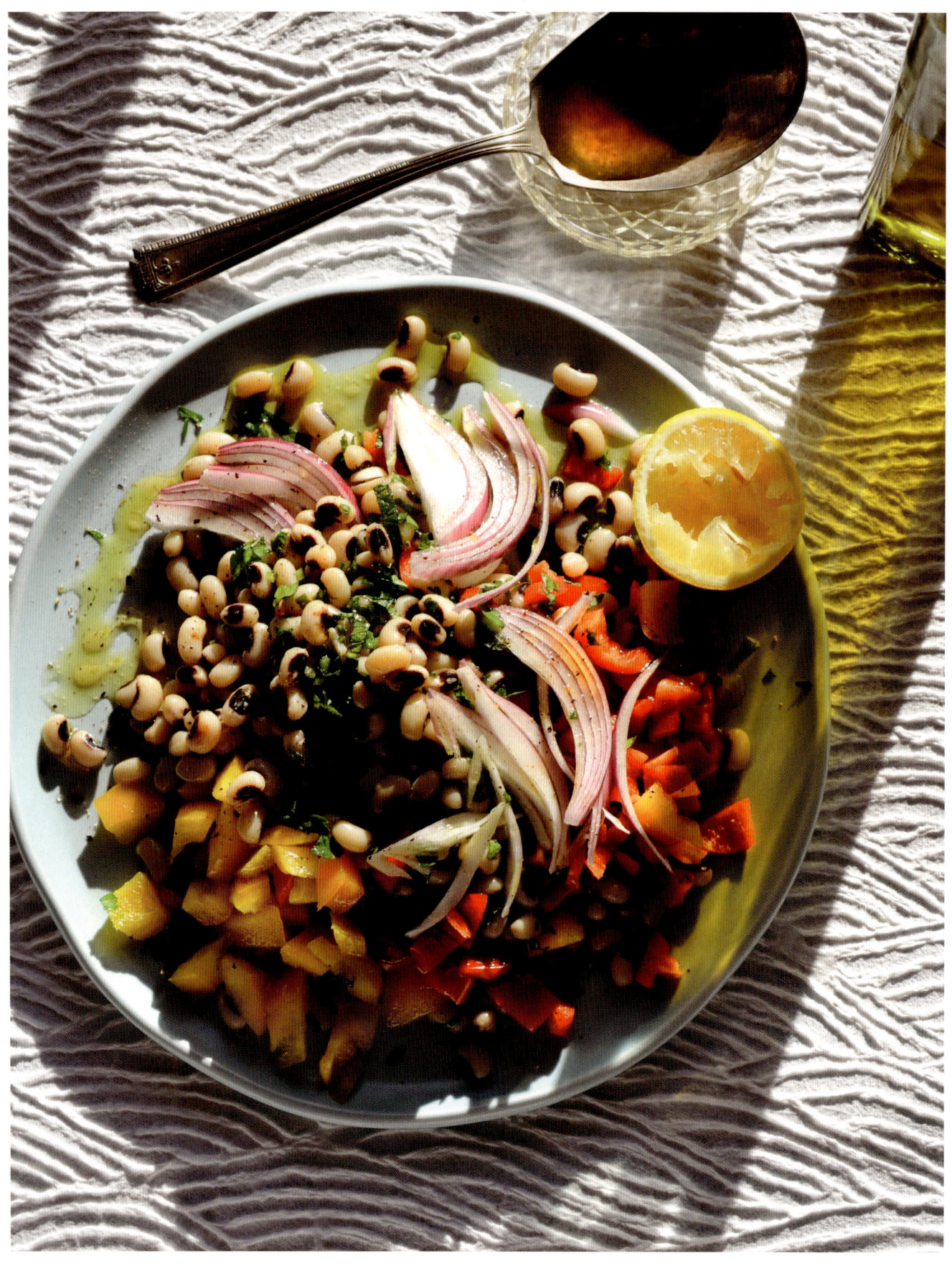

I grew up eating these humble protein-filled black-eyed beans. My mother would cook them in stews or serve them as a cold salad, something she regularly ate as a child back in her village in the Peloponnese. Together with a few other simple ingredients, this salad is not only healthy, but easy to prepare. All the ingredients can be prepped ahead of time and placed in the refrigerator. When ready to eat, add the dressing and toss to combine.

Serves: 3 · 1 hour (plus overnight soaking) · **GLUTEN FREE**

Drain the beans that have been soaking overnight. Place into a saucepan together with the bay leaf and cover with fresh water. Do not add any salt at this stage, otherwise it will toughen the beans and they will not cook. Bring to a boil, and then simmer on low for 35–40 minutes or until beans are soft but not mushy. Rinse under cold water and set aside to cool completely.

In a large bowl, combine all the salad ingredients together with the cooled beans and set aside.

Whisk together the dressing and pour over the salad. Toss and adjust seasoning if needed.

Garnish with some freshly chopped parsley and serve immediately.

Keep covered in refrigerator for up to 2 days.

Σαλάτα με μαυρομάτικα φασόλια

- BLACK-EYED BEAN SALAD -

1 cup black-eyed peas, dried and soaked overnight

1 bay leaf

1 red pepper, chopped

½ yellow or green pepper, chopped

½ cup parsley, chopped

½ cup celery, chopped

¼ cup mint, chopped

½ red onion, thinly sliced

DRESSING

1–2 lemons, juiced

1 lemon, zested

⅓ cup olive oil

Salt and pepper, to taste

Chili flakes (optional)

1 garlic clove, minced (optional)

2 tablespoons runny honey

TO SERVE

3 tablespoons parsley, chopped finely

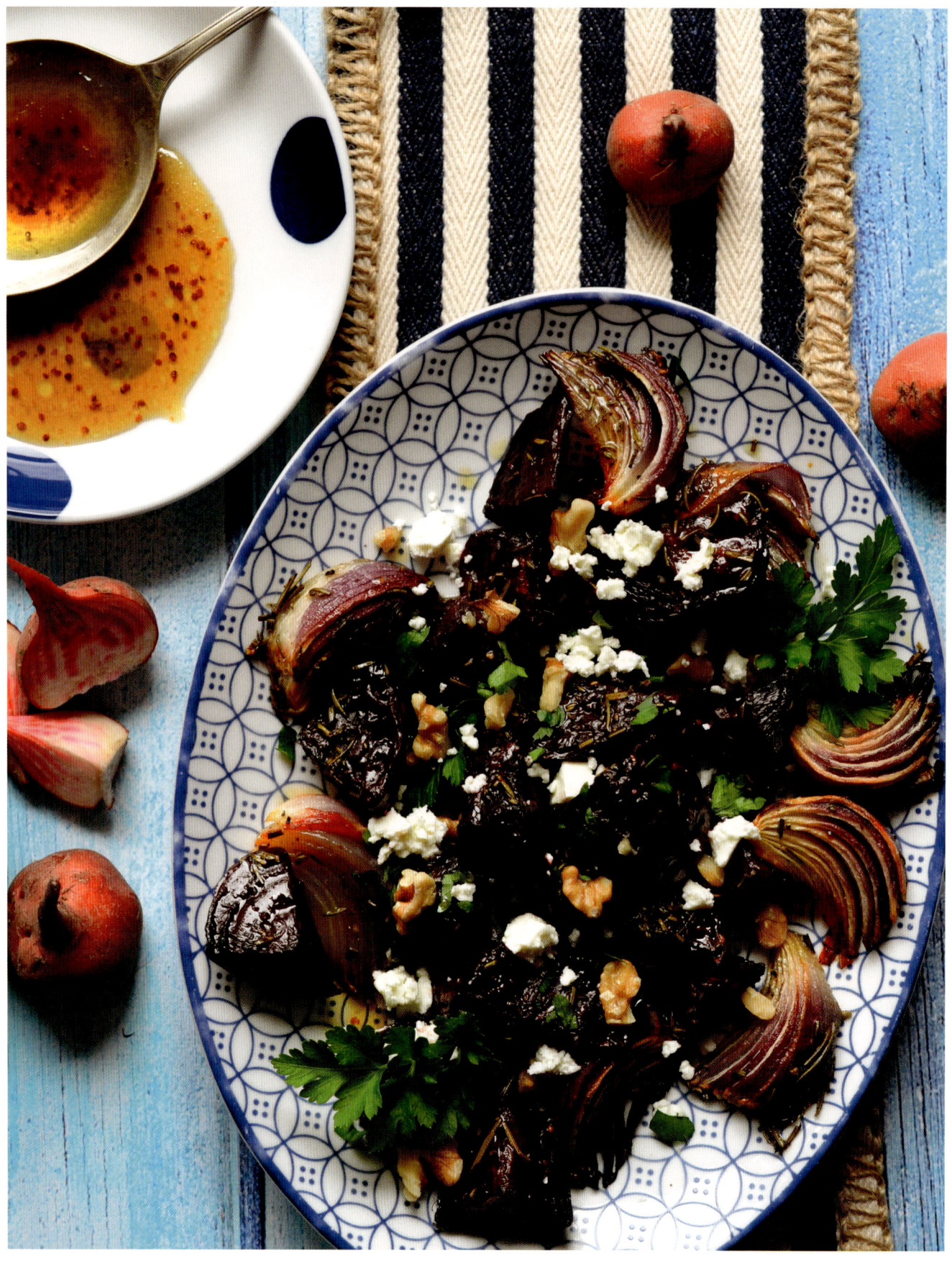

Greeks love beetroots! We boil, roast, steam, or eat them raw. We blanch the leaves and dress them with a simple lemon and olive oil dressing. It is such a simple vegetable and yet so versatile. This recipe is for a warm salad. The beets are boiled then roasted to release a more intense flavor. They are then combined with feta cheese for saltiness, walnuts for added crunch, parsley for freshness, and a sweet mustard honey and olive oil dressing. Best served warm.

Serves: 4 · 50 minutes · GLUTEN FREE

Σαλάτα με ψητά παντζάρια, μαϊντανό και μέλι

- ROAST BEETROOT AND PARSLEY SALAD WITH HONEY DRESSING -

Preheat oven to 180º C/356º F. Line a baking tray with parchment paper.

Place the beetroots into a saucepan covered with fresh water. Bring to a boil, and then simmer on medium heat for 25 minutes or until cooked through but not super soft as they will also be baked.

Drain and place in a bowl together with the onion, ¼ cup olive oil, rosemary, salt, and pepper. Gently mix to coat. Place onto a baking tray and bake for 25 minutes or until the beetroots are incredibly soft and onions have softened and caramelized.

Remove from oven and place on a serving bowl or large platter. Combine the dressing ingredients into a bowl and whisk to combine well. Taste and adjust seasoning if needed. Pour over the salad and gently toss. Scatter parsley, feta cheese, and walnuts over the salad. Serve immediately.

*To roast walnuts, place onto a baking tray and bake for 10 minutes on 200 º C/390º F. Allow to cool, and then roughly chop.

500 g (17.6 oz. or 3–4 medium sized) beetroots, peeled and cut into eighths

1 red onion, cut into eighths

¼ cup olive oil

2 tablespoons rosemary, chopped

Salt and pepper

DRESSING

¼ cup olive oil

½ teaspoon mustard

1 tablespoon balsamic vinegar

2 tablespoons runny honey

1–2 tablespoons water (add only if you prefer a runnier dressing)

Salt, to taste

TO SERVE

¼ cup parsley, finely chopped

½ cup feta cheese, crumbled

½ cup walnuts, roughly chopped and roasted*

Χωριάτικη σαλάτα
- GREEK SALAD -

4 ripe tomatoes, each cut into quarters

½ large cucumber, chopped

½ green bell pepper, sliced thinly

¼ red onion, sliced

¼ cup Kalamata olives

¼ cup extra-virgin olive oil

1½ teaspoons dried oregano

1 tablespoon capers

Salt, to taste

100 g (3.5 oz.) block of feta cheese

I was not intending to add a Greek salad to this book, seeing that I have a recipe in my first publication, *Hellenic Kanella: Memories Made in a Greek Kitchen*. Nonetheless, I changed my mind and decided this book should have the classical Greek salad included. Greek salad does not contain any lettuce. It is made primarily of ripe tomatoes, cucumbers, green peppers, feta cheese, olives, onions, Greek dried oregano, and a good dose of extra-virgin olive oil. Vinegar is optional, as are capers. It is a fresh, exceptionally healthy salad, and, not surprisingly, it is a big part of the Mediterranean diet. It is quick to prepare and consists of ingredients that are usually staples in any kitchen. Make sure not to withhold the amount of olive oil, as this is what makes this salad so delicious. Have plenty of bread to mop up the juices. Always serve this salad using cold vegetables straight from the refrigerator—this makes the salad more refreshing.

Serves: 3 · 10 minutes · GLUTEN FREE

Place the cut tomatoes, cucumber, bell pepper, onion, olives, and capers (if using) in a large salad bowl. Add the olive oil, dried oregano, and salt, and gently mix all the ingredients.

Taste and adjust the seasoning if required. Place the feta cheese on top of the salad in one thick slice. Add more olive oil if the salad is a little dry. Serve the salad immediately with crusty bread.

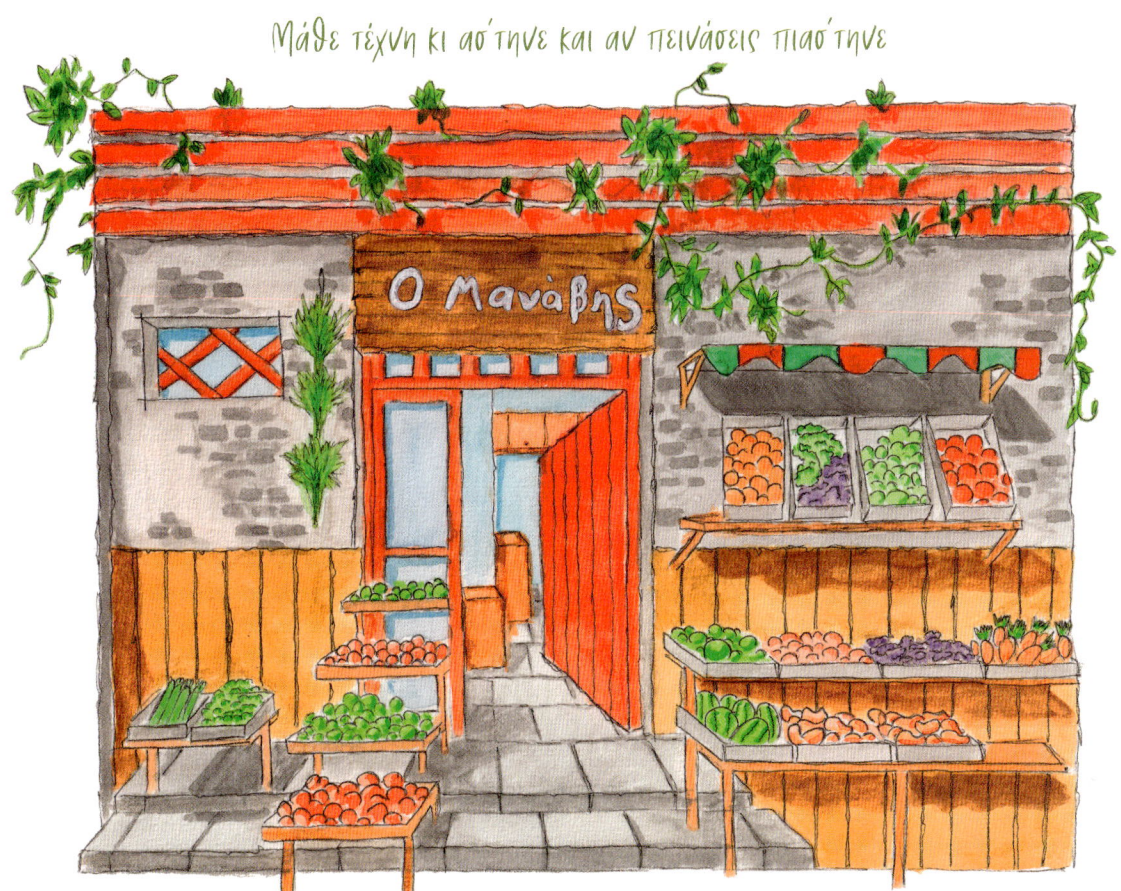

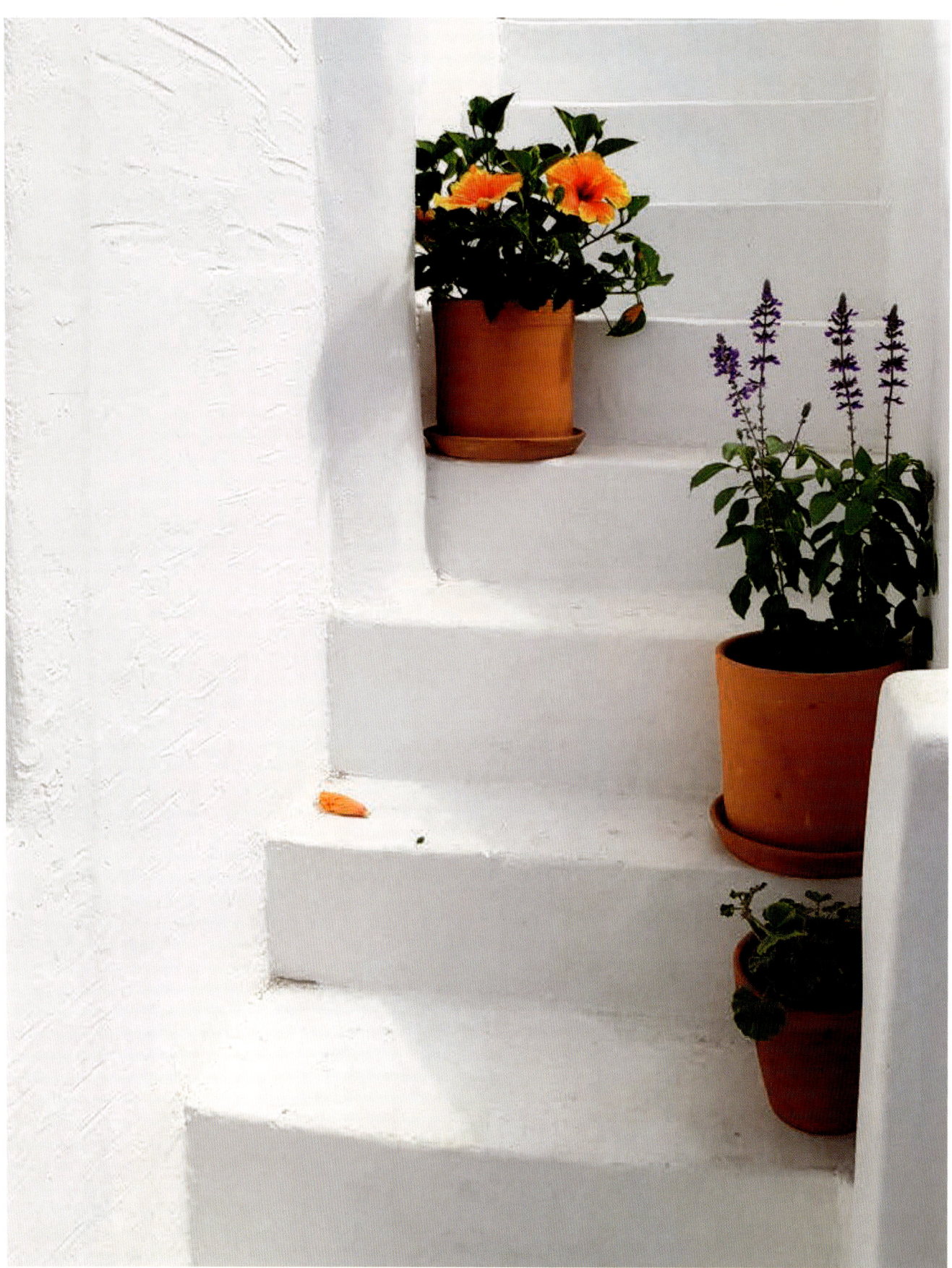

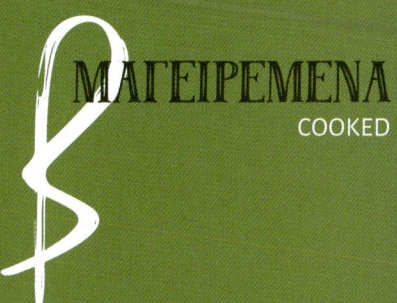

ΜΑΓΕΙΡΕΜΕΝΑ
COOKED

44	**ΠΙΠΕΡΙΕΣ ΦΛΩΡΙΝΗΣ ΜΕ ΤΥΡΙΑ ΚΑΙ ΚΟΛΟΚΥΘΑΚΙΑ** FLORINA PEPPERS WITH CHEESE AND ZUCCHINI (GF)
46	**ΜΕΛΙΤΖΑΝΕΣ ΓΕΜΙΣΤΕΣ ΜΕ ΤΥΡΙ ΚΑΙ ΠΙΚΑΝΤΙΚΗ ΣΑΛΤΣΑ** CHEESE-STUFFED EGGPLANT IN A SPICY TOMATO SAUCE (GF)
48	**ΡΕΒΙΘΑΔΑ ΜΕ ΜΕΛΙ** CHICKPEA STEW WITH HONEY (GF)
50	**ΠΑΤΑΤΕΣ ΓΙΑΧΝΙ ΜΕ ΤΡΑΧΑΝΑ** PATATES GIAHNI ME TRAHANA
52	**ΠΙΚΑΝΤΙΚΕΣ ΠΑΤΑΤΕΣ ΦΟΥΡΝΟΥ** SPICY (NOT HOT) BAKED POTATOES (GF)
54	**ΓΙΓΑΝΤΕΣ ΜΕ ΣΠΑΝΑΚΙ ΣΤΟ ΦΟΥΡΝΟ** LIMA BEANS WITH SPINACH (GF)
56	**ΜΑΝΕΣΤΡΑ ΚΟΛΟΠΙΜΠΙΡΙ** TOMATO AND PASTA SOUP WITH SWEET PAPRIKA
58	**ΣΑΛΑΝΤΟΥΡΜΑΣΙ** FRAGRANT RICE-STUFFED ONIONS WITH PINE NUTS (GF)
60	**ΤΣΟΥΧΤΗ, Η ΜΑΚΑΡΟΝΑΔΑ ΤΗΣ ΜΑΝΗΣ** SPAGHETTI WITH FRIED CHEESE AND EGG
62	**ΝΤΟΛΜΑΔΑΚΙΑ ΜΕ ΣΕΣΚΟΥΛΑ ΣΤΟ ΦΟΥΡΝΟ** BAKED SILVERBEET ROLLS (GF)
66	**ΑΓΙΟΡΕΙΤΙΚΟ ΠΑΣΤΙΤΣΙΟ ΜΕ ΜΑΝΙΤΑΡΙΑ** MUSHROOM PASTITSIO
68	**ΣΤΙΦΑΔΟ ΜΕ ΜΑΝΙΤΑΡΙΑ** MUSHROOM AND ONION STEW (GF)
70	**ΠΑΤΑΤΕΣ ΚΑΙ ΝΤΟΜΑΤΕΣ ΓΕΜΙΣΤΕΣ** STUFFED POTATOES AND TOMATOES (GF)

GF DENOTES GLUTEN-FREE RECIPES

Πιπεριές Φλώρινης με τυριά και κολοκυθάκια

- FLORINA PEPPERS WITH CHEESE AND ZUCCHINI -

Florina peppers are the long, thin variety that get their name from a small mountain town in Florina, Greece. Most people know these peppers as the brined and bottled variety available in European grocery stores. They are the most exported pepper of Greece and uniquely flavorful when roasted. Additionally, while the peppers are in season, tavernas throughout Greece serve a version of them stuffed with various Greek cheeses. The cheese melts and compliments the sweet peppers beautifully. This recipe has the added sweetness of grated zucchini, which is sautéed with onions and olive oil. They are delectable both warm and at room temperature. If you like a little spice, add some chili flakes to the cheese mixture.

Serves: 7 · 1 hour · GLUTEN FREE

---

7 long red peppers
½ cup olive oil, divided
1 small onion, grated
Salt and pepper
1 medium zucchini, grated
2 cups ricotta cheese, crumbled
½ cup feta cheese, crumbled
½ cup kefalograviera cheese, grated*
1½ tablespoons sesame seeds, roasted

TO SERVE

Kalamata olives, sliced
Parsley, chopped
Lemon wedges

Preheat oven to 180° C/356° F.

Wash and remove the tops off the peppers. With a knife, cut lengthwise down one side to create an opening. Remove any seeds and membrane and set aside. Repeat with all the peppers.

Sauté onion in half of the olive oil. Season with salt and pepper. Add the zucchini and continue to sauté for 5 minutes. Place into a bowl and allow to cool slightly. Add in the cheeses. Mix well to combine. With a teaspoon, carefully fill the peppers as much as possible. Place closely side by side onto a baking tray. Pour the remaining olive oil and scatter the sesame seeds over the peppers. Add ¼ cup water to the baking tray.

Bake for 35–40 minutes or until peppers are soft and slightly golden. Remove from the oven and place onto a serving platter. Scatter over olives, parsley, and lemon wedges.

*Kefalograviera cheese can be substituted with Parmesan cheese.

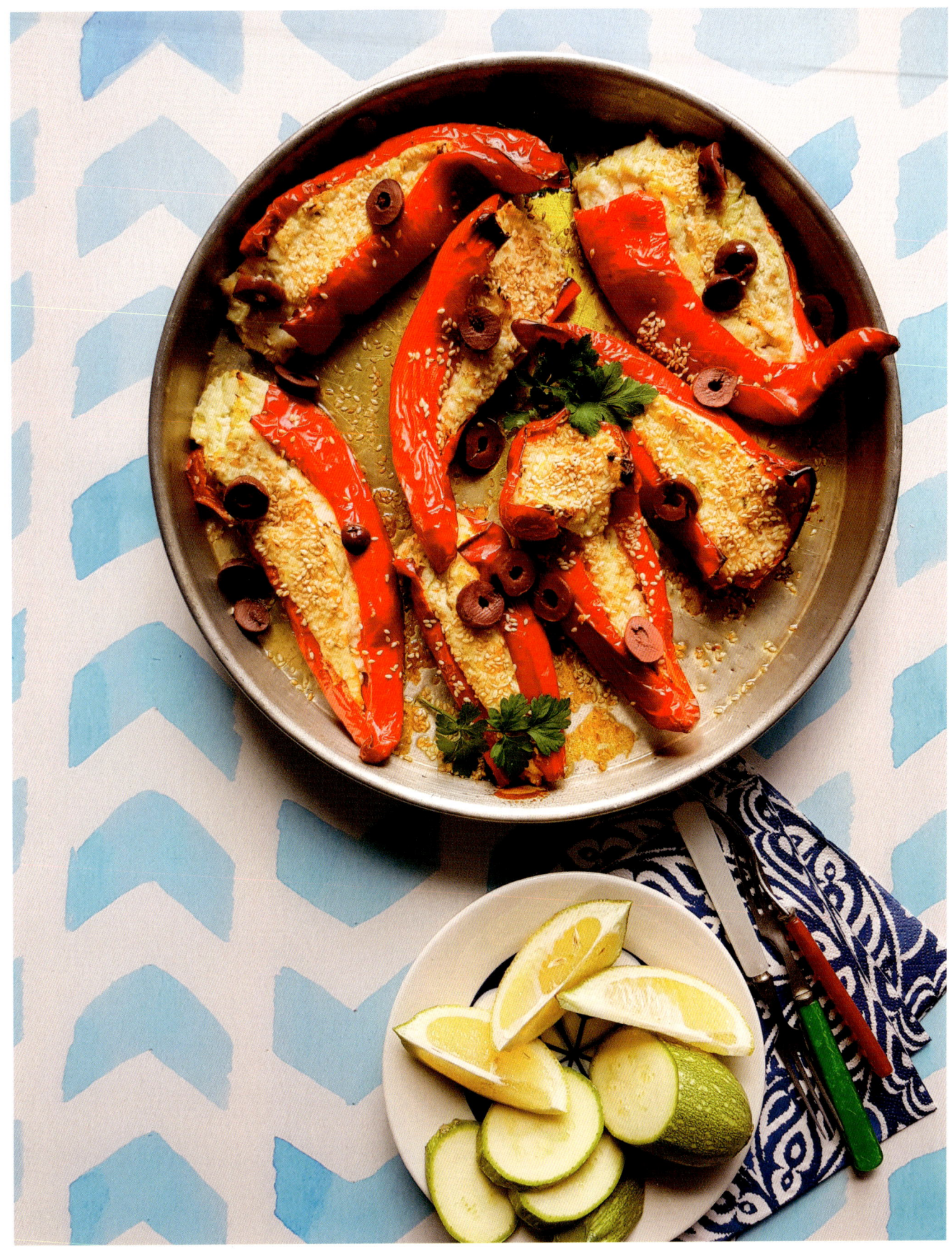

Μελιτζάνες γεμιστές με τυρία και πικάντικη σάλτσα
- CHEESE-STUFFED EGGPLANTS IN A SPICY TOMATO SAUCE -

I have a similar dish in my book *Hellenic Kanella: Memories Made in a Greek Kitchen* of sausages rolled in eggplants and cooked in a cream sauce. This is the vegetarian version, eggplants stuffed with cheeses, baked in a spicy tomato salsa, and topped with roasted pine nuts. The beauty of this dish is that it can be cooked a day in advance (left covered in the refrigerator) and then reheated. The flavors develop and taste better the day after.

Serves: 5 · 1.5 hours · GLUTEN FREE

3 large eggplants

½ cup olive oil, divided

FILLING

1 cup ricotta cheese

1½ cups kefalograviera cheese, divided*

2 tablespoons mint, chopped

½ lemon, juiced

Zest of one lemon

Pepper

TOMATO SALSA

¼ cup olive oil

1 garlic clove, minced

Pinch of chili flakes

2 cups tomato purée

Salt, to taste

2 teaspoons castor (superfine) sugar

¼ cup water

3 basil leaves

7 cherry tomatoes

TO SERVE

Pine nuts, toasted

Preheat oven to 200° C/390° F.

Line a baking tray with parchment paper. Peel the skin off the eggplants (as the skin can be hard) and slice eggplants 1 cm / ½ in. thick (5 slices per eggplant). Place eggplant slices side by side on the baking tray. Brush both sides of the eggplant with olive oil and then sprinkle with salt.

Bake for 30 minutes, turning the eggplants halfway through so that they are golden on both sides. Remove from oven and allow to cool.

Place the filling ingredients into a bowl. Mix, taste, and adjust seasoning as desired. Set aside.

Make the sauce by placing the oil, garlic and chili flakes in a saucepan. Heat until the garlic starts to sizzle. Do not let it burn. Immediately add the tomato purée, salt, sugar, and water. Bring to a boil and then simmer on medium heat for 10 minutes. Remove from heat and add the basil leaves. Taste and adjust seasoning if needed. Set aside.

To assemble, pour the tomato salsa into a baking dish. Add a tablespoon of ricotta mixture onto the widest end of the eggplant, then gently roll up the eggplant and place it seam side down in the pan on top of the salsa. Repeat with all the eggplants. Scatter cherry tomatoes and the remaining ½ cup cheese over the top.

Bake at 200° C/390° F for 30 minutes or until golden and bubbly. Scatter over the roasted pine nuts and serve with a crisp green salad.

*Mozzarella cheese can be substituted for kefalograviera cheese.

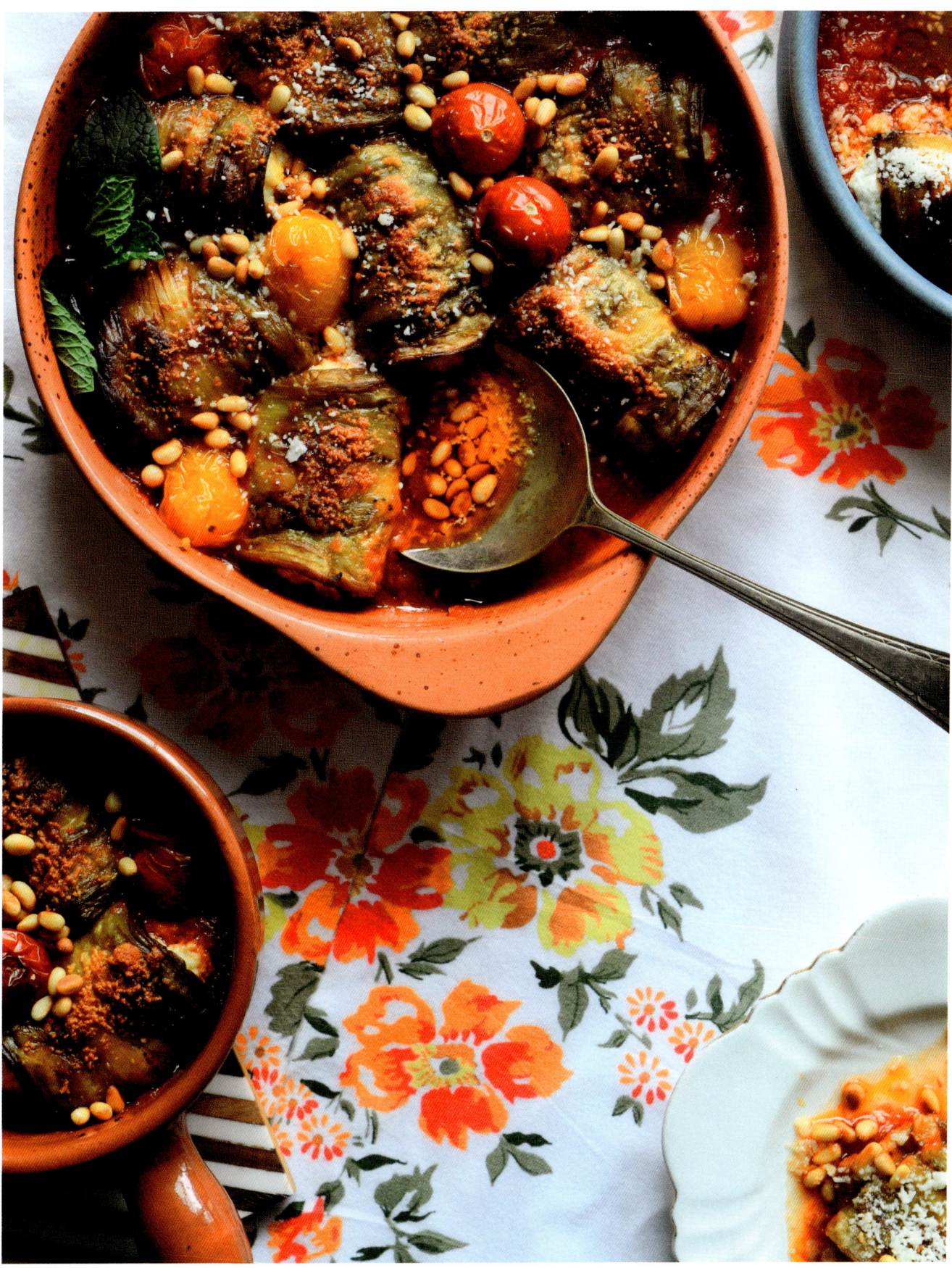

Ρεβιθάδα με μέλι
- CHICKPEA STEW WITH HONEY -

200 g (7.0 oz.) dried chickpeas

½ cup olive oil

1 large onion, grated

1 tablespoon tomato paste

1 cup tomato purée

Salt and pepper, to taste

1 bay leaf

1 tablespoon Greek honey

TO SERVE

Crumbled feta cheese

Chickpea soup is served everywhere in Greece. Some make it white and some red. The white version is flavored with lemon juice and the red with tomatoes. A white version can be found in my first cookbook, *Hellenic Kanella: Memories Made in a Greek Kitchen*. Here I have the alternative version of the red soup with a subtle hint of honey. The sweetness is key to balance the rich tomato base. Though this recipe has few ingredients, it boasts big flavors. An exceptionally good quality olive oil, honey, and tomatoes are key to ensure a beautiful result. Serve with crumbled feta cheese to add some creaminess to the dish.

Serves: 3–4 · 1.5 hours (plus overnight soaking) · GLUTEN FREE

Start the night before by placing dried chickpeas in a bowl of cold water. Allow to stand overnight or at least 8 hours. Drain and place the chickpeas onto a cotton tea towel. Gently rub the chickpeas in the towel to remove any skins (removing the outer skins makes the soup more enjoyable as they can sometimes be tough).

In a pot, heat the olive oil together with the onions and sauté until soft and translucent. Add the tomato paste and tomato purée, stirring to break up the paste. Add the chickpeas, pepper, and bay leaf. Do not add salt until the end as it hardens the chickpeas. Add additional water to cover the chickpeas.

Place a lid half on and simmer for 1 hour or until the chickpeas are fully cooked (still retaining their shape) and the juices have thickened. Check periodically to ensure the water does not totally evaporate. Add salt and honey, mixing well. Taste and adjust seasoning if needed.

Serve in bowls with crumbled feta cheese and an extra drizzle of honey (if desired).

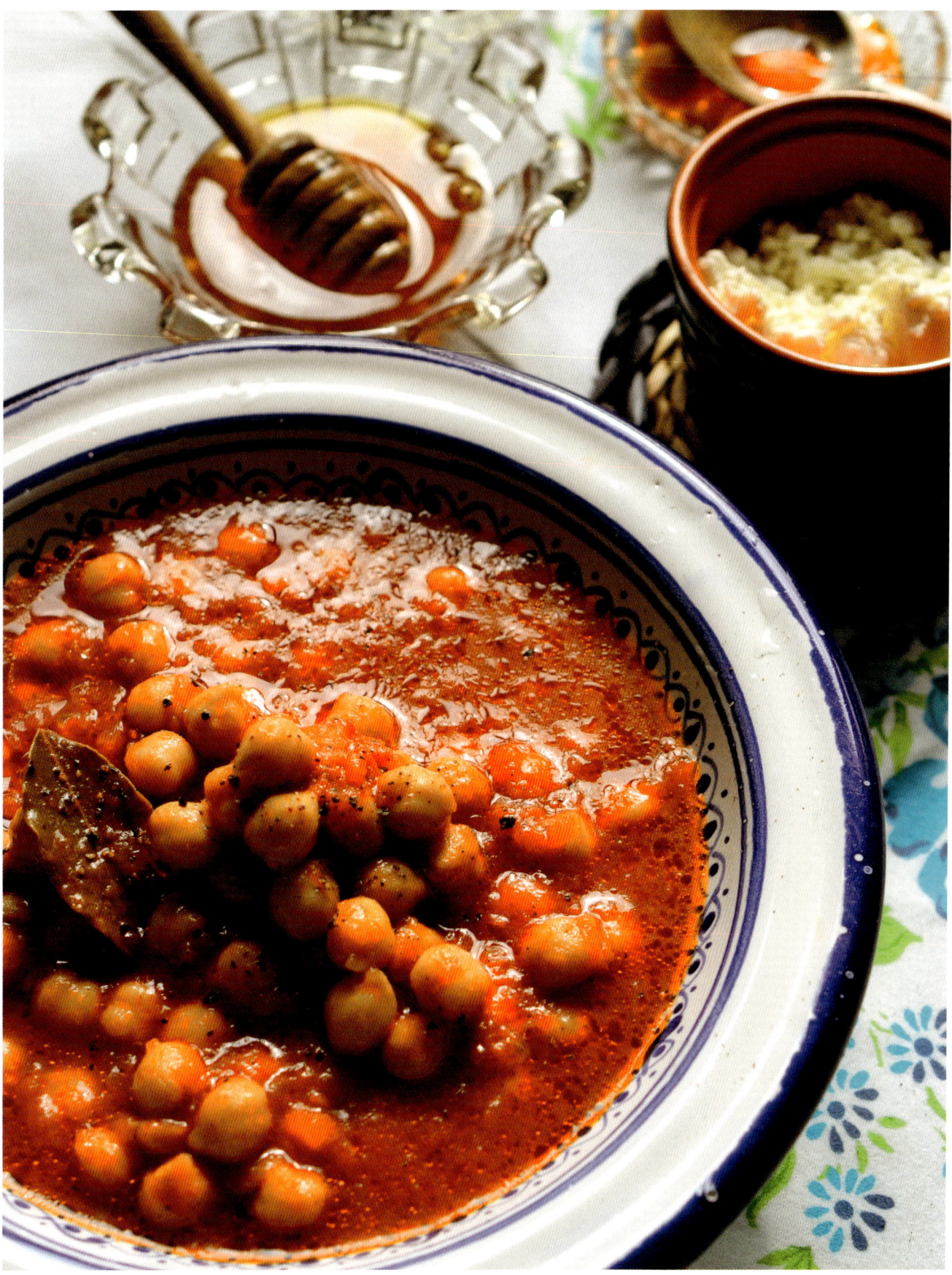

Πατάτες γιαχνί με τραχανά
- PATATES GIAHNI ME TRAHANA -

½ cup olive oil

1 large onion, minced

1 large carrot, sliced thinly

6 medium size potatoes, peeled and quartered

1 tablespoon tomato paste

1 teaspoon castor (superfine) sugar

5 cherry tomatoes, halved

2 bay leaves

5 allspice berries

1 teaspoon cinnamon powder

Salt and pepper, to taste

½ cup white wine

3 cups (750 ml) water

1 cup trahana*

TO SERVE

Parmesan or kefalograviera cheese*

This recipe comes from the Peloponnese. My mother, being from this region, used to cook with trahana very often as I was growing up. I love the consistency that this small ingredient gives to dishes. Trahana can be made several ways—with cracked wheat or bulgur, salt, flour and yogurt or sour milk. It resembles a small pasta and aids as a thickener to soups and stews. I like to think of it as in between the texture of rice and pasta. In this stew, it gives a great soft texture and balance to the potatoes. The combination of spices makes this dish very aromatic.

Serves: 4 · 45 minutes

Place oil in a large pan with the onion and sauté until soft and translucent. Add carrot and potatoes and sauté for 5 minutes. Add the tomato paste, sugar, tomatoes, bay leaves, allspice berries, cinnamon powder, salt, pepper, and wine. Mix and allow it to cook for 3 minutes. Add the water and place a lid on the pan.

Cook for 20–25 minutes on medium heat or until potatoes are cooked through. Taste the liquid at this point and ensure it is well seasoned. Adjust as needed.

Add the trahana over the mixture without stirring. Ensure there is plenty of liquid still in the pan. If not, add ½ cup boiled water. Bring to a boil and then simmer for 3 minutes with the lid on. Turn heat off, keeping the lid on pan, and allow the trahana to soak in the juices and cook with the residual heat, roughly 10 minutes.

Serve with a generous amount of grated Parmesan or Greek kefalograviera cheese.

*Trahana and kefalograviera cheese can be purchased from European grocers.

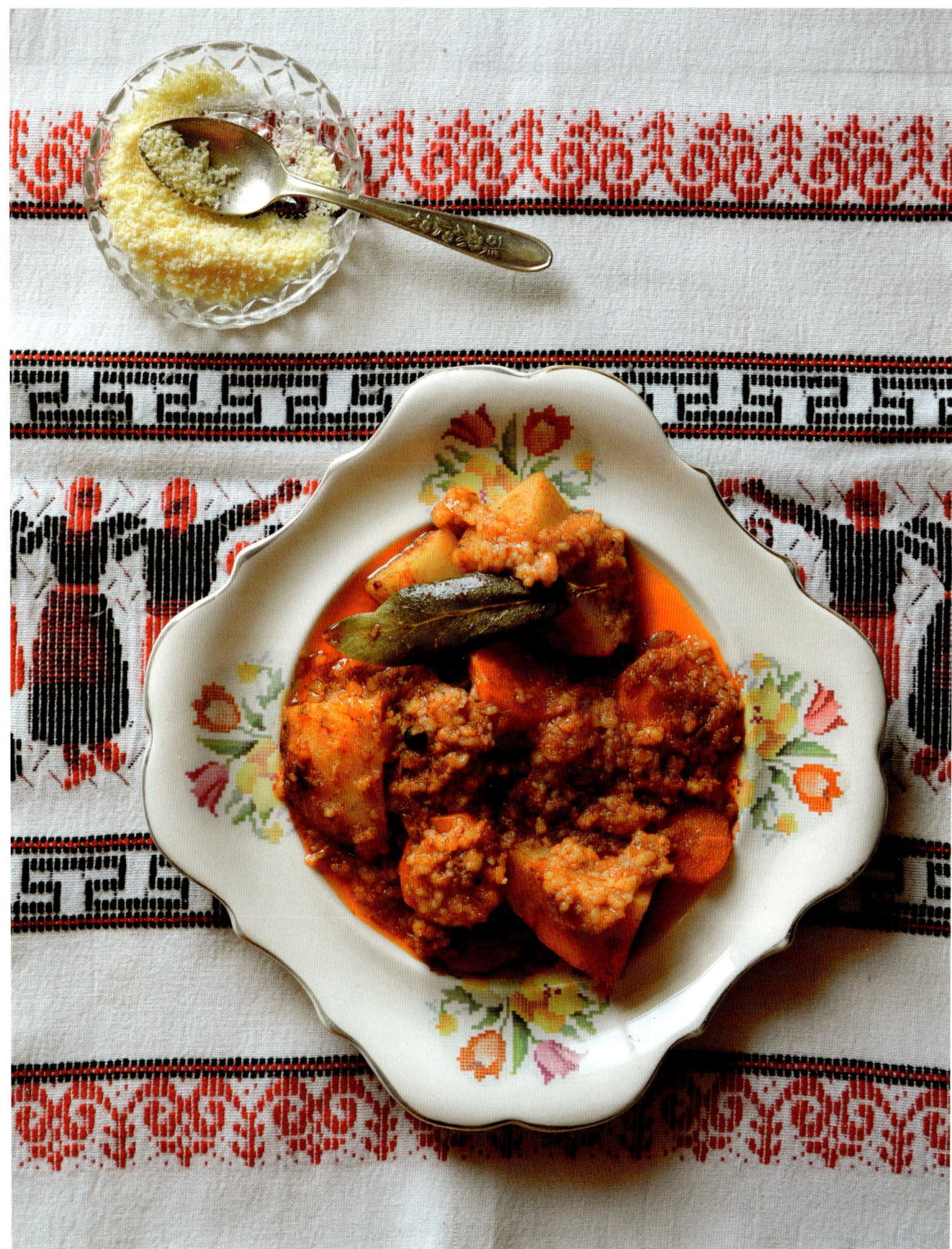

Πικάντικες πατάτες φούρνου
- SPICY (NOT HOT) BAKED POTATOES -

This is another recipe from the Peloponnese showcasing baked potatoes with wine and spices. Cinnamon is a common ingredient used in many savory and sweet dishes. This dish is a great alternative to the classic lemon baked potatoes that are commonly eaten on mainland Greece. It is simple to prepare and deliciously flavored. Serve as a side.

Serves: 4 · 1.5 hours · GLUTEN FREE

6 potatoes (700 g or 24.6 oz.), quartered

¾ cup white wine

⅓ cup olive oil

6 garlic cloves, skin on

4 bay leaves

1 tablespoon tomato paste, diluted in 1 cup water

5 allspice berries

1 teaspoon sweet paprika powder

Salt and pepper, to taste

1 cinnamon stick

½ cup water

Preheat oven to 180° C/356° F.

Place all the ingredients onto a baking dish and mix so that the potatoes are coated.

Bake for 50 minutes or until potatoes are fully cooked, golden, and the oil has risen to the top.

Serve immediately with a protein or a side salad.

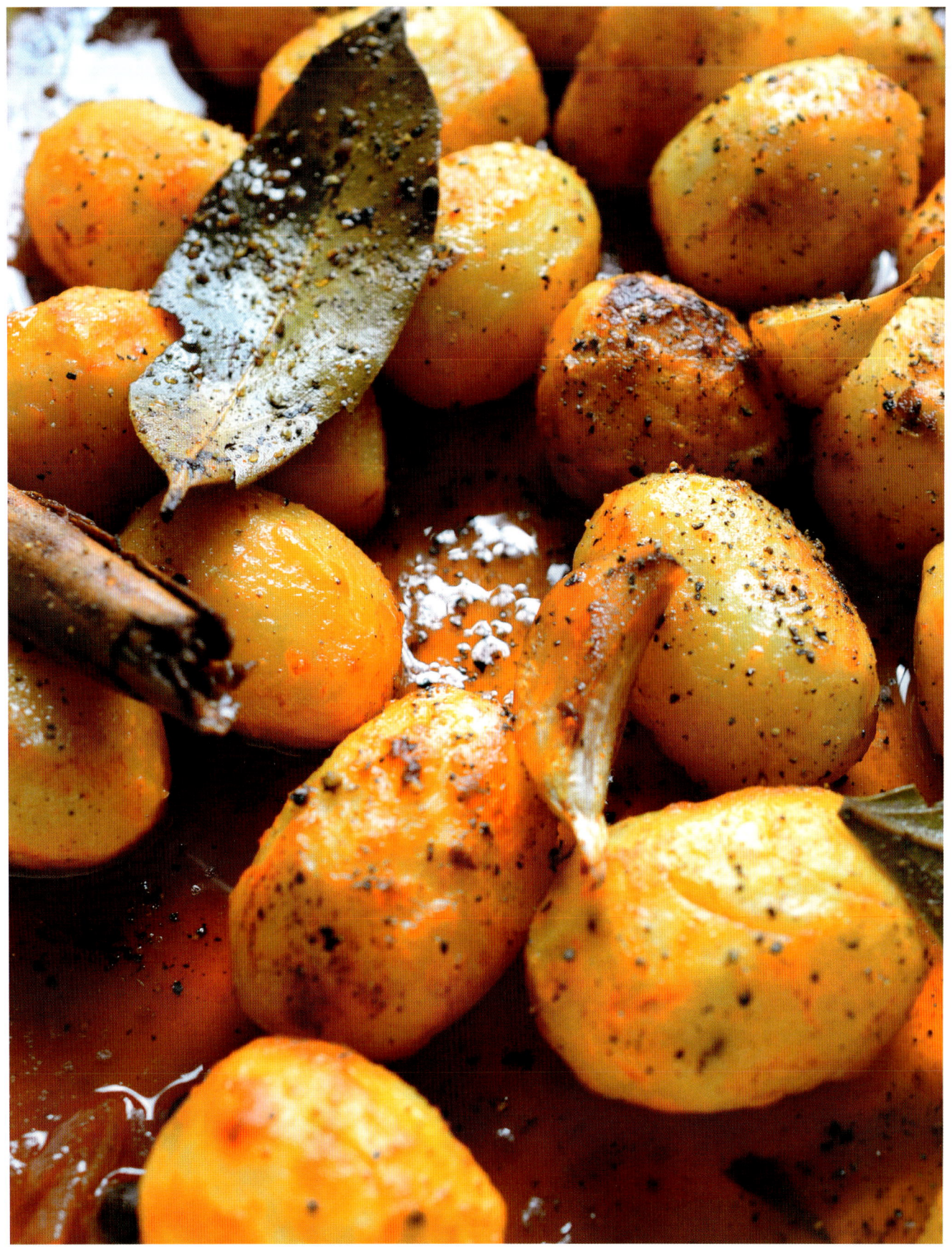

Γίγαντες με σπανάκι στο φούρνο
- LIMA BEANS WITH SPINACH -

In most regions of Greece, *gigantes* are classically made with a tomato-based sauce (see my book *Hellenic Kanella: Memories Made in a Greek Kitchen* for the recipe). This recipe, however, differs as it is prepared the traditional Messinian way from southern Greece. Beans are cooked together with spinach and fresh herbs. The spinach wilts considerably but still compliment the beans nicely. A splash of fresh lemon juice right at the end adds a touch of freshness—simple and healthy.

Serves: 3–4 · 1.5 hours (plus overnight soaking) · GLUTEN FREE

---

1 cup (200 g or 7.0 oz.) lima beans, dried*

1 bay leaf

½ cup olive oil

1 onion, sliced

½ tablespoon tomato paste

1 cup spring onions, finely chopped

½ cup white wine

Salt and pepper, to taste

1 teaspoon castor (superfine) sugar

½ teaspoon chili flakes, optional

250 g (8.8 oz.) spinach, roughly chopped

1 lemon, juiced

¾ cup feta cheese, crumbled

Place the lima beans in a bowl covered with fresh water to soak overnight or a minimum of 10 hours. Drain and add to a pot covered with fresh water. Do not add any salt at this stage as this hardens the beans. Add the bay leaf and bring to a boil, and then simmer for 30–40 minutes or until fork tender. Reserve ½ cup of water, and then drain beans and set aside.

Preheat oven to 200° C/390° F.

Heat oil in a saucepan with sliced onion and sauté until soft. Add tomato paste (mixing well to incorporate), spring onions, wine, salt, pepper, sugar, chili flakes if using, and cook for another minute. Remove from heat.

Place the spinach on the bottom of the baking dish. Top with the lima beans, and then add the onion mixture. Do not stir. Add the ½ cup reserved bean water.

Bake for 20 minutes covered, then uncover and stir to combine. Taste and adjust seasoning if needed. It may require a little more salt and pepper.

Bake for a further 10 minutes or until the juices have evaporated and beans are golden. Juice one lemon and pour over the top. Crumble over feta cheese and return to oven for 10 minutes or until it melts.

Serve warm with some crusty bread.

*One cup uncooked beans equals approximately 2½–3 cups cooked beans.

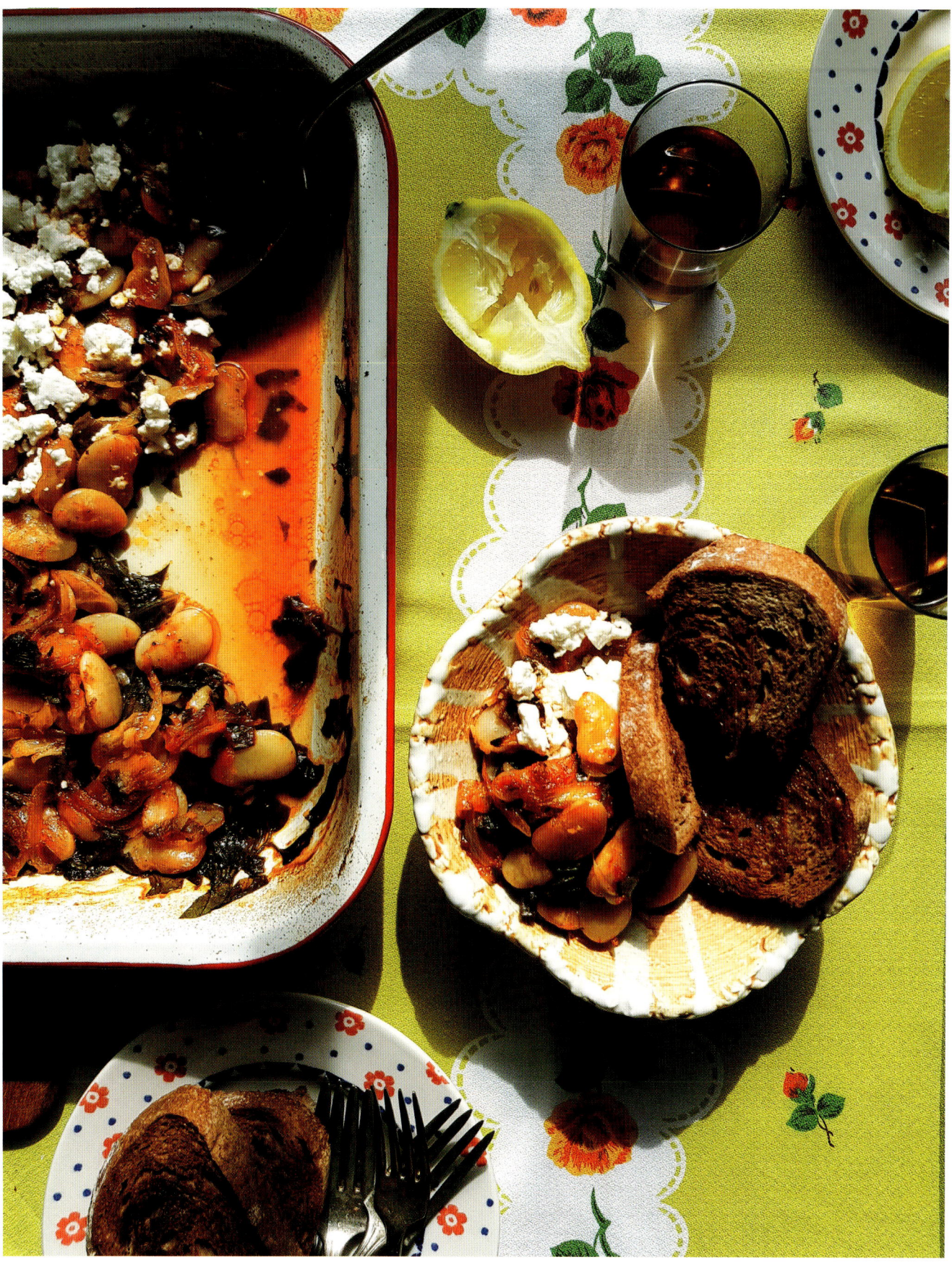

Μανέστρα κολοπίμπιρι
- TOMATO AND PASTA SOUP WITH SWEET PAPRIKA -

¼ cup olive oil

1 large onion, grated

2 cups tomato purée

1 liter water, boiled

Salt and pepper, to taste

1 teaspoon sweet paprika

1 cinnamon stick

1 bay leaf

2 teaspoons castor (superfine) sugar

300 g (10.5 oz.) medium kritharaki pasta* (also known as orzo pasta)

TO SERVE

Greek mizithra cheese, grated*

A quick to prepare and delicious Corfiot soup with Byzantian influences. *Kolopibiri* comes from the Venetian word *collu pimpiri*, meaning "with pepper." Sweet or hot paprika can be used according to your preference but not with any stinginess. Do not be shy to add more if desired. I recall my mother cooking this soup often when my siblings and I wanted soup in a flash. Serve with grated Greek cheese. The soup will thicken when cold. If you prefer it to be soupier, add another ½ cup water when cooking.

Serves: 6 · 35 minutes

Heat the oil in a saucepan. Sauté the onion until translucent. Add tomato purée, water, salt, pepper, paprika, cinnamon stick, bay leaf, and sugar and stir to mix through. Bring to a full boil, and then lower heat to a simmer. Add the pasta and stir for a minute or two to ensure the pasta does not stick to the bottom of the saucepan. Stir every few minutes thereafter as well.

Allow the pasta to cook as directed on package (roughly 10–12 minutes). Taste the soup and adjust seasoning if needed. Once the pasta is cooked, remove from heat, cover with a lid and allow pasta to thicken in the juices, about 10 minutes. Remove cinnamon stick.

Serve warm or hot with a good helping of Greek cheese.

*Parmesan cheese can be used in place of mizithra cheese.

*Kritharaki pasta can be purchased from European grocers.

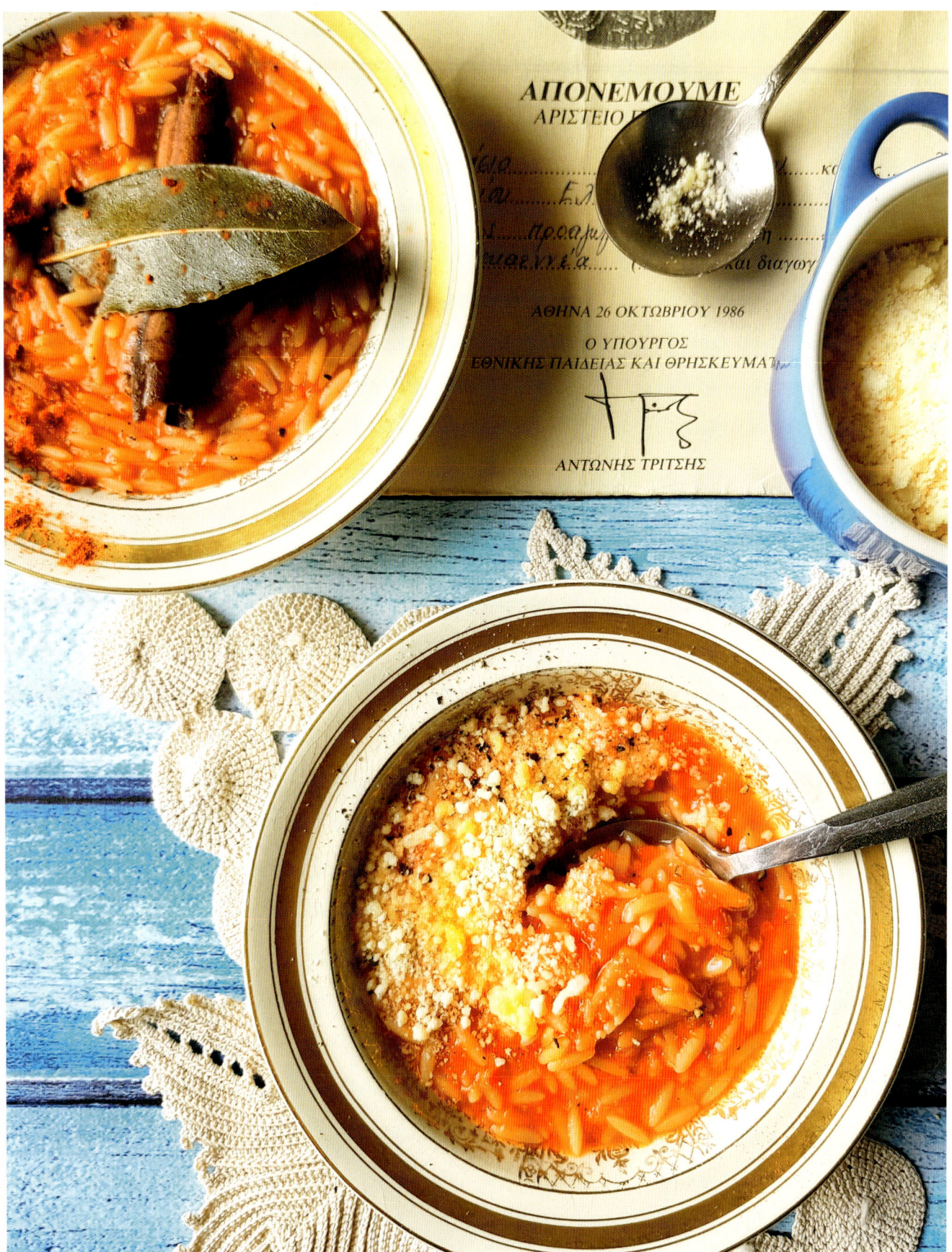

Σαλαντούρμασι

- FRAGRANT RICE-STUFFED ONIONS WITH PINE NUTS -

This recipe is from Kastelorizo, a small and remote treasure island in the Aegean Sea found at the southernmost part of the Dodecanese. It is also located close to the southern coast of Turkey, hence the influence of flavors used in this recipe such as the cumin and pine nuts. Eaten either as a meze (starter) or main, this recipe is sure to impress. Once baked, the onions become super soft and caramelized.

Serves: 3–4 • 1.5 hours • GLUTEN FREE

---

8 medium onions (white or red), or large banana shallots

¾ cup olive oil, divided

2 garlic cloves, minced

Salt and pepper, to taste

1 cup tomato purée

1 cup arborio rice

1 teaspoon cumin powder

1 teaspoon cinnamon powder

¼ cup pine nuts, toasted

½ cup parsley, chopped

¼ cup mint, chopped

1 tablespoon white vinegar

TO SERVE

Parsley, chopped

Pine nuts, roasted

Preheat oven to 200° C/390° F.

Cut off the top and bottom of the onions. Take each one and slit open lengthwise, cutting halfway down the center (be careful you do not cut all the way). Fill a pot with water and bring to a boil. Gently add the onions and cook for 10 minutes or until the flesh starts to soften but onions still hold their shape. Drain, and when cool enough to handle, separate the layers by removing the outer skins first, reserving the inner part. Chop the small inner onion and set aside.

In a sauté pan, heat ¼ cup olive oil. Add the chopped onion and garlic and sauté for 3 minutes. Add salt, pepper, and tomato purée. Cook for a further 3 minutes, and then remove from heat and place into a large bowl. Add the rice, cumin powder, cinnamon powder, pine nuts, herbs, salt, and pepper and mix well to combine.

Fill each layer of onion with a spoonful of the mixture and roll up gently to encase the filling. Place tightly into a baking dish. Pour the vinegar and the remaining ½ cup olive oil over the onions.

Bake covered for 30 minutes, and then uncover and bake for a further 30 minutes or until the onions are slightly golden and caramelized.

Serve with some chopped parsley and extra pine nuts.

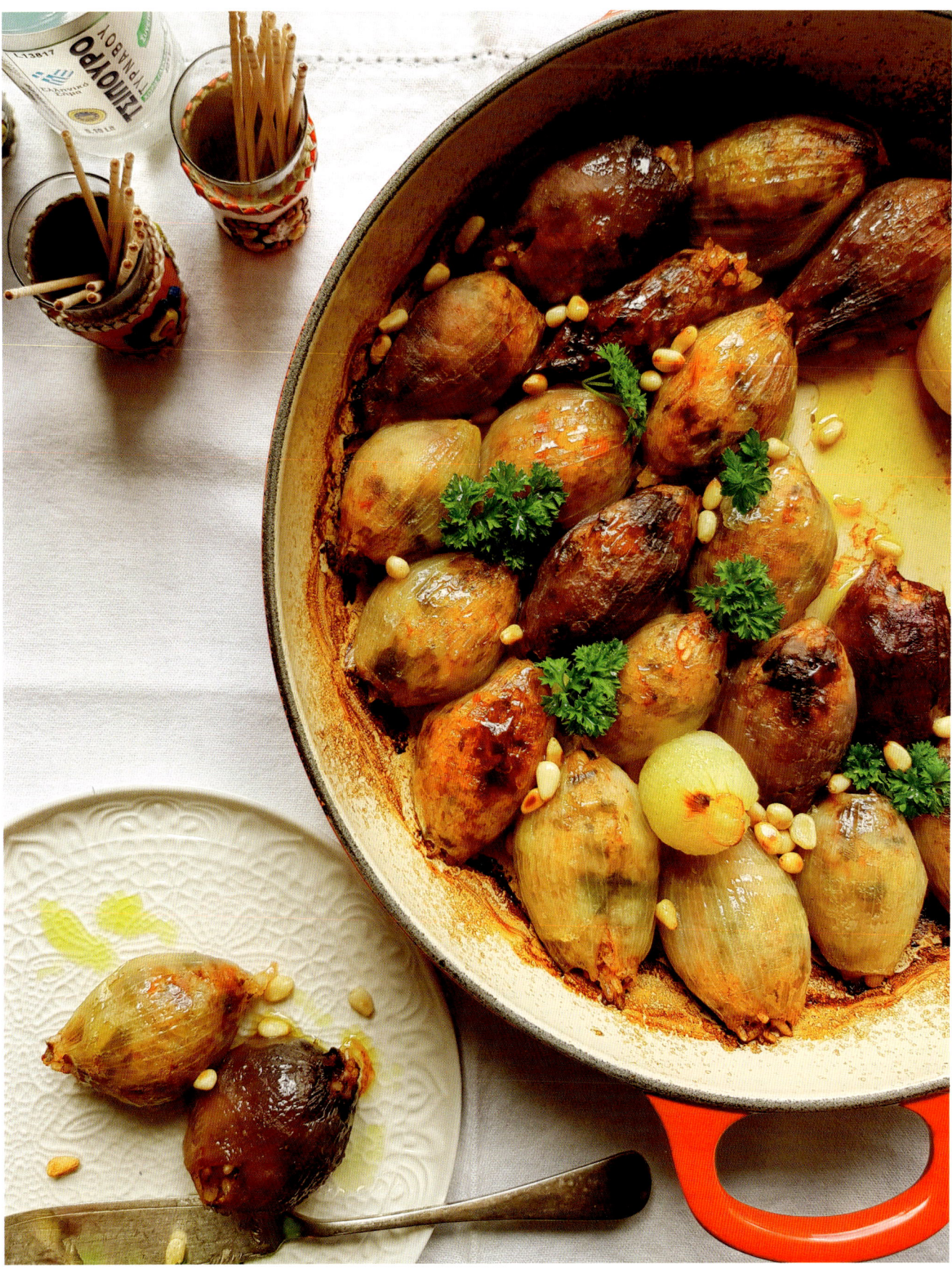

Τσουχτή η Μακαρονάδα της Μάνης

- SPAGHETTI WITH FRIED CHEESE AND EGG -

This may not sound too fancy, but it is comfort and fast food in a bowl. If you enjoy eating pasta, cheese, and eggs, this recipe is for you. Use mizithra cheese, which is a salt-dried cheese made from sheep and goat's milk. From the region of Mani in the Peloponnese, this dish is usually made using thick tubular pasta, but I have opted for spaghetti, though any pasta you fancy will do. For additional flavor—and if you are a garlic lover—sauté 1–2 minced garlic cloves and add them to the oil while it heats up.

500 g (17.6 oz.) spaghetti or fettuccini (Greek brand preferably)

½ cup olive oil

250 g (8.8 oz.) mizithra cheese, grated*

Salt and pepper, to taste

4 whole eggs

TO SERVE

Additional mizithra cheese*

Black pepper

Serves: 4 · 20 minutes

Boil pasta as instructed on packet. A few minutes prior to draining the pasta, add the olive oil to a large frying pan. Heat it until it starts to become aromatic. Add the cheese and fry, stirring until it is slightly colored.

Drain pasta and add it to the hot cheese and oil. Mix through so that the pasta is coated well. Divide onto four serving plates.

In the same frying pan, add a few tablespoons oil, and then crack the four eggs into the oil (no need to heat the oil first). Cover and allow the eggs to fry on medium heat until the egg whites are cooked but the yolk is slightly runny. Season with salt and pepper. Using a spatula, gently remove eggs and place over the pasta (one per serving).

To serve, sprinkle with a little more grated cheese and black pepper. Serve warm.

*Mizithra cheese is the best variety for this recipe and can be purchased from Mediterranean grocers.

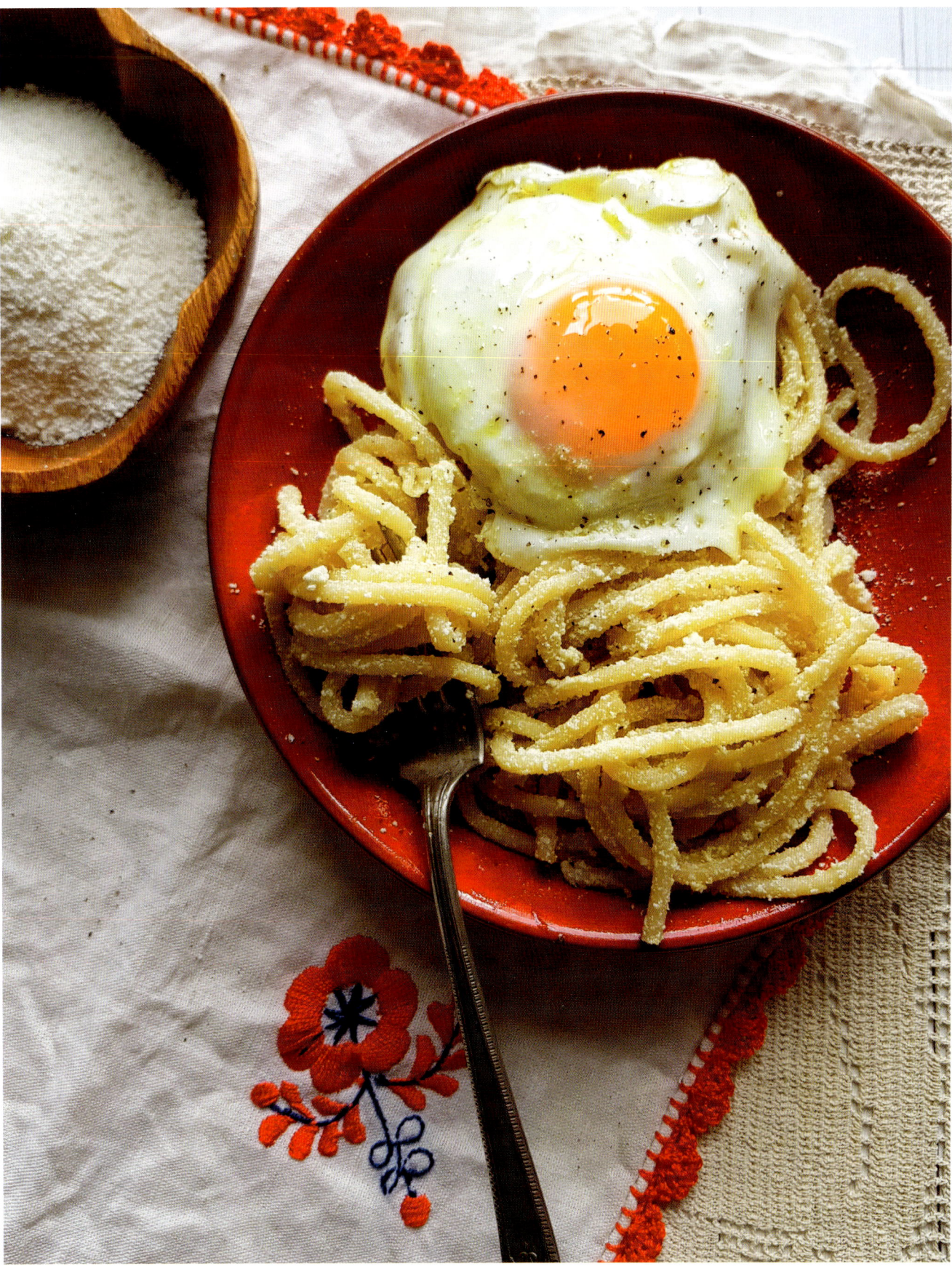

Ντολμαδάκια με σέσκουλα στο φούρνο

- BAKED SILVERBEET ROLLS -

Dolmades are eaten throughout Greece, traditionally made with vine leaves. The word *dolma* comes from the Turkish word for "stuffed." These can also be made with any large leafy vegetable such as silverbeet or Swiss chard. Using the same method, the leaves are blanched and filled with a rice and herb mixture. Dolmades are usually made on the stove top, but in this case, they are baked. Serve with a fresh squeeze of lemon juice and Greek yogurt.

Serves: 5 · 2 hours · GLUTEN FREE

---

800 g (28.2 oz.) silverbeet leaves (approximately 2 large bunches)

FILLING

1 onion, grated

½ cup spring onion, chopped

1½ cups long-grain rice

½ cup parsley, finely chopped

½ cup mint, finely chopped

½ cup olive oil

Salt and pepper, to taste

TOP

2 lemons, juiced

2 bay leaves

Salt, to taste

1 cup tomato purée

¼ cup olive oil

TO SERVE

Squeeze of lemon juice

Yogurt

Preheat oven 180º C/350º F.

Place the filling ingredients into a bowl and mix to combine. Set aside.

Wash the silverbeet leaves, and then remove the veins (the thick stalk in the middle) using kitchen scissors. If the leaves are large, cut into two. Bring a pot of water to a boil. Add leaves to the boiling water, a few at a time, to soften, about 2–3 minutes. Remove and allow to cool.

Line the bottom of a baking tray with silverbeet leaves. This helps the dolmades not to burn. Now take a softened silver beet leaf and place 1 teaspoon of the filling into the center. Gently fold in the sides and roll up tightly. Repeat with all the silverbeet leaves. Place the filled rolls into the tray seam side down and huddled close together, preferably all in one row.

Add the lemon juice, bay leaves, salt, tomato purée, and olive oil. Pour enough water to just cover the rolls. Cover with aluminum foil or lid and bake for 1 hour or until rice is cooked and juices evaporated.

Serve immediately with a squeeze of lemon juice and a dollop of yogurt.

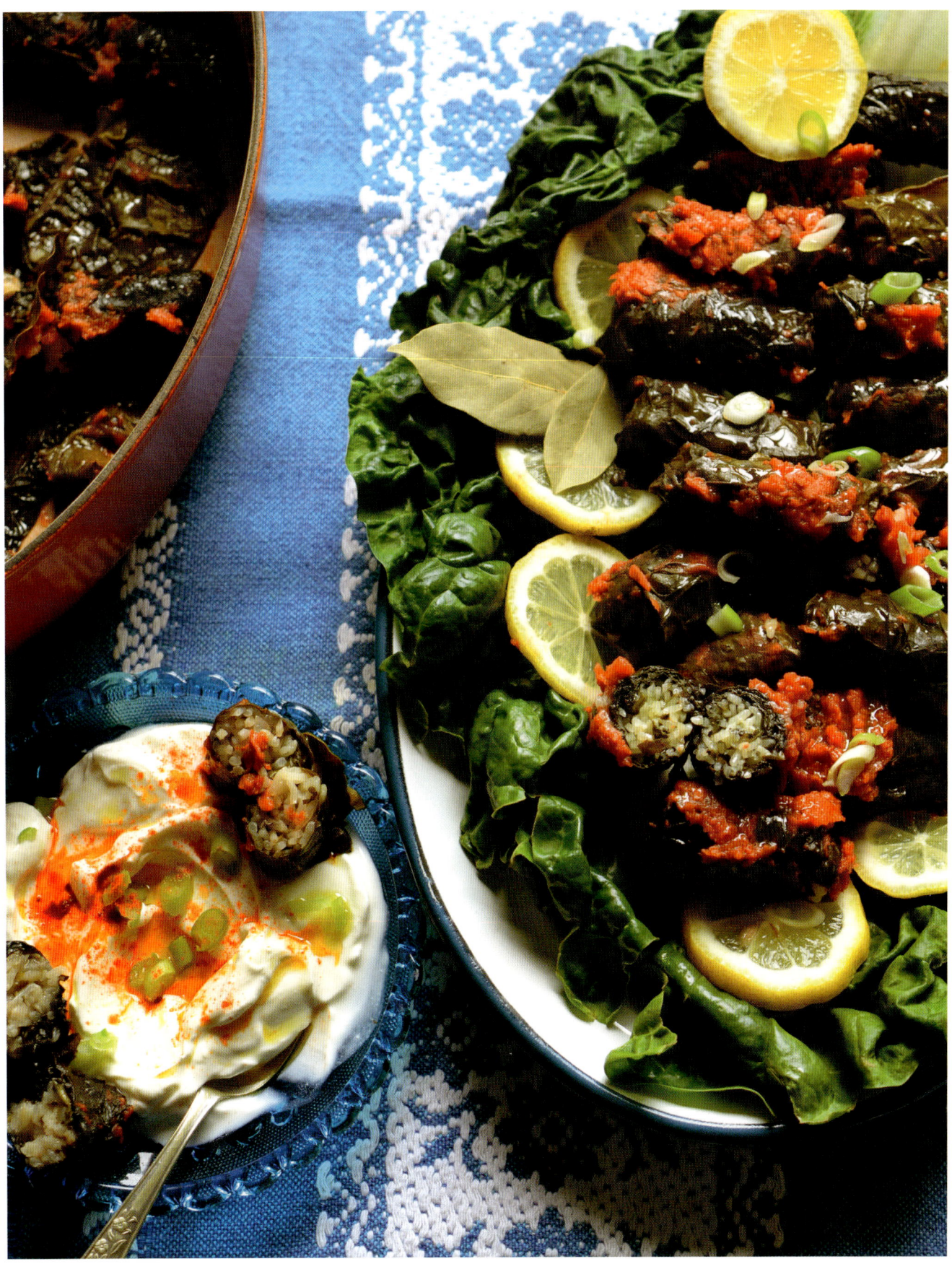

MANITAPIA
MUSHROOMS

Wild mushrooms are quite common in various regions of Greece, boasting a few different varieties. In northern Greece, and more specifically in the city of Greneva, mushrooms are a staple vegetable, and so much so that they have an annual mushroom festival, the largest festival of this sort in Europe. Mushrooms grow well due to the oak forests and wet weather, which is essential for mushrooms to sprout. Hunting expeditions for fungi are very popular in this region. Factories also process mushrooms into oil, soups, and desserts. Households in this region make use of fresh and dried mushrooms throughout the year. In the autumn and spring, mushrooms grow well in Kozani, where the humidity is higher and the temperatures are mild.

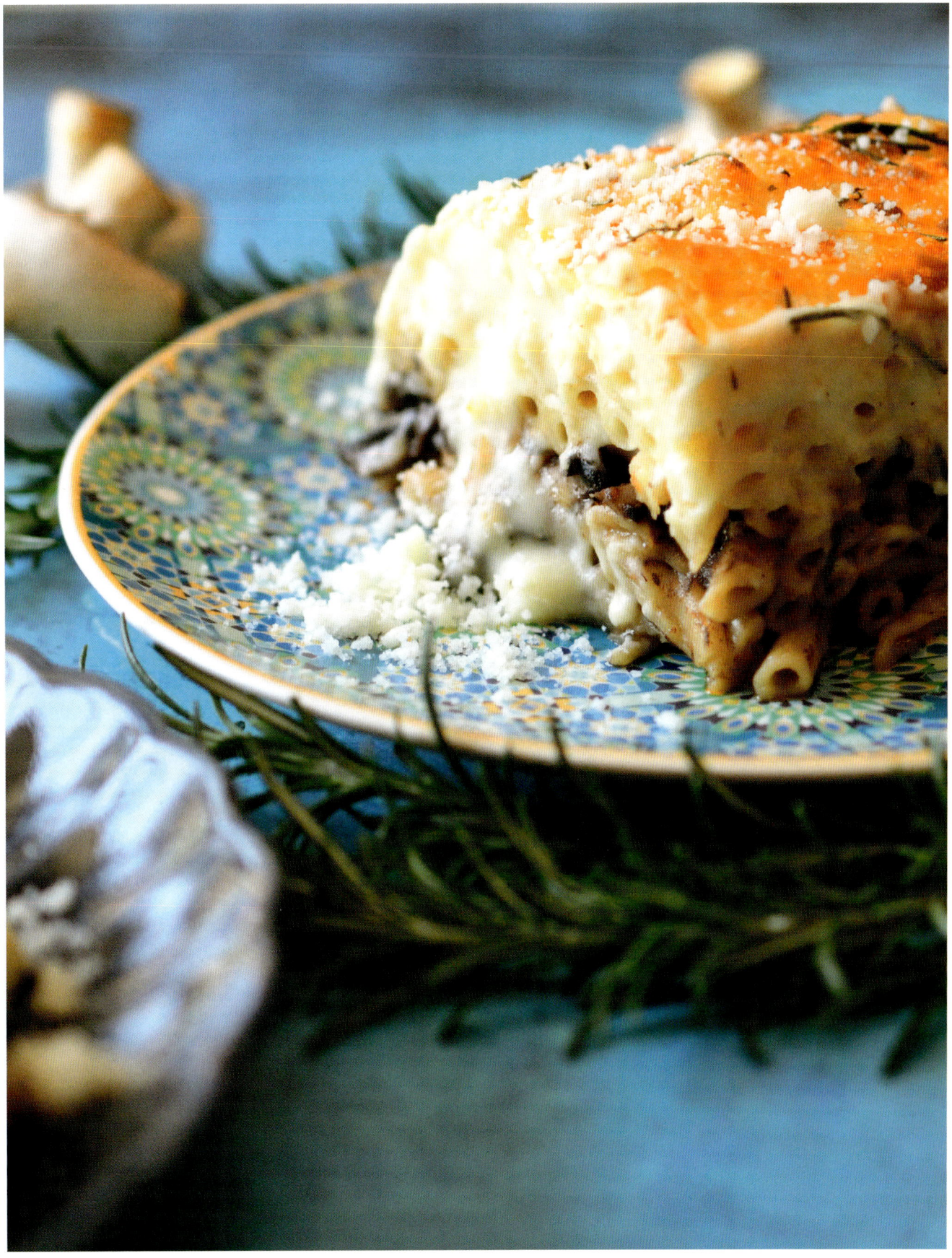

Mushroom Pastitsio, page 66-67.

Αγιορείτικο παστίτσιο με μανιτάρια
- MUSHROOM *PASTITSIO* -

½ cup olive oil

1 medium onion, chopped finely

1½ tablespoons rosemary, chopped, plus a few more sprigs for topping

500 g (17.6 oz.) button mushrooms, sliced

1 teaspoon cinnamon powder

¾ cup tomato purée

Salt and pepper, to taste

2 teaspoons castor (superfine) sugar

1 cup sweet white wine

300 g (10.5 oz.) spaghetti for *pastitsio**

1 ¼ cup kefalograviera cheese, grated and divided*

Pastitsio, as most know, is a pasta-bolognaise dish topped with a béchamel sauce. This *pastitsio*, however, is a vegetarian version, which comes from a repertoire of monastic recipes substituting the meat with mushrooms for fasting purposes. My skepticism was very quickly overcome once I cooked and ate this version. I was intrigued at how flavorful and delicious it was. Ensure you use the correct size baking dish so that the ratios of each layer are balanced. The amount of pasta may seem small, but it is perfect for this size dish. Ensure you use a sweet wine for this recipe and fresh mushrooms.

Serves: 9 · 2 hours

Heat the olive oil and onion in a large pan and sauté until soft. Add the rosemary and cook for 3 minutes, and then add mushrooms and cook for 5 minutes or until slightly colored. Add cinnamon powder, tomato purée, salt, sugar, pepper, and white wine. Cook on medium heat until the liquid has mostly evaporated and the oil has risen to the top, approximately 10–15 minutes. If it is drying out, add a little water. You do not want a very dry mixture. Taste and adjust seasoning. It should taste a little oversalted.

Boil pasta as directed on the packet. Drain and add half the pasta to a baking tray (26x26x7 cm or 10x10x3 in.). Sprinkle ¼ cup cheese over the pasta, and then top with the mushroom sauce. Add the remaining pasta and another ¼ cup cheese over the top.

To make white sauce, place flour in a bowl with water to create a runny batter, whisking to remove any lumps. Set aside.

In a pot, heat the milk, egg, and salt, whisking well to combine. Once it is hot, pour in the flour batter, whisking continuously to remove any lumps until the sauce thickens. This should take about 10 minutes or until the sauce reaches boiling point.

Remove white sauce from stove and add the nutmeg and ½ cup cheese. Taste and adjust seasoning if needed. Pour the sauce on top of the spaghetti. Sprinkle the extra ¼ cup cheese and the rosemary stalks over the casserole.

Bake at 200° C/390° F for 1 hour or until golden. Remove and allow the pastitsio to sit for 30 minutes before serving. Serve with a Greek salad.

*Kefalograviera cheese can be purchased from international grocers or substituted with Parmesan cheese.

*Spaghetti for *pastitsio* can be purchased from international grocers. You could also substitute a thick tubular pasta.

WHITE SAUCE

1 cup all-purpose flour

1 cup water

900 ml (31.6 fl. oz.) whole milk

1 egg, whisked

Salt, to taste

1 teaspoon nutmeg, ground

1 teaspoon salt

TO SERVE

Greek Salad (recipe on page 40)

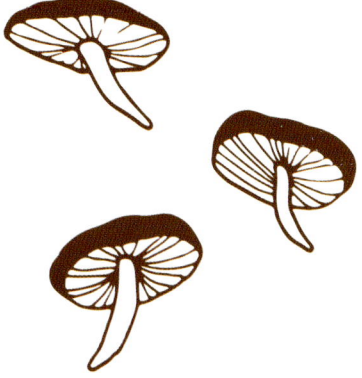

Στιφάδο με μανιτάρια
- MUSHROOM & ONION STEW -

This hearty stew will satisfy vegetarians and meat-eaters alike. It is exceptionally tasty as the onions cook down and become super sweet. The wine reduces, and the added spices give a unique flavor. The mushrooms in this recipe can substitute for meat any day. Trust me, this recipe is a keeper if you love mushrooms.

Serves: 4 · 1.5 hours · GLUTEN FREE

Ingredients:

- ¾ cup olive oil
- 1 kg (35.2 oz.) pearl (pickling) onions, peeled
- 4 garlic cloves, sliced
- 500 g (17.6 oz.) mushrooms, quartered
- Salt, to taste
- 1 teaspoon castor (superfine) sugar
- 1 teaspoon oregano, dried
- 1 cup red wine
- 2 cups tomato purée
- 6 whole peppercorns
- 5 pimento berries
- 8 cloves, whole
- 1 cinnamon stick
- 2 bay leaves
- Chili flakes (optional)
- 2 tablespoons honey

In a saucepan, heat the olive oil, and then add the onions and brown for 8 minutes. Remove with a slotted spoon and set aside.

In the same pot, add the garlic, mushrooms, salt, pepper, sugar, oregano, and sauté for 5 minutes. The mushrooms will shrink. Add the wine and cook for a further 3 minutes. Now add the onions and all the remaining ingredients except the honey. Ensure everything is covered with juices. If not, add some water or extra wine to just cover.

Cover and cook on low heat for 40–60 minutes or until the liquid has thickened and evaporated by half and the onions are very soft.

Remove from stove and add the honey. Gently stir, being careful not to break up the onions. Taste and adjust seasoning if needed.

Serve with mashed potato, rice, pasta, or on its own with crusty bread to mop the juices.

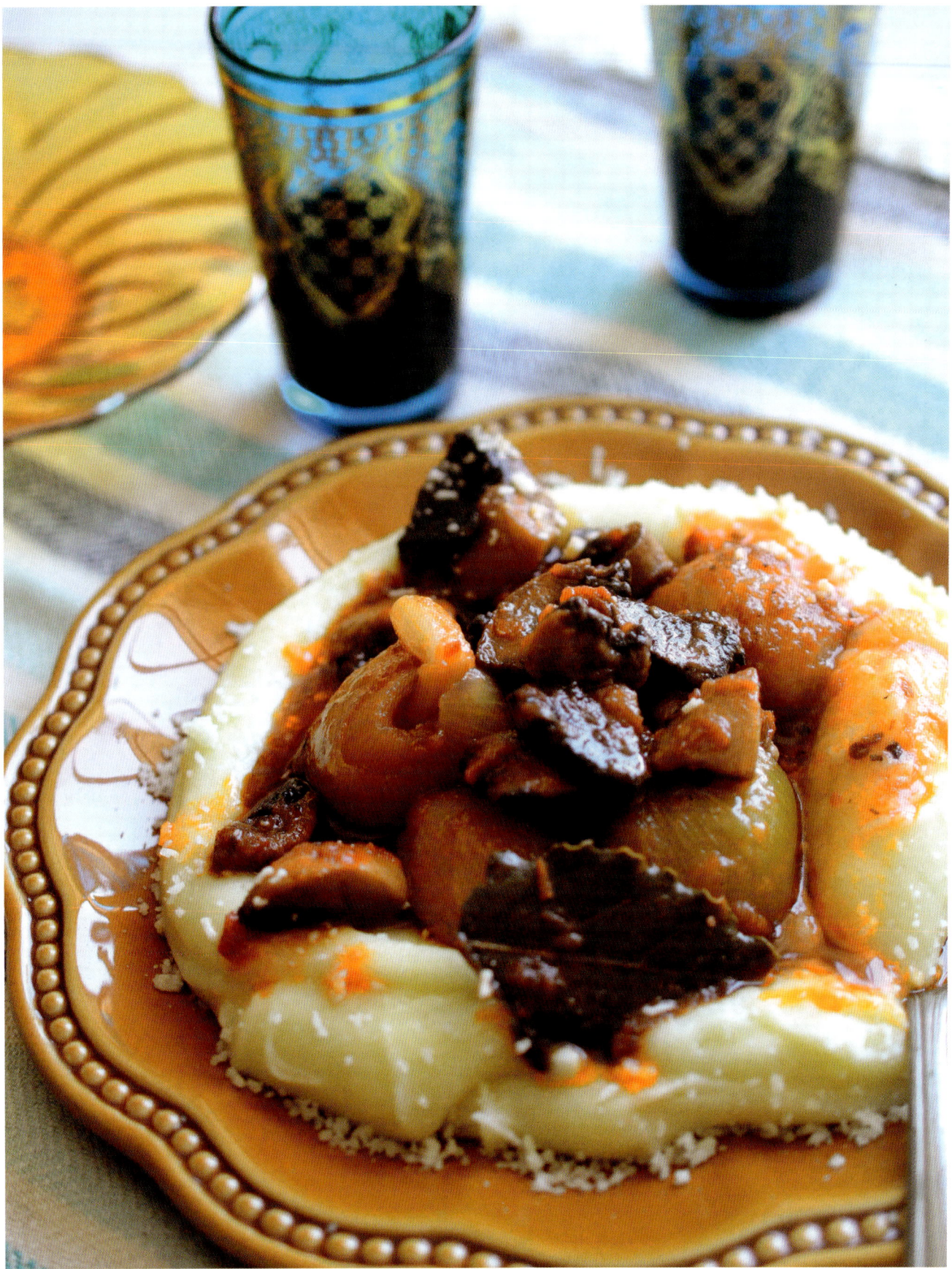

Πατάτες και ντομάτες γεμιστές
- STUFFED POTATOES AND TOMATOES -

6 medium ripe tomatoes

3 medium potatoes

1½ cups olive oil, divided

2 large onions, diced

2 garlic cloves, chopped

1½ cups medium-grain rice

½ cup parsley, finely chopped

½ cup mint, finely chopped

½ cup dill, finely chopped

2 tablespoons tomato paste

1 tablespoon tomato ketchup

1½ teaspoon salt

1½ teaspoon black pepper

½ cup pine nuts, roasted

2 additional large potatoes, peeled and quartered

½ cup tomato purée

1 cup water

I would have to say that for me, the ultimate comfort vegetarian dish would be stuffed vegetables of any sort. They scream summer, but also everything Greek cuisine epitomizes. This dish is simple, nutritious, and easy to make. Gemista means "stuffed." In this recipe, I have used the classic tomatoes and potatoes, but feel free to use zucchini, eggplant, or peppers (as pictured). You could also stuff vine leaves, which are delicious. Brined or fresh vine leaves rolled up can be added to the baking tray and cooked together. I enjoy these most the day after they are made. The juices are delicious mopped up with crusty bread.

Serves: 4 people · 1.5–2 hours · GLUTEN FREE

Preheat oven to 210º C/410º F.

Wash the tomatoes. Slice off the top of the tomatoes and scoop out the flesh (do not discard the top—put it back once you've hollowed out the tomato). Put the tomatoes in a baking dish and season the insides with a pinch of salt. Blend the tomato flesh in a food processor and set aside.

Peel potatoes and slice a top layer off. With a spoon or apple corer, hollow out the potatoes.

Sauté the onions and garlic in half of the olive oil until they are soft. Add the blended tomato and cook for about 6 minutes. Pour this mixture into a large bowl and add the rice, parsley, mint, dill, tomato paste, ketchup, salt, pepper, and pine nuts. Mix the ingredients well and taste to ensure it is well seasoned.

Spoon this mixture into the tomatoes and potatoes. Place the additional quartered potatoes between the tomatoes. Combine tomato purée and 1 cup of water in a bowl. Mix well and pour around the tomatoes. Pour the remaining olive oil over the top.

Bake uncovered for approximately 1½ hours. The juices will evaporate by half, and a lovely layer of oil will be left at the bottom of the pan.

Serve the stuffed veggies with feta cheese and olives. If you have leftovers, they are just as wonderful the next day.

Make-ahead tip: Wash the tomatoes and scoop out the insides one day prior to baking. Arrange them in a baking dish, cover the dish with plastic wrap, and refrigerate the tomatoes until you are ready to fill them.

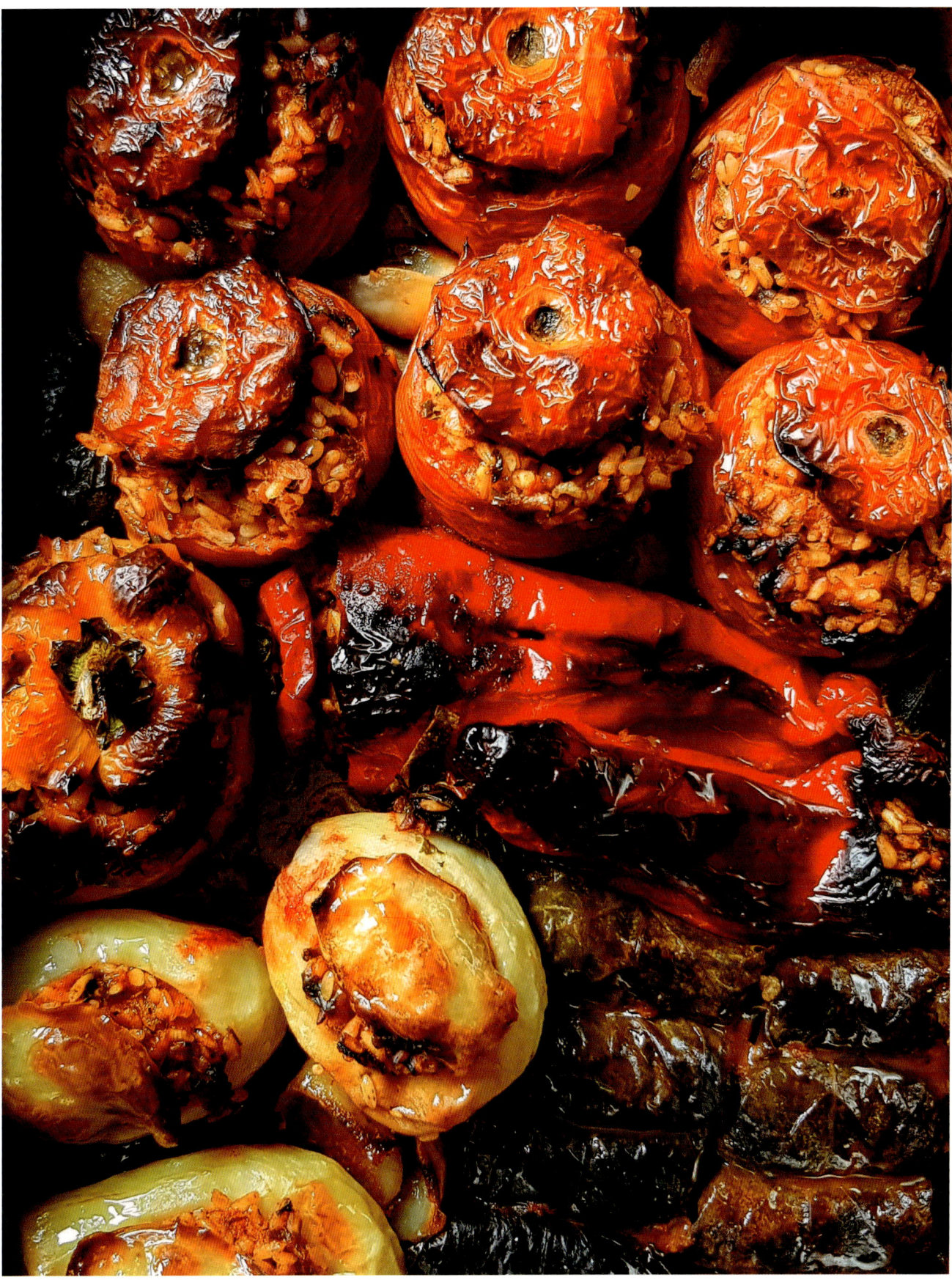

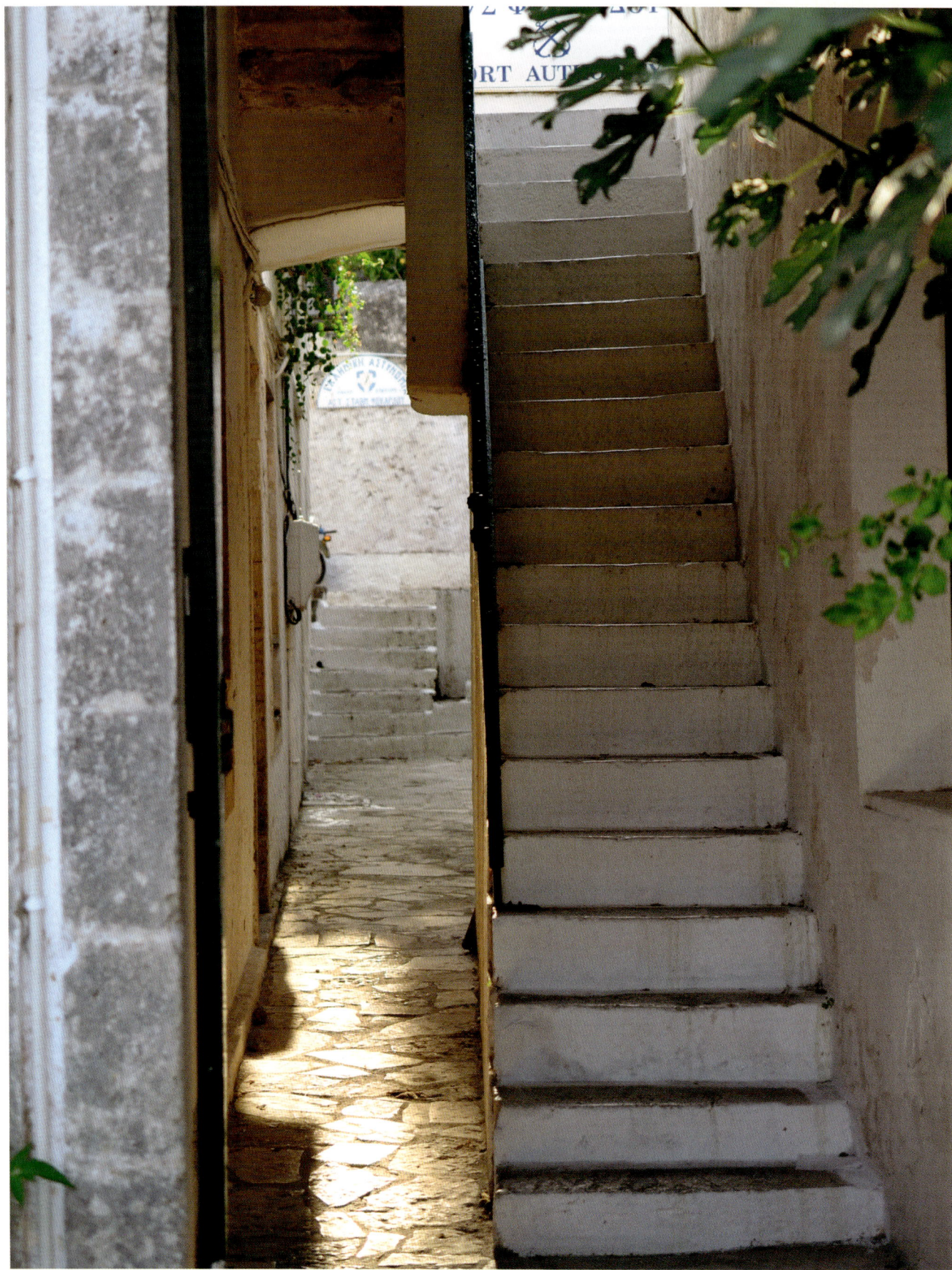

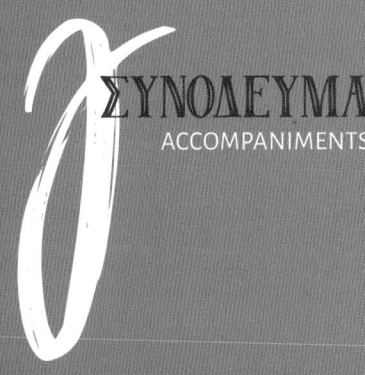

ΣΥΝΟΔΕΥΜΑ
ACCOMPANIMENTS

75 **ΡΕΒΙΘΙΑ ΜΕ ΚΑΣΤΑΝΑ**
CHICKPEAS WITH CHESTNUTS (GF)

77 **ΠΑΤΖΑΡΟΣΑΛΑΤΑ**
BEETROOT AND FETA DIP (GF)

78 **ΣΥΡΙΑΝΗ ΚΑΠΑΡΟΣΑΛΑΤΑ**
CAPER MASH FROM SYROS (GF)

79 **ΜΑΪΝΤΑΝΟΣΑΛΑΤΑ**
PARSLEY DIP (GF)

81 **ΤΣΙΓΑΡΕΛΙ ΜΕ ΑΥΓΑ**
GREENS WITH EGGS AND FETA CHEESE (GF)

82 **ΝΤΟΛΜΑΔΑΚΙΑ ΓΙΑΛΑΝΤΖΙ**
VINE LEAVES STUFFED WITH RICE, CURRANTS, AND PINE NUTS (GF)

83 **ΠΡΑΣΑ ΜΕ ΔΑΜΑΣΚΗΝΑ**
LEEKS WITH PRUNES AND WHITE WINE (GF)

85 **ΑΓΡΙΑ ΣΠΑΡΑΓΓΙΑ ΜΕ ΑΥΓΑ**
WILD ASPARAGUS WITH EGGS (GF)

87 **ΚΟΥΝΟΥΠΙΔΙ ΓΙΑΧΝΙ ΜΕ ΣΤΑΦΙΔΕΣ**
CAULIFLOWER STEW WITH SPICES AND RAISINS (GF)

88 **ΚΟΛΟΚΥΘΟΚΕΦΤΕΔΕΣ**
ZUCCHINI FRITTERS

89 **ΤΗΓΑΝΙΤΕΣ ΠΑΤΑΤΕΣ**
OLIVE-OIL FRIED POTATOES (GF)

GF DENOTES GLUTEN-FREE RECIPES

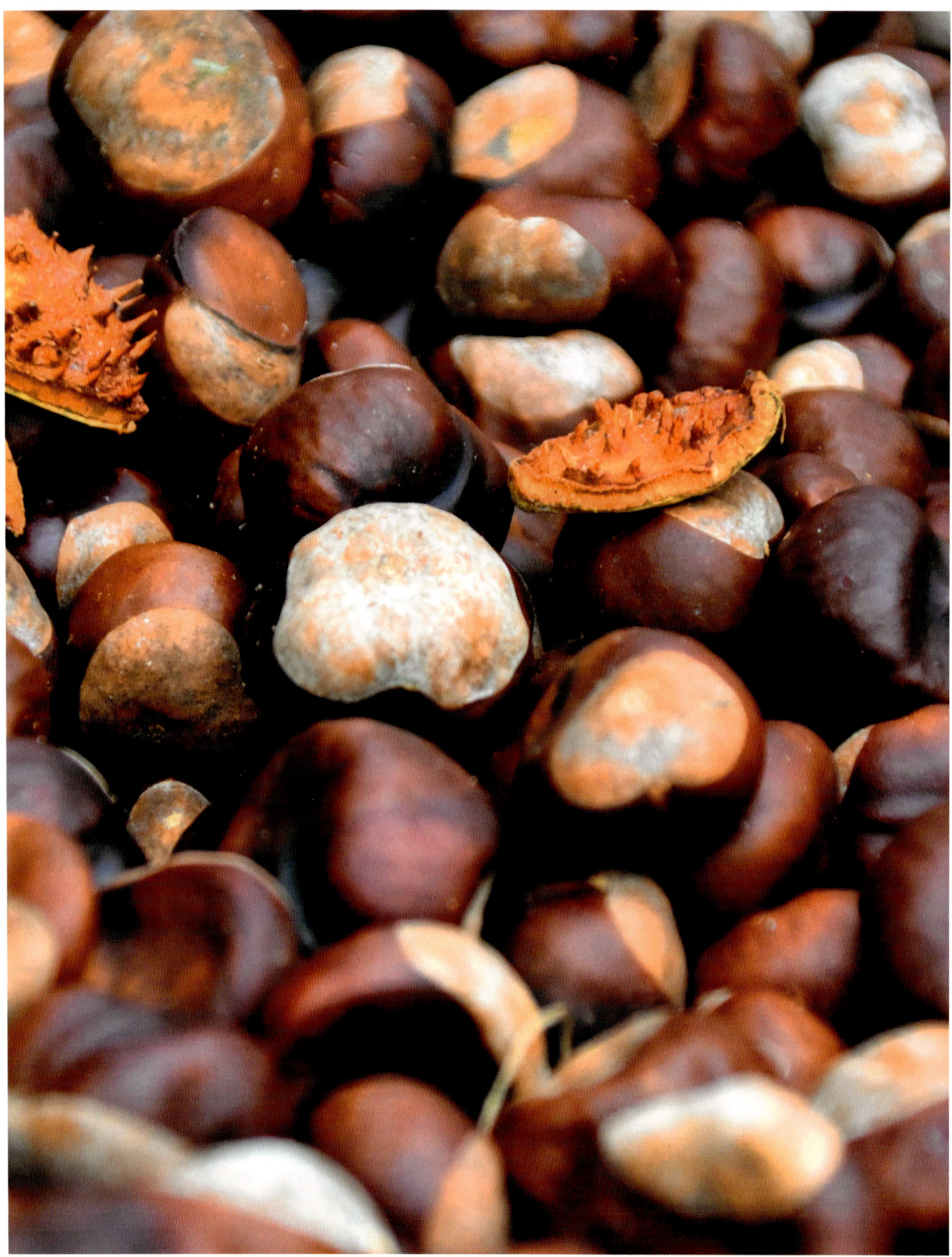

A delightful winter dish from the area of Arkadías in the Peloponnese. Chestnuts grow plentifully in this region. When chestnuts are in season, a chestnut festival is held in honor of this amazing produce. This dish is rich, so it is best served as a starter. It is known as "a poor man's food," yet it is full of flavor and nutrients.

Serves: 4 · 2 hours (plus overnight soaking)
· GLUTEN FREE

Place dried chickpeas in a bowl and cover with fresh water. Allow to soak a minimum 10 hours or overnight. Drain and add to a pot covered with fresh water and the halved onion. Bring to a boil, and then simmer on low heat for 30–50 minutes or until chickpeas are cooked through but not falling apart. Drain chickpeas and set aside to cool. Alternatively, use canned chickpeas that have been drained. Just go straight to the step below.

Place chickpeas together with all the remaining ingredients (except the chestnuts) into a baking dish. A clay pot works perfectly for this recipe, but any heavy dish that has a sealing lid will work. Mix well. Cover with a lid (or alternatively with foil) and bake for 1 hour at 180° C/356° F.

Uncover and add the chestnuts, mixing gently to not mash up the chickpeas. Cook for a further 20 minutes so that the chickpeas become slightly golden and juices evaporate.

Serve immediately with a sprinkle of extra chopped parsley and a lemon wedge on the side.

*To peel chestnut skins, score the chestnuts with a cross and place onto a baking tray. Bake at 160° C/320° F for 25–30 minutes. Remove from oven. Allow to cool slightly (only enough to handle), and then peel skins off while warm.

Ρεβίθια με κάστανα
- CHICKPEAS WITH CHESTNUTS -

1 cup (190 g or 6.7 oz.) dried chickpeas
(if canned, omit first step)

1 large onion, halved

200 g (7.0 oz.) whole chestnuts, skin off*

2 tomatoes, quartered

¾ cup olive oil

¾ cup white wine

Salt and pepper, to taste

½ lemon, juiced

1 tablespoon parsley, chopped

1 teaspoon sweet paprika powder

TO SERVE

Lemon wedge

Parsley, chopped

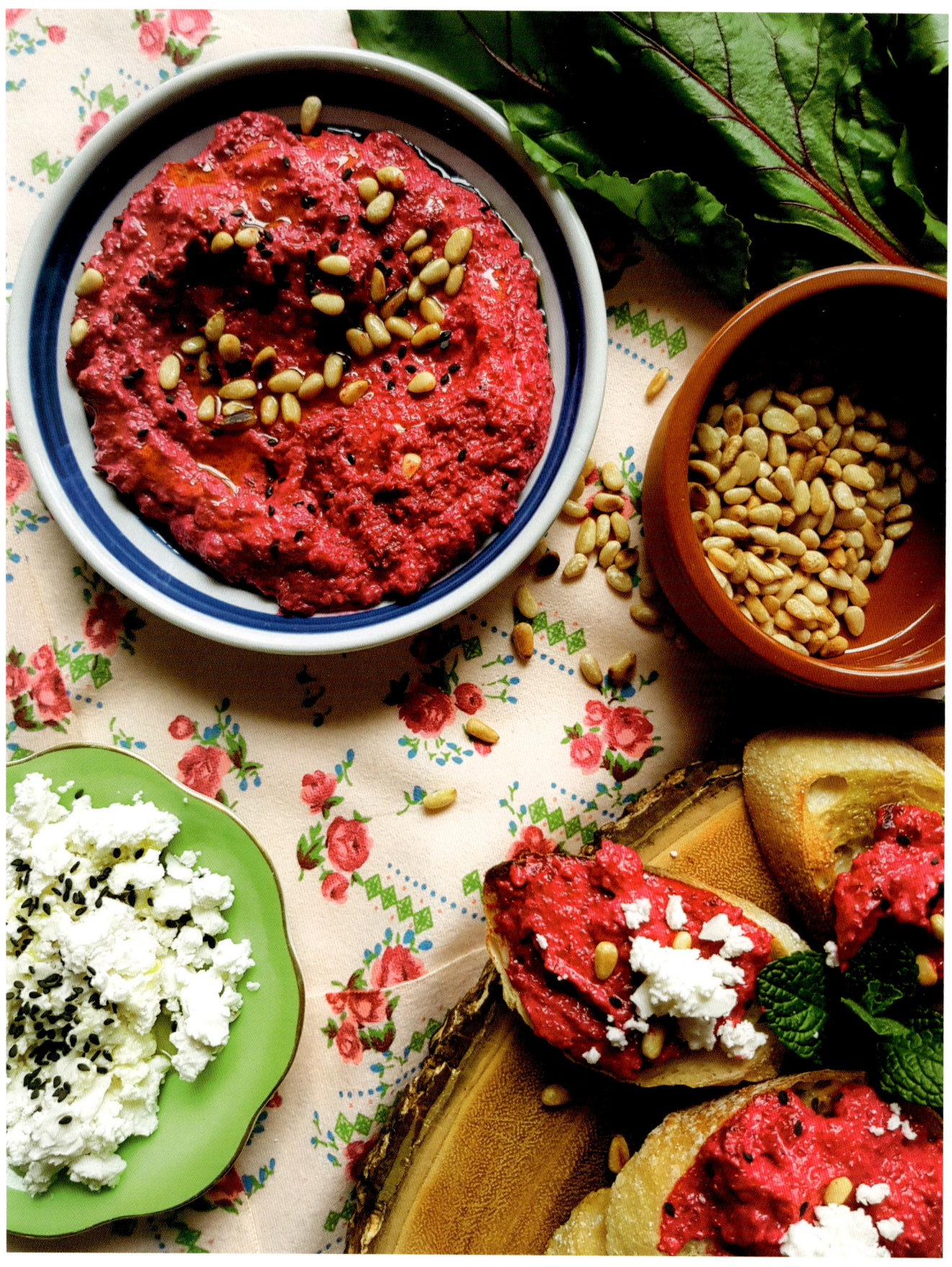

Beetroot and feta dip is a popular meze throughout central Greece and beyond. Most tavernas have a variation of a beetroot dip, some with garlic, dairy, and others vegan and the like. I prefer this version as I enjoy yogurt and feta combined with the beets. This version has a tanginess and a great texture. The color is so lively, and the taste is intensified by the roasting of the beets. This is a fabulous dip to prepare days in advance and have refrigerated until required. As with all vegetables, ensure the beets are in season for optimum flavor. For some variance, you could add 1–2 tablespoons of tahini paste for a sesame-beetroot dip. Mix well and serve.

Makes: 3 cups · 1 hour · GLUTEN FREE

Take a large piece of aluminum foil that is big enough to enclose the beets and place onto a counter. Place a sheet of parchment paper over the top. Put the quartered beetroot onto the paper together with the rosemary, 3 tablespoons olive oil, and some salt. Enclose the foil to make into a parcel, ensuring it is closed completely. Place on a baking tray and roast at 200° C/390° F for 45 minutes or until the beets are soft. Set aside to cool.

Put the cooled beets in a food processor. Add the remaining olive oil, yogurt, feta, and salt. Pulse until a smooth texture is achieved. Taste and adjust seasoning. It should have a nice salty taste. Add more cheese if desired. Refrigerate for a minimum 2 hours before serving.

Keeps refrigerated for up to 3 days.

TIP: To avoid red hands when peeling beetroots, submerge and peel them in a bowl of water.

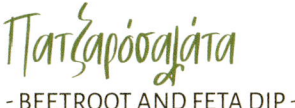

Πατζαρόσαλάτα
- BEETROOT AND FETA DIP -

800 g (28.21 oz.), 3–4 medium beetroots peeled and quartered

1 sprig rosemary

½ cup olive oil, divided

¾ cup yogurt

250 g (8.8 oz.) feta cheese

Salt, to taste

TO SERVE

Feta cheese, crumbled

Pine nuts, roasted

Mint leaves

Olive oil

Συριανή Καππαροσαλάτα
- CAPER MASH FROM SYROS -

3 large potatoes (650 g or 22.92 oz.), peeled and quartered

¼ cup olive oil

Juice of one lemon

Salt and pepper, to taste

¾ cup capers, rinsed and drained

TO SERVE

Parsley, chopped

This is a traditional mash from the island of Syros, combining boiled potatoes and capers (a prominent ingredient grown in this region). I must admit this mash has become one of my favorites. It pairs wonderfully well with seafood. It is best to purée it in a food processor to achieve a smoother texture (Picture on page 110).

Serves: 3–4 · 35 minutes · GLUTEN FREE

Place potatoes into a saucepan covered with water. Add 1 tablespoon salt and boil potatoes until soft.

Drain, place into a food processor, and pulse 1–2 times.

Now add the oil, lemon, salt, pepper, and capers. Pulse until a smooth dip has been achieved.

Taste and adjust seasoning. Add a little more olive oil if the mash is very dry.

Serve topped with some additional chopped parsley.

Keeps refrigerated 1–2 days. If it has thickened add more olive oil.

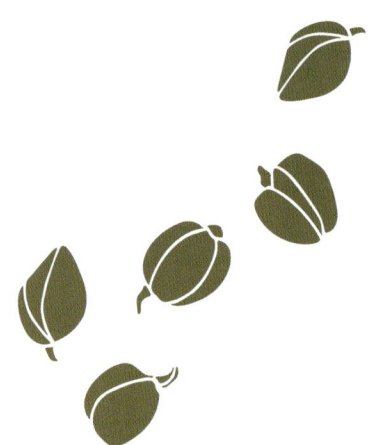

Another classic dip from the island of Syros is this creamy parsley dip, or parsley salad, as Greeks call it. It is very similar to the caper mash on previous page, but the main ingredient and flavor is the parsley. You can make this recipe without the potato if you like. The result will be more like a salsa than a dip, or reminiscent of an Italian salsa verde. Serve on some crusty oiled bread or as a side for seafood.

Serves: 3–4 · 25 minutes · GLUTEN FREE

Soak the bread in ½ cup water. After 10 minutes, remove the bread and squeeze out any excess water with your hands. Place the bread into a bowl and set aside.

Place the potato in a saucepan filled with water and boil until soft. Remove potato with a slotted spoon and set aside.

In a food processor, combine the parsley, onion, garlic, oil, capers, salt, pepper, the juice of one lemon, soaked bread, and the boiled potato. Pulse until smooth. Taste and adjust seasoning. It should have a balance of salt and sour. If it is too thick, add a little more oil and pulse again.

Serve with some whole capers and an extra squeeze of lemon juice. Cover and leave in the refrigerator for at least an hour before serving.

*Substitute gluten-free bread if preferred or omit entirely.

Μαϊντανοσαλάτα
- PARSLEY DIP -

1 cup day-old bread, crusts removed, cut into small pieces*

1 large potato, peeled and quartered

1 cup parsley, chopped

½ small onion, minced

½ garlic clove, minced

¼ cup olive oil

2 tablespoons capers

Salt and pepper, to taste

1–2 lemons, juiced, to taste

TO SERVE

Capers, whole

Lemon juice

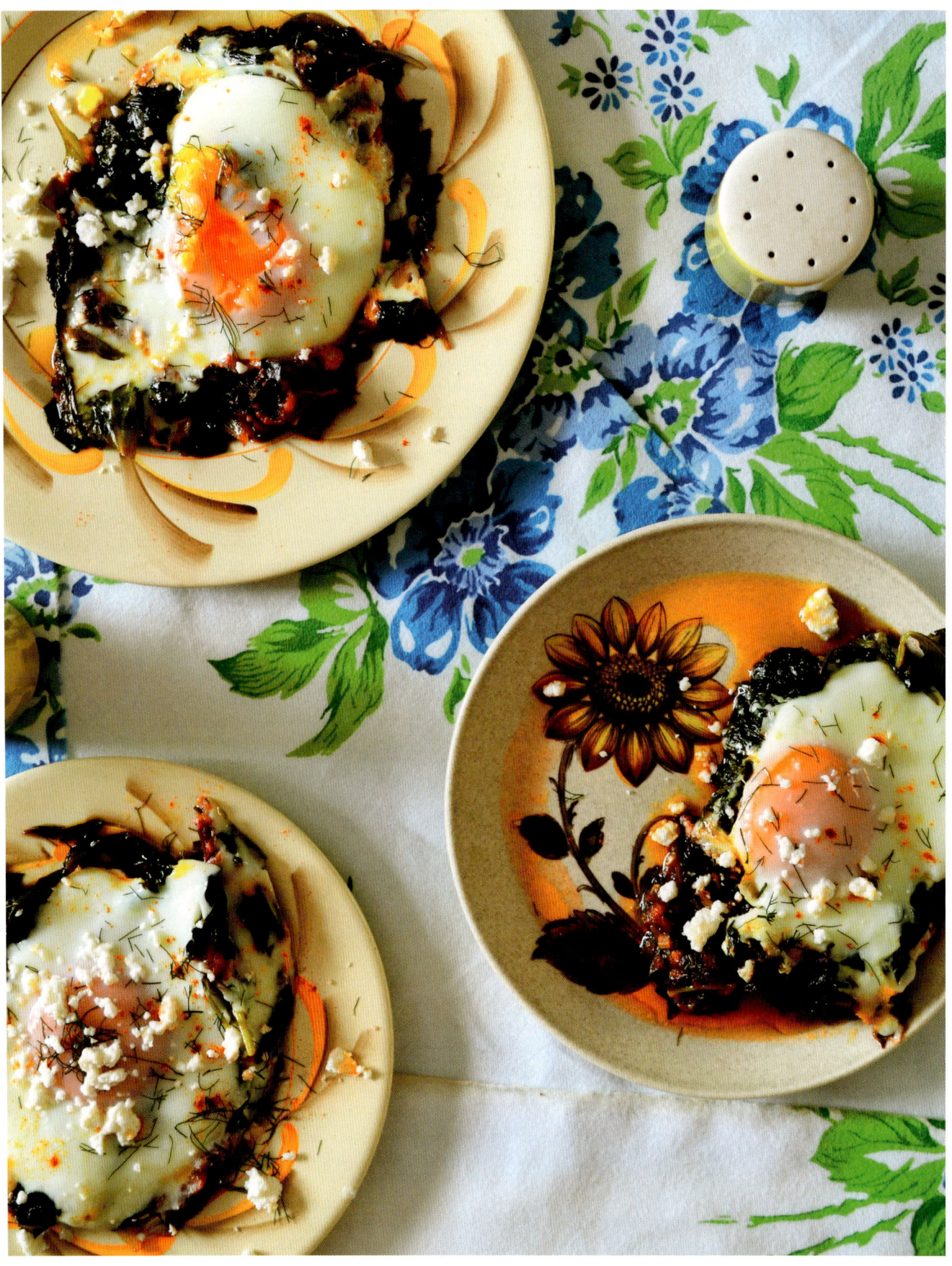

Tsigareli comes from the Greek word *tsigarizo*, meaning "to sauté." It is a Corfiot recipe and an Ionian Islands favorite. Wild greens are sautéed in plenty of olive oil, herbs, tomato, onions, and cayenne pepper or chili flakes. Once the greens are wilted, eggs are cracked over the top, cooked to one's liking, and then covered with crumbled feta cheese. The dish can be eaten for breakfast, brunch, lunch, or even dinner with a side of baked potatoes or fish. I have substituted wild greens with the more common and accessible year-round greens.

Serves: 4 · 20 minutes · GLUTEN FREE

Heat the oil in a sauté pan. Add the greens and allow to wilt on medium heat for about 5 minutes. Do not add any liquid. Add the spring onions, parsley, dill, mint, tomato purée, and cayenne pepper and season with salt and pepper. Place a lid on the saucepan and cook for 15 minutes or until the oil has risen to the top.

Crack the eggs on top of the greens. Return the lid and cook for another 5 minutes or until the egg whites are cooked and the yolk is slightly runny. Remove from heat.

Crumble feta cheese over the top and serve.

Τσιγαρέλι με αυγά
- GREENS WITH EGGS AND FETA CHEESE -

¼ cup (60 ml) olive oil

450 g (15.87 oz.) green leafy vegetables (silverbeet, spinach), washed and roughly chopped

½ cup spring onions, chopped

¼ cup parsley, chopped

1 tablespoon dill, chopped

5 mint leaves, chopped

1 cup tomato purée

½ teaspoon cayenne pepper or chili flakes (optional)

Salt and pepper, to taste

4 whole eggs

TO SERVE

Feta cheese, crumbled

Ντολμαδάκια Γιαλαντζί

- VINE LEAVES STUFFED WITH RICE, CURRANTS, AND PINE NUTS -

Dolmadakia (ντολμαδάκια) are the quintessential meze dish. Herbs and rice are delicately rolled in vine leaves and left to simmer on the stove. To finish the dish, a good squeeze of lemon juice and olive oil are added. There are slight differences to the stuffing depending on where you are in Greece. This is a classic version from the south with the addition of raisins and pine nuts.

Makes: 70 pieces • 1.5 hours • GLUTEN FREE

---

500 g (17.6 oz.) vine leaves, preserved in brine

2 cups medium-grain rice

2 cups spring onion, finely chopped

1 large onion, diced

½ cup mint, finely chopped

½ cup parsley, finely chopped

½ cup dill, finely chopped

¼ cup pine nuts (optional)

¼ cup currants (optional)

1½ cups olive oil, divided

1 teaspoon salt

1 teaspoon black pepper

2½ cups boiling water

2 lemons, freshly squeezed

TO SERVE

Yogurt

Squeeze of lemon

Soak the vine leaves in a bowl of cold water for 30 minutes. This will wash off any excess salt. Drain the leaves and layer one row on the bottom of a saucepan. This will protect the *dolmadakia* from sticking to the bottom of the saucepan.

Place the rice, spring onions, onion, mint, parsley, dill, pine nuts, currants, ¾ cup of the olive oil, salt, and pepper in a bowl. Taste a little of the rice to see if there is enough seasoning. Adjust if needed.

Lay each leaf stem side up and place 1 teaspoon of the rice mixture in its center. Fold the leaf by bringing the sides together, and then roll the leaf to enclose the rice in the leaf. Place each dolmadaki close together seam side down in the pan.

Pour the remaining ¾ cup olive oil, boiled water, and lemon juice into the pot. Place a plate that is smaller than the diameter of the pot on top of the *dolmadakia* so that they don't puff up and open while cooking. Place a lid on the pot and simmer over low heat for about 35 minutes or until the water is absorbed and the rice is cooked through. If you are finding that the water is absorbing too quickly, just keep adding a little more boiling water until the *dolmadakia* are cooked.

Take the pan off the heat and remove lid. Place a clean tea towel on top, and then cover with the lid. This will allow the steam to be completely absorbed by the towel. *Dolmadakia* can be kept refrigerated for up to 3 days.

Serve them with yogurt and an additional squeeze of lemon.

A classic recipe from Epiros. Sweet prunes are added to leeks and potatoes. It is a peasant-style dish cooked on the stove—*giahni* style, as they say in Greek. It boasts intense sweet and sour flavors. The leeks get cooked down to release natural sweetness. Sweet wine, bay leaf, prunes and potatoes are then added. The concept of sweet and sour in Greek food has long existed. Dried fruits or sweeteners such as honey or grape must (or *petimezi*) have always been added to dishes such as this. Grab yourself a loaf of crusty bread and enjoy.

Serves: 4 · 45 minutes · GLUTEN FREE

In a wide saucepan, heat the olive oil with the onion and sauté until translucent. Add the leeks and potatoes and cook for 2–3 minutes. Pour in wine and cook for a further 3–5 minutes for the alcohol to evaporate. Now add all other ingredients except the prunes. Cook covered on low to medium heat for 15–20 minutes or until potatoes are half cooked.

If the liquid is evaporating too quickly, add another ¼ cup water to the pan. Add the prunes (but do not mix). With the lid on, cook for a further 10–15 minutes or until potatoes are fully cooked. Taste and adjust seasoning. It should be sweet and a little tart. Remove from heat, cover, and let it stand for around 10 minutes.

Serve with crusty bread or omit for a gluten-free meal.

Πράσα με δαμάσκηνα

- LEEK WITH PRUNES AND WHITE WINE -

¼ cup olive oil

½ medium onion, grated

3 leeks, cleaned and cut into 3 cm (1.1 in.) pieces

2 medium potatoes, peeled and cut into bite-size pieces

¼ cup sweet white wine

½ cup tomato purée

1 bay leaf

1 cinnamon stick

1 teaspoon castor (superfine) sugar

1 tablespoon red or white vinegar

Salt and pepper, to taste

½ cup water

15 pitted prunes, whole

THE GARDEN

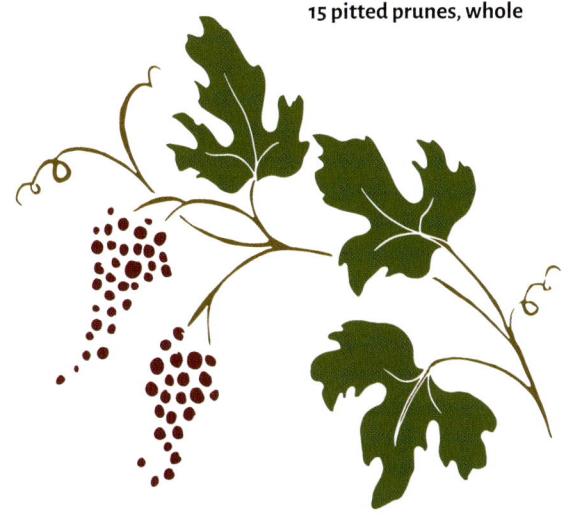

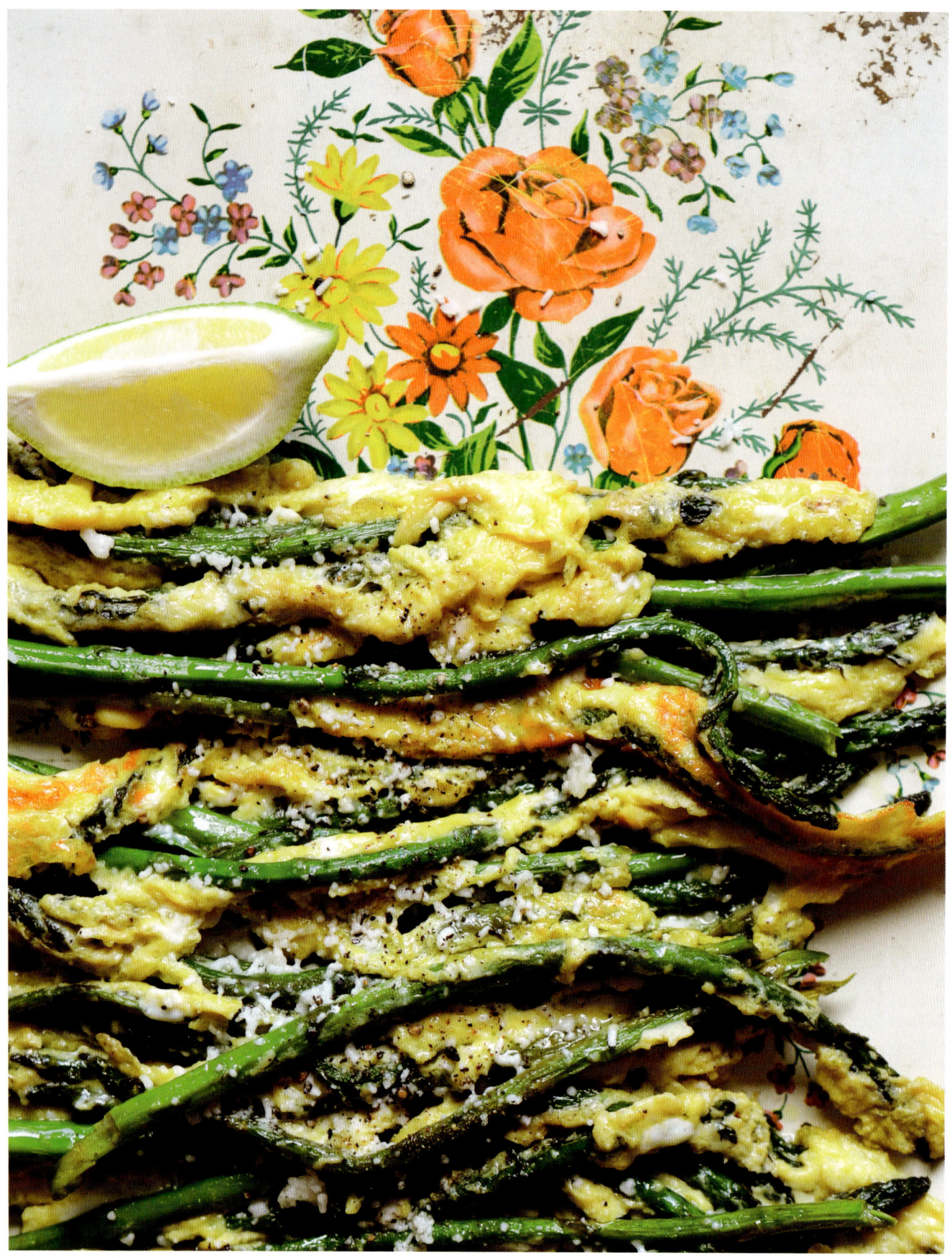

Usually, one does not associate asparagus with many Greek meals, yet in the region of Pilio (central region of Greece), this recipe is a favorite with the locals. In Pilio, asparagus is grown in abundance and generally eaten very simply. Asparagus are either boiled then tossed in some olive oil and lemon juice (*ladolemono*) or vinegar (*ladoxilo*) or quickly fried and added to scrambled eggs. It can be eaten as a side or a main meal. The asparagus must be in season, preferably the thin variety, otherwise the asparagus will taste woody.

Serves: 2 · 15 minutes · GLUTEN FREE

Heat the olive oil in a wide saucepan. Add the asparagus, salt, and pepper and sauté with lid on until softened, around 10 minutes. Taste to ensure they are not hard.

Place the eggs in a bowl together with the milk and a little salt. Whisk to combine well. Pour over the asparagus and allow to cook without turning for 30 seconds, and then gently toss to evenly coat the asparagus with egg. Remove from heat once the eggs are cooked.

Serve on a platter with a squeeze of lemon juice and topped with cheese. Serve immediately.

*Kefalograviera cheese can be purchased from European grocers. Parmesan cheese can be substituted.

Άγρια σπαράγγια με αυγά
- WILD ASPARAGUS WITH EGGS -

⅓ cup olive oil

220 g (7.7 oz.) asparagus, woody ends trimmed

Salt and pepper, to taste

3 eggs, beaten

2 tablespoons whole milk

TO SERVE

Squeeze of lemon juice

2 tablespoons kefalograviera cheese*

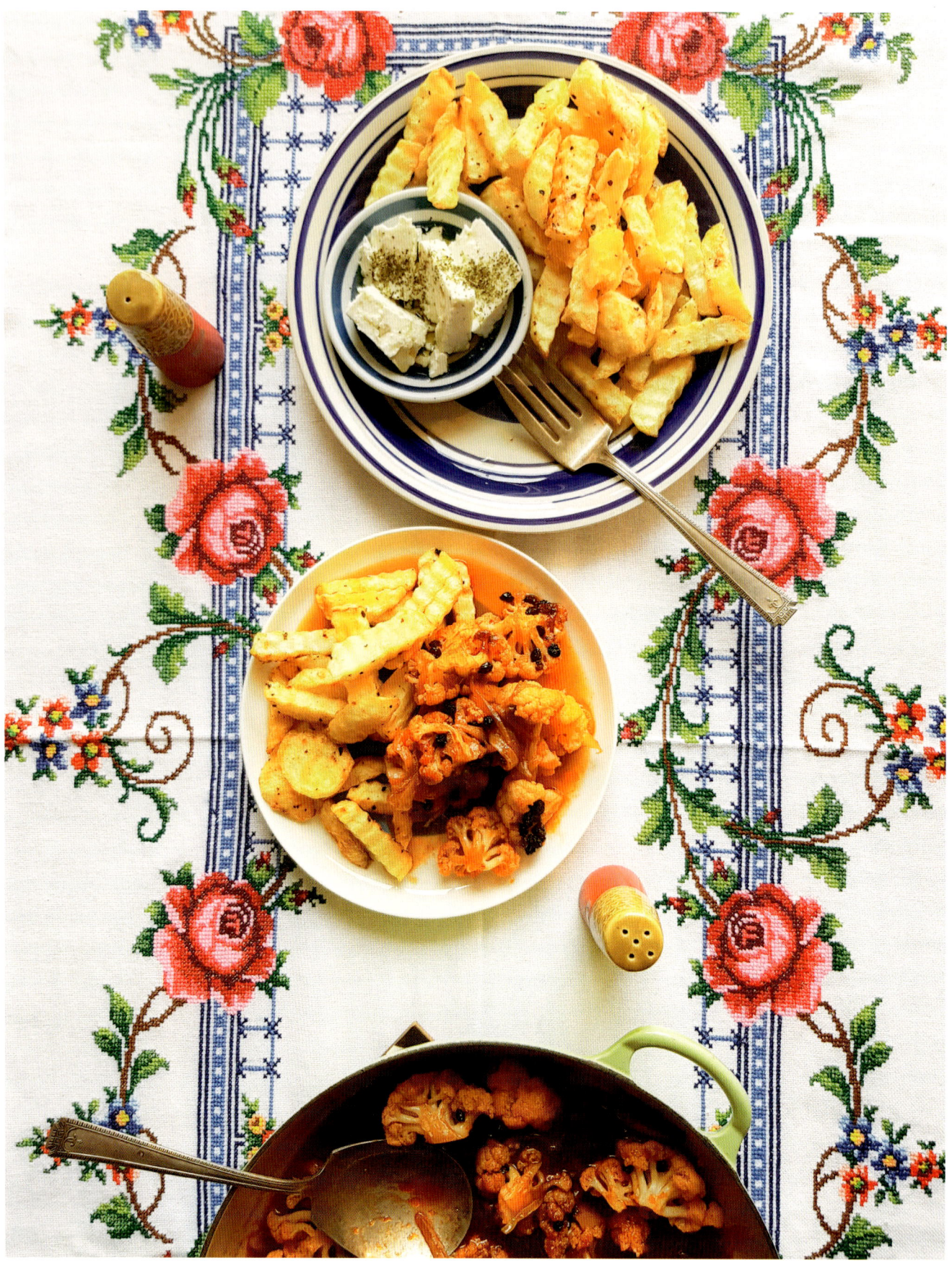

Cauliflower is one of those vegetables that either turns heads in disgust or in pleasure. Though seemingly bland on its own, cauliflower is such that, with a few spices, sweet grape must, and some low and slow cooking, it becomes the star of a meal. This is a traditional recipe throughout Greece. It is very flavorsome. You can keep it a little saucier or let it cook for longer to have a drier stew. Various names exist depending on which region of Greece you are from, such as κουνουπίδι γιαχνί (*giahni*), κουνουπίδι κοκκινιστό (*kokkinisto*), κουνουπίδι καπαμά (*kapama*). It can be eaten hot or at room temperature as a side or with rice.

Serves: 4 · 1 hour · GLUTEN FREE

Use a wide saucepan that has a lid. Heat the olive oil together with the onion and sauté until soft. Add the tomato paste, cinnamon stick, cloves, red wine, sugar, allspice, salt, and pepper. Cook for 3 minutes, and then add the cauliflower florets. Pour enough water to half cover the cauliflower. Place the lid on the saucepan and simmer on low to medium heat for around 30 minutes or until the cauliflower is soft. Remove the lid, taste the juices, and adjust seasoning at this point if needed.

Cook for a further 20 minutes or until the juices have thickened by less than half (this is so that it is not too saucy). Add *petimezi* and the raisins, stirring to incorporate. Continue to cook with the lid off for a further 5 minutes or until the sauce has thickened.

Serve warm with rice or fried potatoes.

*Petimezi is also known as grape must and can be purchased from European grocers. Runny honey can be used as a substitute.

Κουνουπίδι γιαχνί με σταφίδες
- CAULIFLOWER STEW WITH SPICES AND RAISINS -

½ cup olive oil

1 small onion, sliced

2 tablespoons tomato paste

1 cinnamon stick

5 cloves, whole

½ cup red wine

1 teaspoon castor (superfine) sugar

3 allspice berries, whole

Salt and pepper, to taste

1 medium cauliflower head, washed and separated in medium-sized florets

¼ cup *petimezi** or sweet balsamic vinegar

¼ cup raisins

TO SERVE

Fried potatoes (recipe on page 89)

Or steamed rice

THE GARDEN

Κολοκυθοκεφτέδες
- ZUCCHINI FRITTERS -

5–6 large zucchini, grated

3 tablespoons breadcrumbs

5 tablespoons all-purpose flour

1 teaspoon baking powder

3 tablespoons semolina flour

¼ cup dill, finely chopped

¼ cup mint, finely chopped

¼ cup spring onions, finely chopped

2 whole eggs, lightly whisked

100 g (3.5 oz.) feta cheese, crumbled

¼ cup Parmesan cheese (optional)

Pinch of salt and pepper

Olive oil for frying

TO SERVE

Lemon wedges

Yogurt

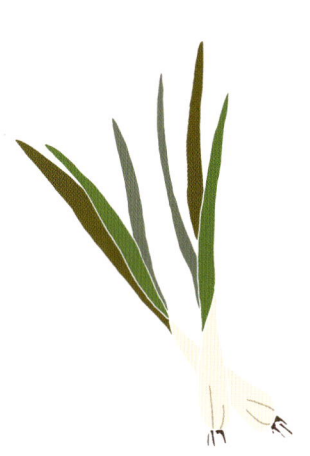

Kolo-kitho-kefte-des (κολοκυθοκεφτέδες) is a mouthful to say, but they are a delightful mouthful to eat! The word translates as *kolo-kithi*, meaning "zucchini," and *keftedes*, meaning "meatball—thus a "zucchini meatball." They are not your everyday fritter. These are packed with herbs and cheeses and then shallow fried in olive oil. They have a crispy exterior and a gooey soft center. They can be eaten as a snack or as a side with a Greek salad.

Serves: 20 · 40 minutes

Grate the zucchini and place in a strainer with 1 teaspoon salt. Mix well and set aside for 30 minutes so juices can be released. After 30 minutes, squeeze out any extra moisture with your hands and place into a bowl.

To the zucchini, add the breadcrumbs, flour, baking powder, semolina, dill, mint, spring onions, eggs, feta, Parmesan, salt, and pepper. Mix until all the ingredients are incorporated. Do not overmix, otherwise you will have dense fritters. The batter should be thick and sticky and hold its shape when formed into a fritter. If the batter is too wet, add a little more flour.

Heat the oil in a shallow wide pan until very hot. Add spoonfuls of the mixture into the oil. The hot oil ensures the fritters cook quickly and do not become soggy. Cook the fritters in batches without overcrowding the pan (I do 4 fritters per batch). Add more oil if it is too dry. Cook 3–4 minutes each side until golden and crispy. Transfer to a plate lined with paper towels.

Serve with a side of yogurt and lemon wedges. Can be eaten cold or hot.

Yes, potatoes fried in olive oil. There are plenty of myths suggesting that olive oil is not good for frying. Truth be told, olive oil is ideal for frying, and it's better for you. There are many oils and fats that, once heated, release unhealthy toxins. The difference and the benefit of frying with olive oil is that it undergoes no significant structural alteration when heated, and it also retains its nutritional value. Its high smoking point (210°C/410°F) is significantly greater than the perfect temperature for frying food (180°C/356°F).

The smell, the taste, the crunch of perfect fried potatoes definitely cannot be resisted. Remember to heat the oil adequately so that the potatoes retain their crunchy exterior.

Serves: 2 · 45 minutes · GLUTEN FREE

Cut the potatoes and season them with salt. Heat the oil in a wide pan. Place 1 potato in the oil; if it sizzles, the oil is ready for frying.

Gently add potatoes to the hot oil and fry them, turning once or twice throughout the cooking process so that they brown up evenly. Drain the potatoes and place them on a plate.

Immediately sprinkle with oregano. Serve hot.

Τηγανιτές πατάτες
- OLIVE-OIL FRIED POTATOES -

Light olive oil for frying (enough to fill your pan ¼ of the way)

2 large potatoes, peeled and cut into fries about 1 cm (0.4 in.) wide

Salt, to taste

1 teaspoon dried oregano

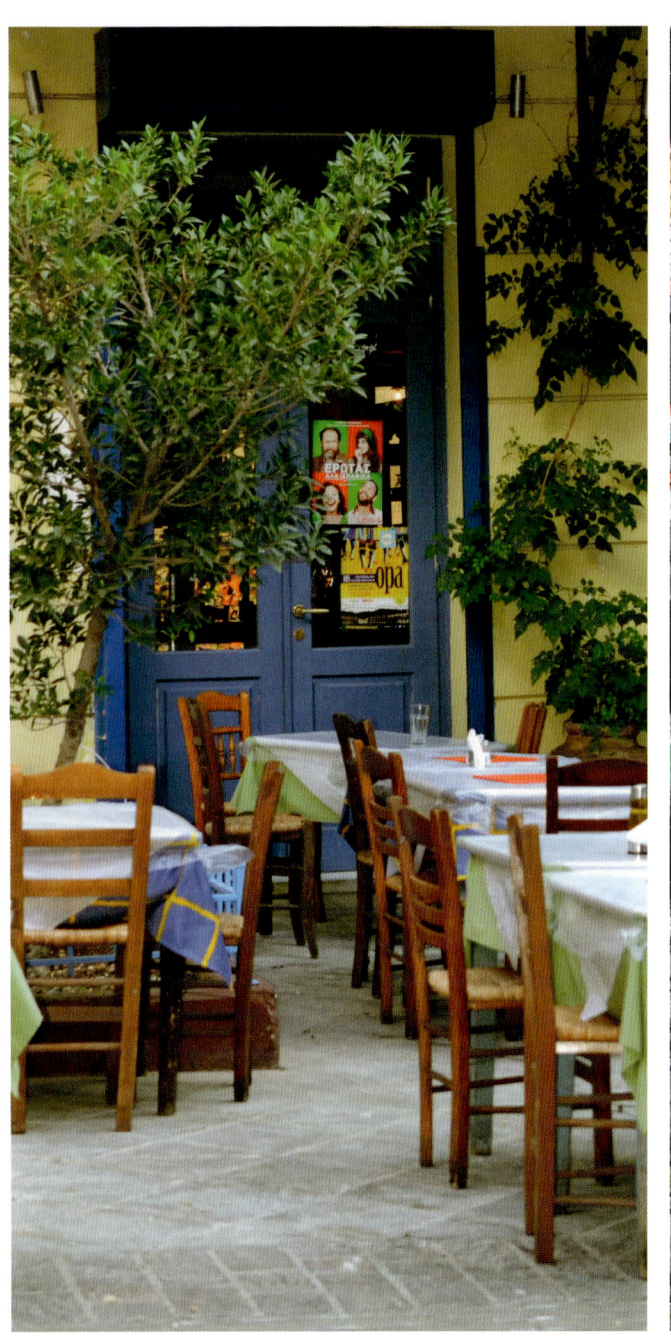
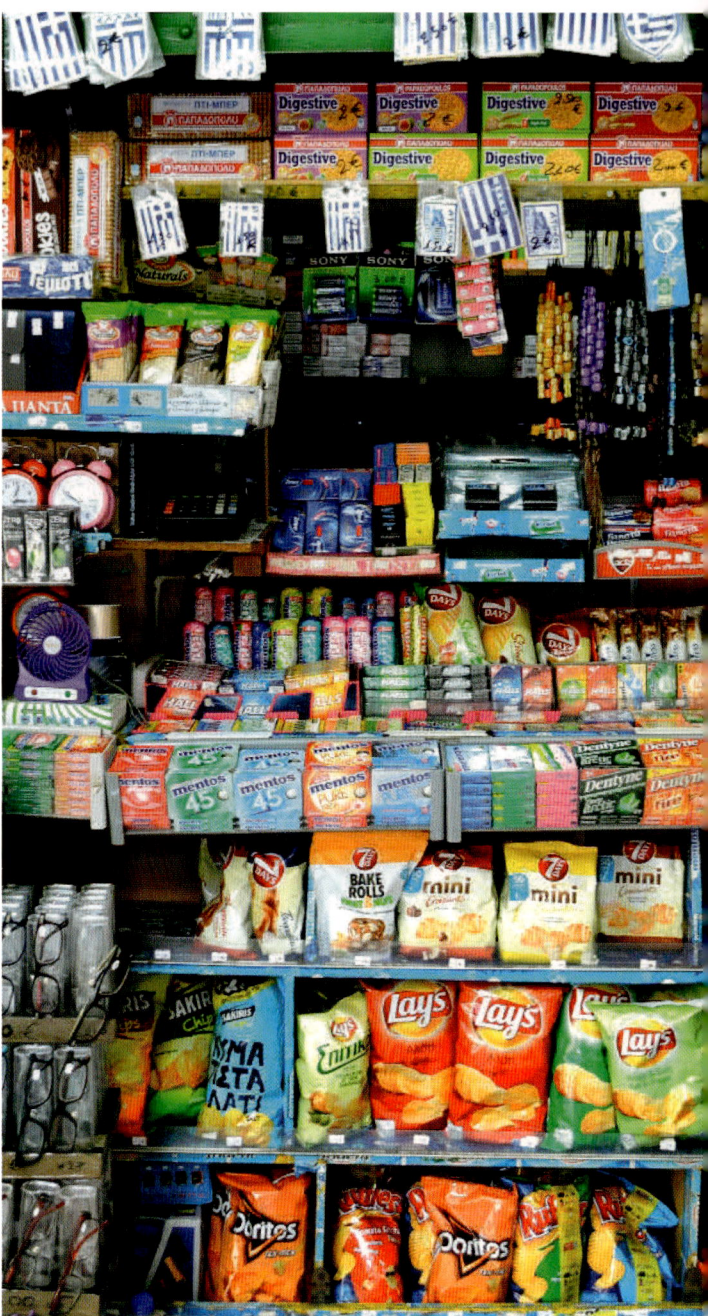

ΚΑΡΕΚΛΑΔΙΚΟ
ΕΠΙΣΚΕΥΕΣ ΚΑΤΑΣΚΕΥΕΣ
Β. ΑΘΑΝΑΣΟΠΟΥΛΟΣ · ΤΗΛ 3249998
ΚΑΡΕΚΛΕΣ · ΤΡΑΠΕΖΙ

ΚΑΦΕΣ
ΛΟΥΜΙΔΗ
ΠΑΠΑΓΑΛΟΣ

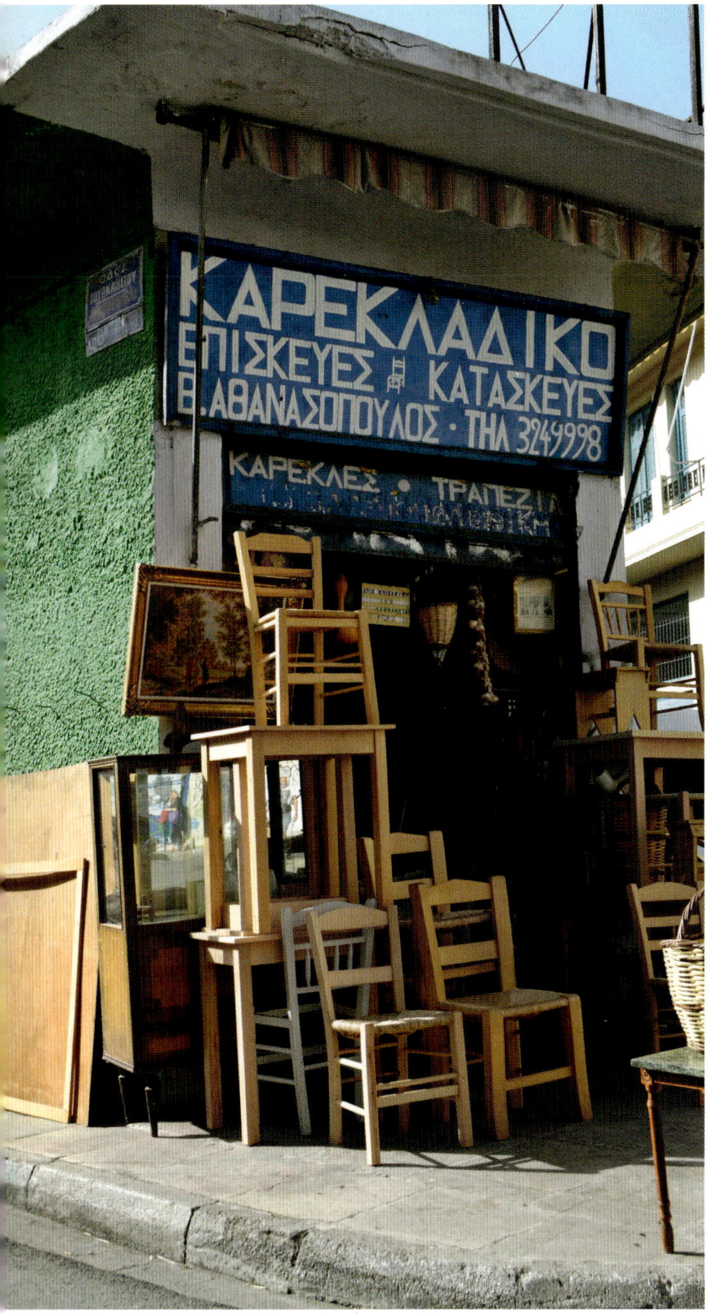

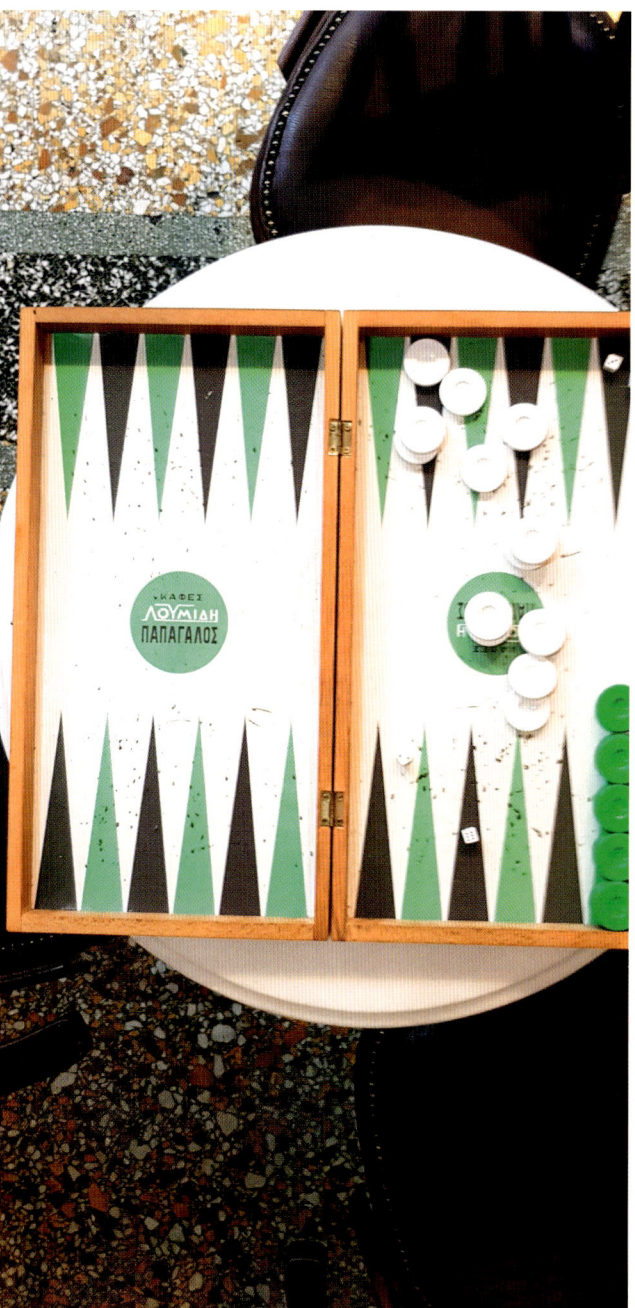

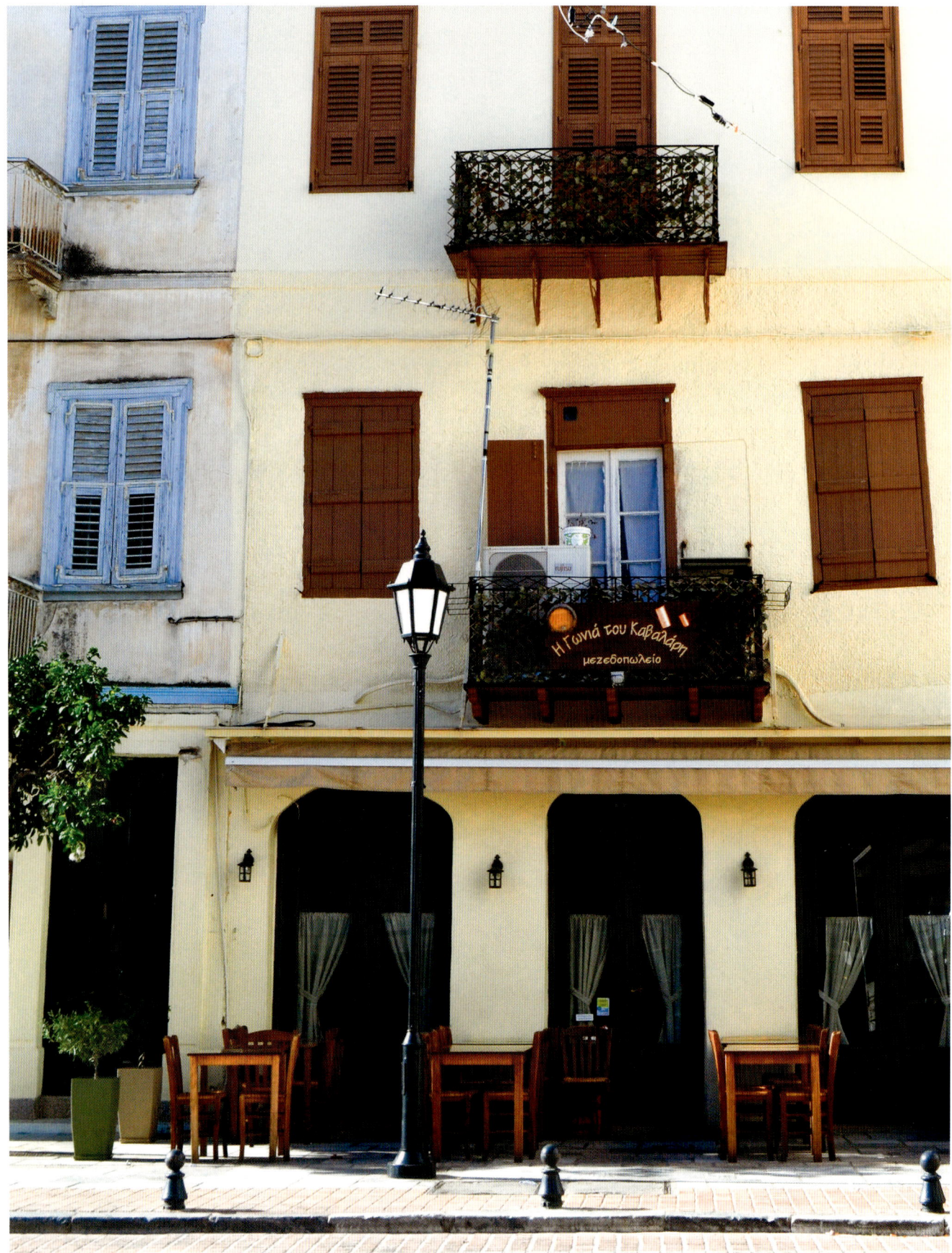

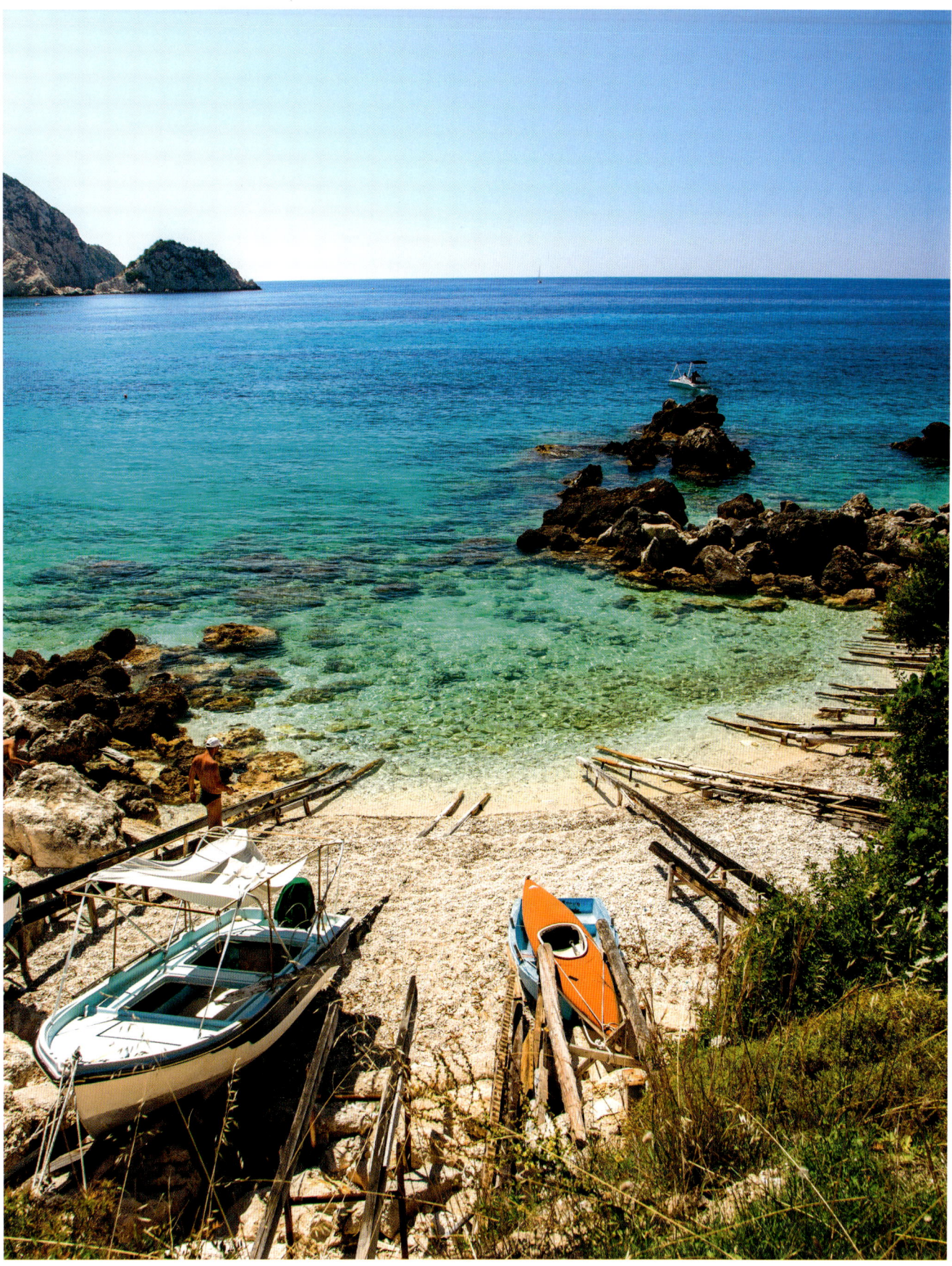

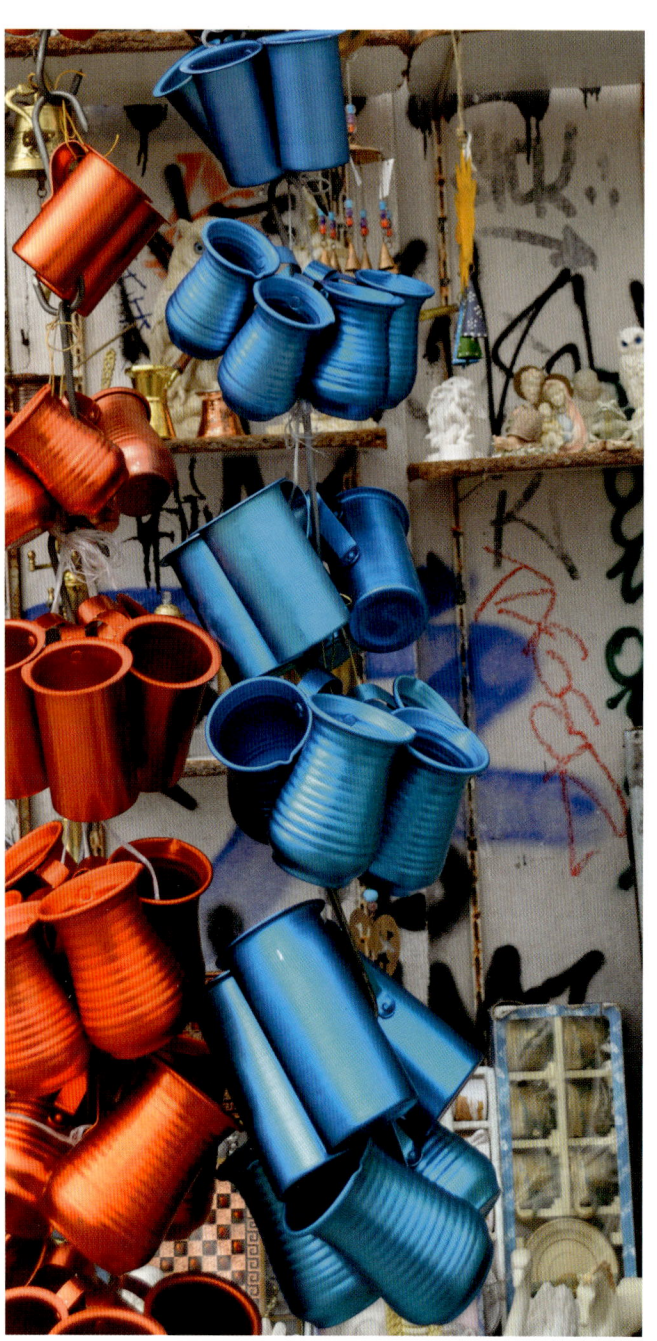
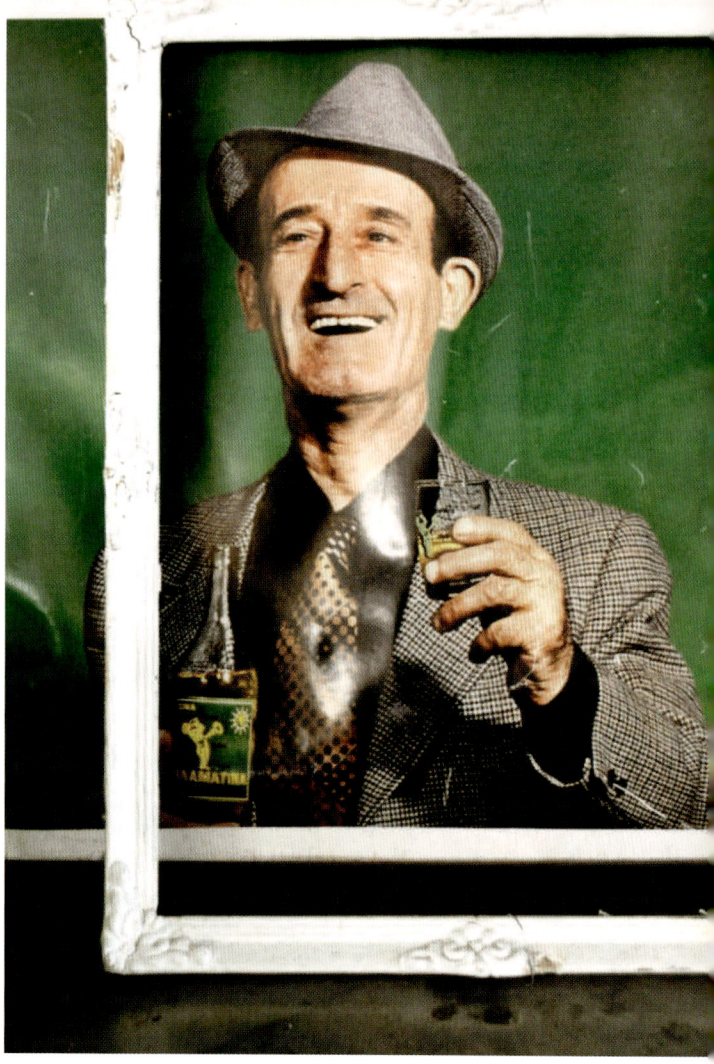

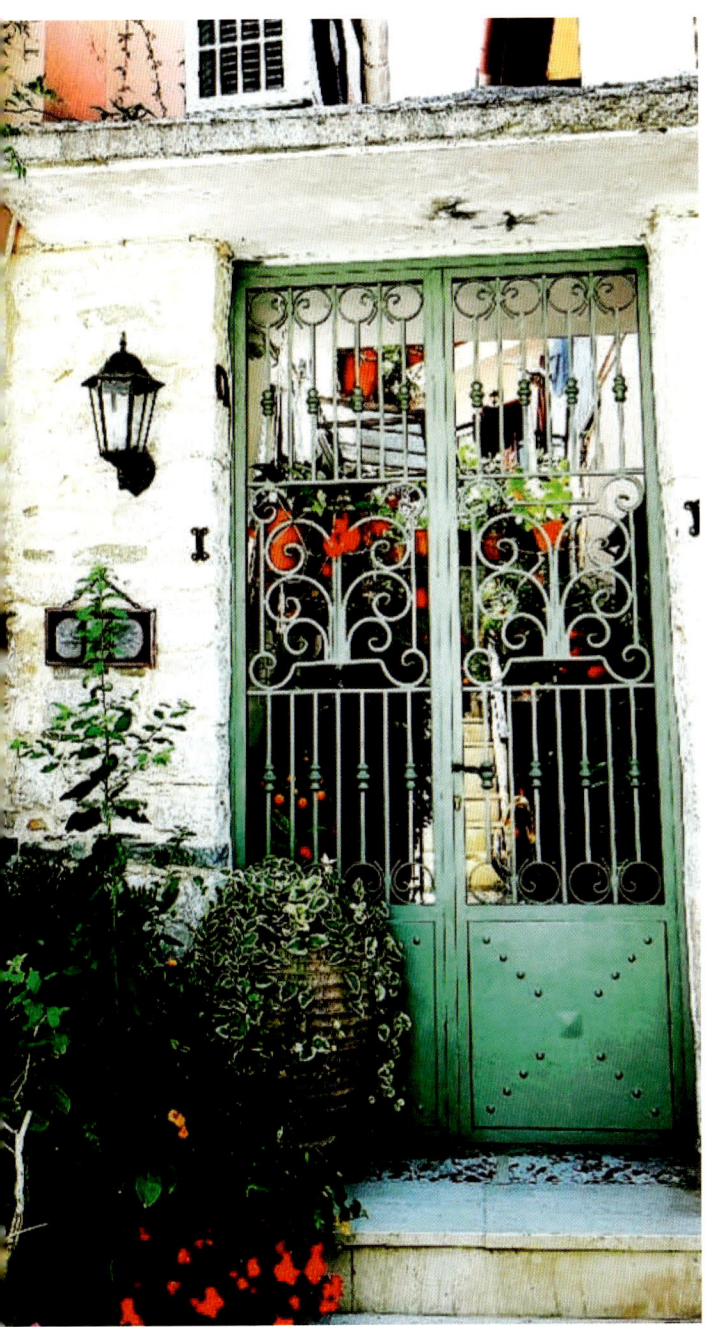
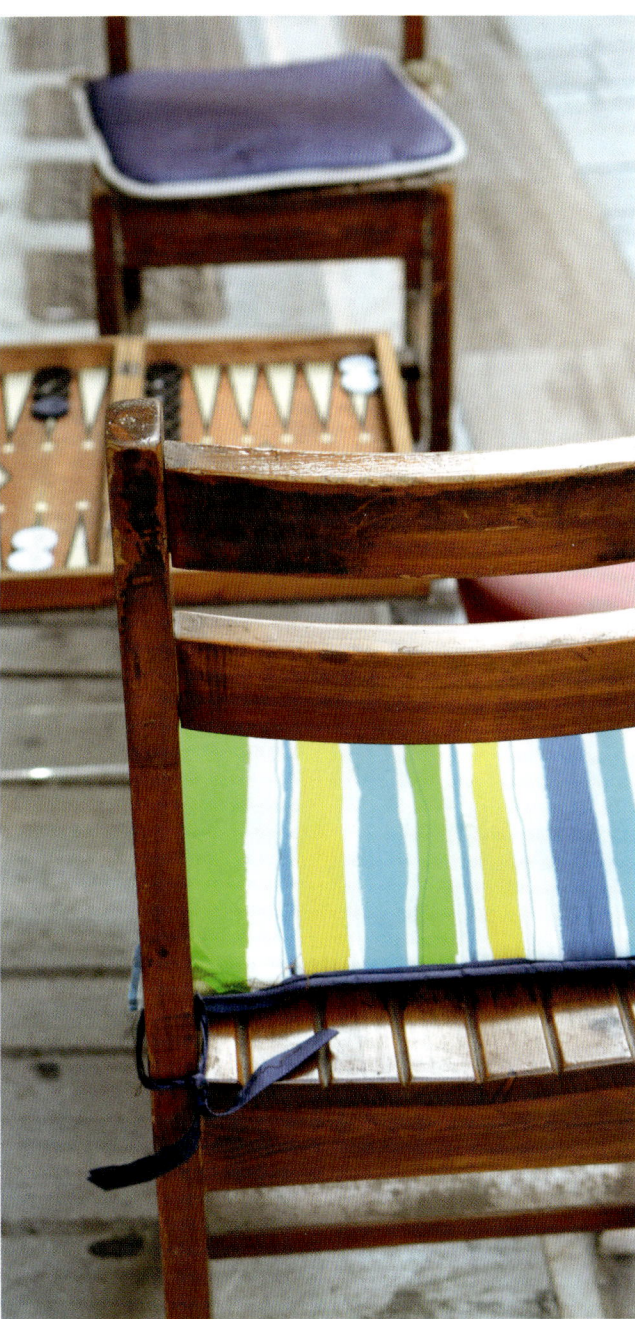

The only true wisdom
is in knowing you know nothing.
— SOCRATES

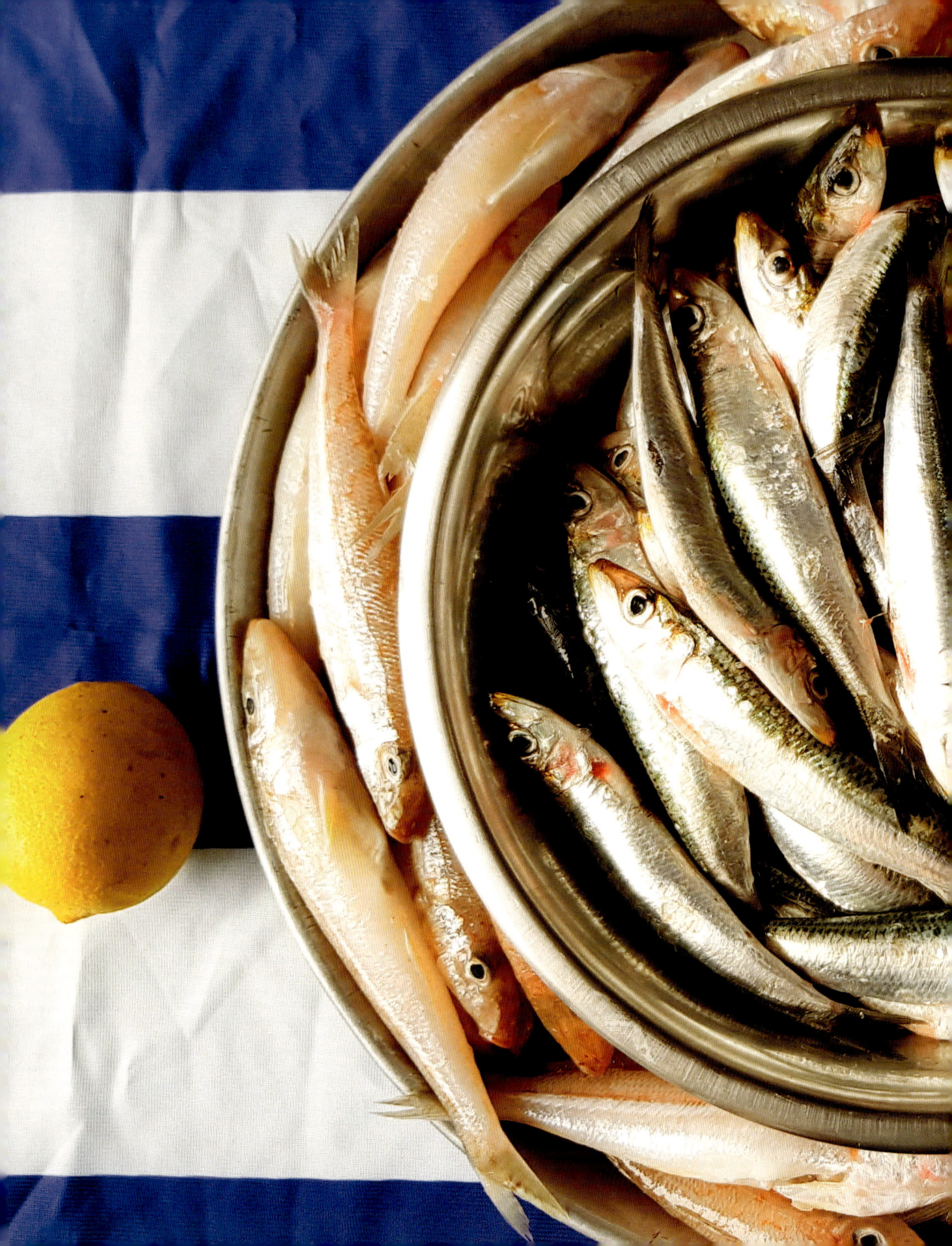

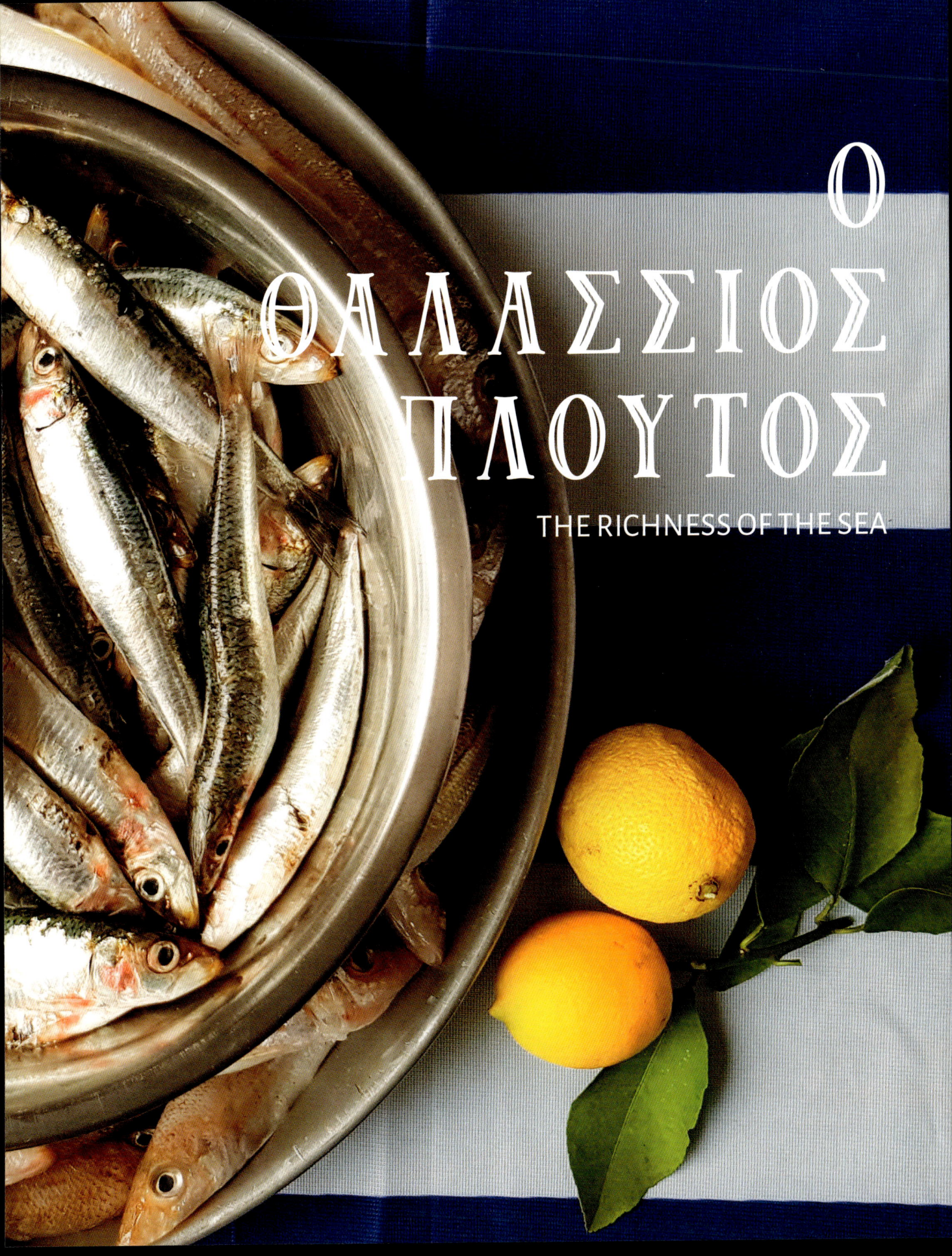

Ο ΘΑΛΑΣΣΙΟΣ ΠΛΟΥΤΟΣ

THE RICHNESS OF THE SEA

Ο ΘΑΛΑΣΣΙΟΣ ΠΛΟΥΤΟΣ

THE RICHNESS OF THE SEA

The sea, with its intoxicating emerald and turquoise color, salty foam, and warmth from the Mediterranean sun, boasts a treasure chest of creatures around Greece.

The most caught and consumed come from the Aegean Sea, though there are approximately 250 marine creatures around Greece. The most frequent fish eaten are sardines (σαρδέλες), sea bream (τσιπούρα), sea bass (λαβράκι), anchovy (γαύρος) and mussels (μύδια). Even though these varieties are some of the cheapest to buy, they do boast some of the highest omega 3-fatty acids. Fish being so widely available in Greece is the reason it is eaten so frequently as the main source of protein. It is affordable, local, lean, healthy, and easy to cook.

Fish is more commonly eaten with heads and tails intact. It boasts more flavor when cooking, and once you get the hang of eating it this way, you will probably never go back to just fillets of fish. In this chapter, I have added both fillets and whole fish, as I wanted to retain the originality of the recipes.

When shopping for fish, ensure they smell like the sea and not "fishy." The eyes should be shiny (not muggy), scales shiny and intact, and the gills must be bright red.

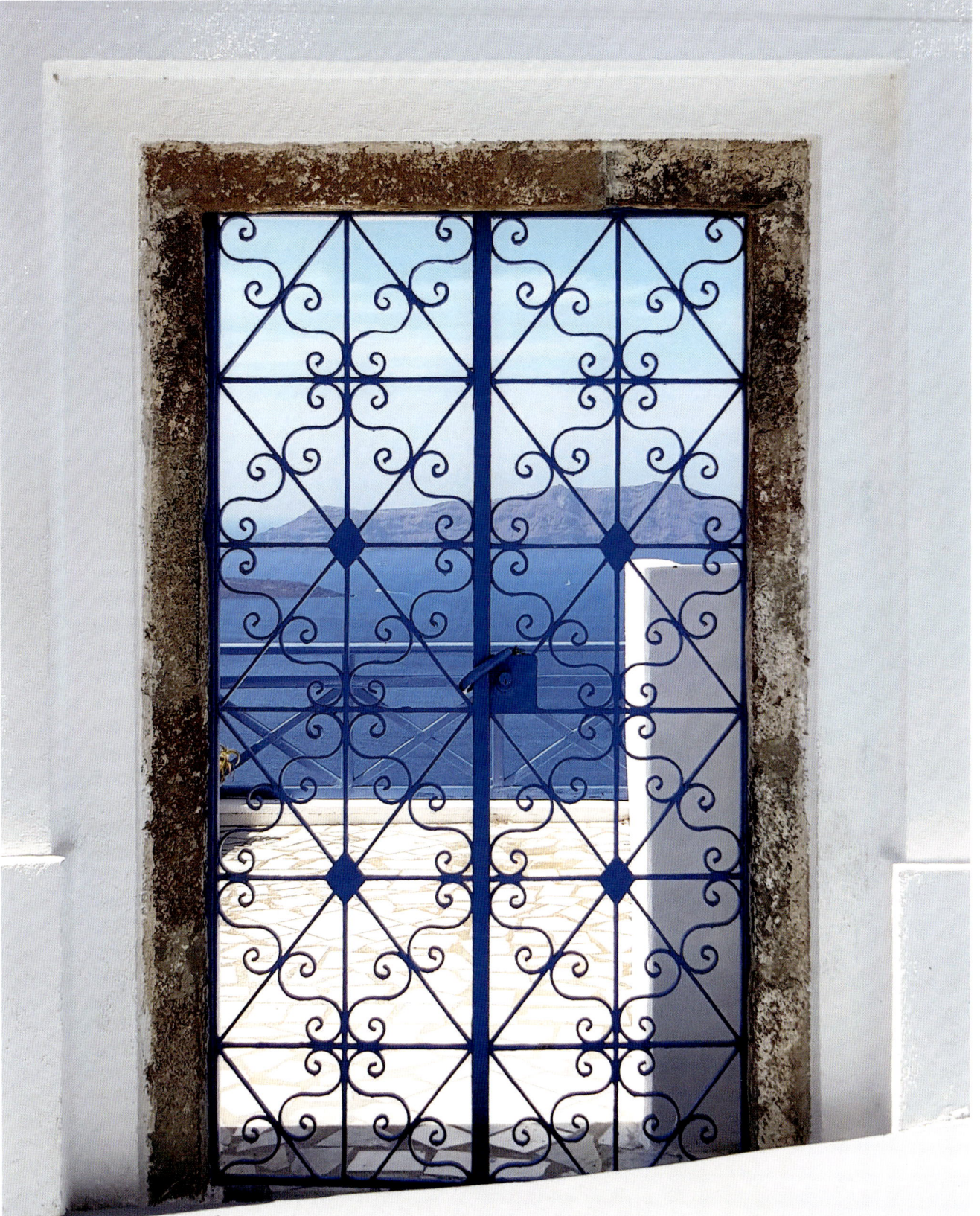

ψάρια και οι εποχές τους

ΙΑΝΟΥΑΡΙΟΣ
Μπαρμπούνι, λούφαρει, αστακοί, στρείδια και κτένια.

ΦΛΕΒΑΡΗΣ
Λαβράκι και κέφαλος

ΜΑΡΤΙΟΣ
Κέφαλος, λαβράκι, μπαρμπούνια, κουτσομούρα, μαυρόψαρο, σκορπίνα

ΑΠΡΙΛΙΟΣ
Ψαριά για βράσιμο - αστακός, καβούρι, καλκάνι.

ΜΑΪΟΣ
Καλκάνι, το πίσι, σαρδέλα, χελιδονόψαρο, κοκωβιό.

ΙΟΥΝΙΟΣ
Χελιδονόψαρο, μουρούνα, λαβράκι, αστακός, κουτσομούρα, μπαρμπούνια.

ΙΟΥΛΙΟΣ
Λυθρίνι, σαρδέλα, σαβρίδι, καβούρι, μαρίδα, αθερίνα, πίσι, καλαμαράκι, καβούρια.

ΑΥΓΟΥΣΤΟΣ
Μπαρμπούνι, γλώσσα, μαρίδα, αθερίνα, κολιό, ξιφίας.

ΣΕΠΤΕΜΒΡΙΟΣ
Σε αφθονία - ξιφίας, μπαρμπούνια, κουτσομούρα, κολιός, μαρίδες, σπάροι.

ΟΚΤΩΒΡΙΟΣ
Παχιά ψάρια – παλαμίδα, τορικι το οποίο γίνεται η λακέρδα.

ΝΟΕΜΒΡΙΟΣ
Αστακοί, στρείδια, μύδια, σκουμπρί.

ΔΕΚΕΜΒΡΙΟΣ
Αστακοί, στρείδια, μύδια, σκουμπρί.

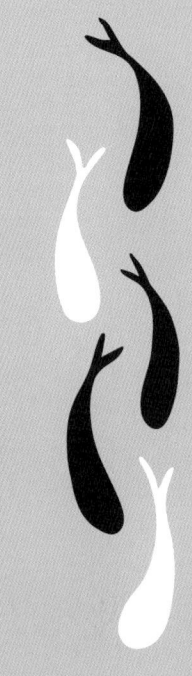

ΓΙΓΑΝΤΕΣ ΜΕ ΧΤΑΠΟΔΙ, ΜΕΛΙ ΚΑΙ ΠΟΡΤΟΚΑΛΙ
102   LIMA BEANS WITH HONEY AND ORANGE OCTOPUS (GF)

ΣΑΒΟΡΟ ΨΑΡΙ ΜΕ ΠΕΤΙΜΕΖΙ ΚΑΙ ΣΤΑΦΙΔΕΣ
104   *SAVORO*, SWEET AND SOUR WHITING

ΜΠΑΚΑΛΙΑΡΟΣ ΚΟΚΚΙΝΙΣΤΟΣ ΜΕ ΠΙΠΕΡΙΕΣ
106   COD STEW WITH CAPSICUMS (GF)

ΣΑΡΔΕΛΕΣ ΠΑΝΤΡΕΜΕΝΕΣ
108   MARRIED SARDINES (GF)

ΤΡΑΓΑΝΕΣ ΣΑΡΔΕΛΕΣ ΦΟΥΡΝΟΥ
110   CRISPY BAKED SARDINE ROLLS

ΧΤΑΠΟΔΙ ΣΤΙΦΑΔΟ
112   OCTOPUS STIFADO (GF)

ΑΓΙΟΡΕΙΤΙΚΕΣ ΜΠΑΜΙΕΣ ΜΕ ΨΑΡΙ ΣΤΟ ΦΟΥΡΝΟ
114   BAKED FISH WITH OKRA (GF)

ΜΠΑΚΑΛΙΑΡΟΣ ΤΣΙΛΑΔΙΑ
116   BAKED COD WITH FRIED POTATO, ZUCCHINI, AND RAISIN SALSA

ΓΑΡΙΔΕΣ ΣΑΓΑΝΑΚΙ ΜΕ ΛΕΜΟΝΙ, ΜΑΡΑΘΟ ΚΑΙ ΤΥΡΙ ΦΕΤΑ
118   PRAWN *SAGANAKI* WITH LEMON, FENNEL, AND FETA CHEESE (GF)

ΓΕΜΙΣΤΕΣ ΣΑΡΔΕΛΕΣ ΣΕ ΑΜΠΕΛΟΦΥΛΛΑ
120   STUFFED SARDINES WRAPPED IN VINE LEAVES (GF)

ΣΚΟΡΔΑΛΙΑ ΜΕ ΧΤΑΠΟΔΙ ΚΑΙ ΜΕΛΙ
122   ROASTED GARLIC MASH AND HONEY OCTOPUS (GF)

GF DENOTES GLUTEN-FREE RECIPES

Γίγαντες με χταπόδι, μέλι και πορτοκάλι

- LIMA BEANS WITH HONEY AND ORANGE OCTOPUS -

The classic lima bean stew around Greece known as *gigantes* has no meat nor fish. This recipe, on the other hand, has its roots from Mani in the Peloponnese and incorporates octopus. I absolutely love the char on the octopus when it gets baked in the oven. It has a grilled flavor yet still retains moisture. The addition of honey in this stew is intriguing, adding a subtle sweetness to the dish. It is served as a main meal. Lima beans are legumes and are packed with protein, fiber, iron, and other nutrients.

**Serves: 5 · 2 hours (plus overnight soaking)
· GLUTEN FREE**

---

2 cups lima beans, dried

3 bay leaves, divided

1 kg (35.2 oz.) octopus, cleaned and beak removed

3 tablespoons runny honey

1 piece of orange rind

¾ cup olive oil

1 large onion, diced

1 garlic clove, minced

1 teaspoon castor (superfine) sugar

Salt and pepper, to taste

1 tablespoon tomato paste

2 large red bell peppers, sliced thinly

½ cup white wine

Place the dried lima beans in a bowl covered with fresh water to soak overnight or a minimum of 10 hours. Do not add any salt as it hardens the beans. Drain and add to a pot covered with fresh water and a bay leaf. Bring to a boil, and then simmer for 30–40 minutes or until fork tender. Do not overcook as they will continue to cook in the oven. They should still retain a bite to them at this stage. Drain and set aside.

Place the whole octopus with the honey and orange rind in a saucepan. On low heat, simmer for around 30 minutes. Do not add any liquid as the octopus will release its own juices. Once cooked, set it aside. Do not discard the juices.

Preheat oven to 180° C/350° F.

In a sauté pan, heat the oil with the onion and sauté until soft and translucent. Add the garlic, sugar, salt, pepper, and the tomato paste. Cook for 1 minute and set aside. In a baking tray, place the drained beans, bay leaves, peppers, wine, the onion mixture, and a little more salt and pepper. Mix. Now place the octopus on the top together with all its juices. Ensure there is enough liquid to cover the beans at least halfway up. If not, add an additional 1 cup water.

Bake uncovered for 1 hour or until juices have thickened, octopus is charred, beans are fully cooked, and oil has risen to the top. Serve warm with crusty bread.

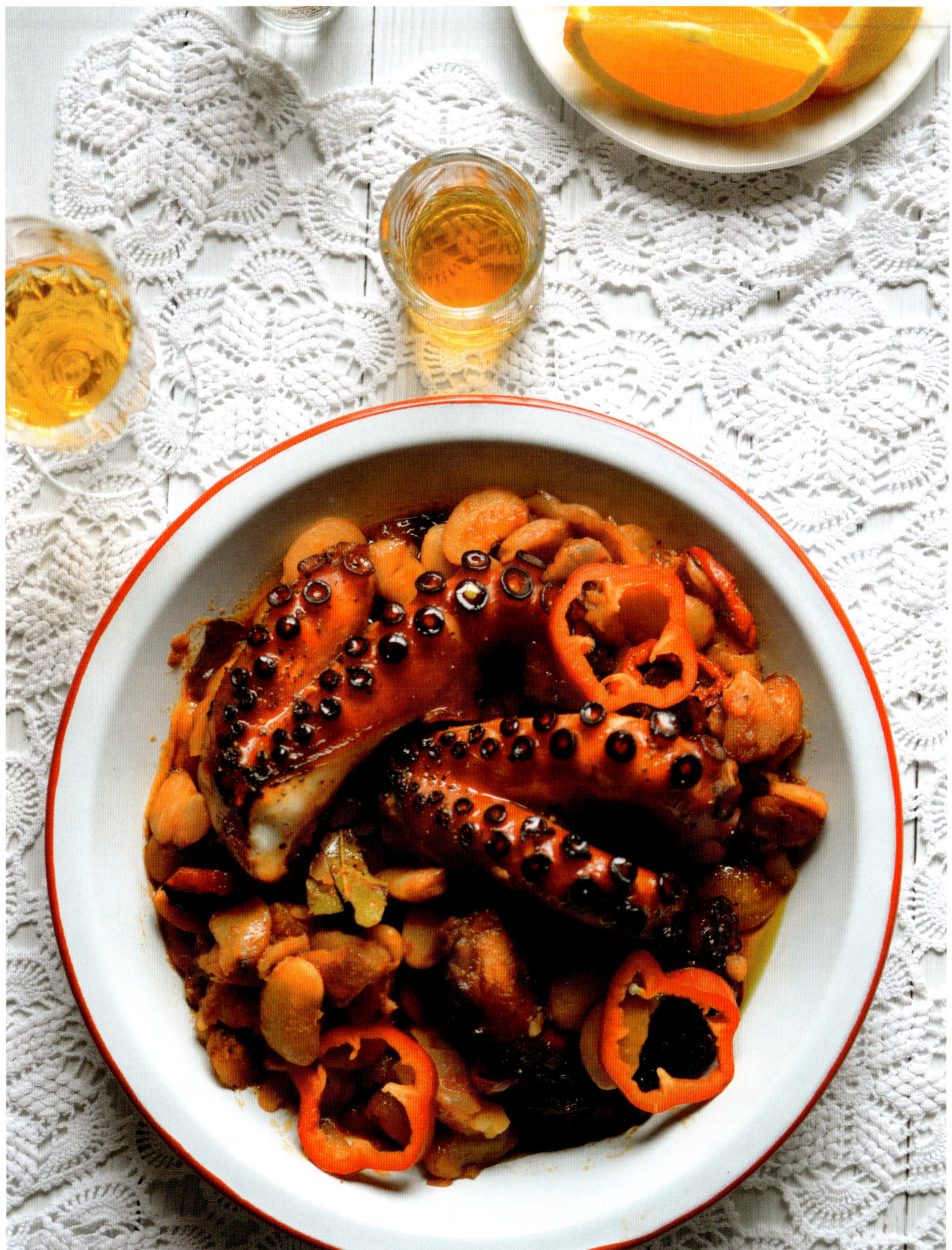

Σαβόρο ψάρι με πετιμέζι και σταφίδες
- SAVORO, SWEET AND SOUR WHITING -

Savoro is the name of fried fish topped with an absolute delight of a sauce made from grape must, rosemary, garlic, and raisins. It originates from Corfu. The sauce has an intriguing intense flavor of sweet and sour. Traditionally, the sauce is poured over the fish, though you could have it served as a dipping sauce on the side. If you prefer, you can thin out the sauce by adding a little more water.

Serves: 4 · 1 hour

1 kg (35.2 oz.) whiting, cleaned and gutted, head and tail intact*

1 cup all-purpose flour

Salt

Olive oil, for frying

SAUCE

4 tablespoons olive oil

2 garlic cloves, minced

2 tablespoons all-purpose flour

1 tablespoon rosemary, chopped

1 cup water

4 tablespoons grape must (petimezi)*

2 tablespoons red wine vinegar

1 cup raisins

Salt, to taste

Place the fish, flour, and salt into a clean plastic bag. Close bag and shake to ensure the fish are covered in flour. Set aside.

Add enough oil in a large frying pan to cover the bottom of the pan (about 1 cm / 0.4 in. deep). Heat the oil. To test if it is ready, drop a sprinkle of flour in. If it sizzles, it is ready. Gently shake off any excess flour from the fish and drop into the hot oil. Do not overcrowd the pan; only fry a few at a time. Allow to brown well on one side and then turn to cook the other side. Do not keep turning—you should only need to do it once. Remove and place on paper towel to drain any excess oil.

In another saucepan, make the sauce. Heat the oil with the garlic until it starts to sizzle. Add the flour, whisking continuously for 1 minute, and then add all the other ingredients (except raisins). Continue to whisk on a medium heat until the sauce thickens. Taste and adjust seasoning if needed. Add the raisins and mix. Remove from heat. Place fish on a serving platter with the sauce either on the side or spooned over the fish.

Serve immediately.

*Grape must can be purchased from European grocers. Boneless fish can also be used.

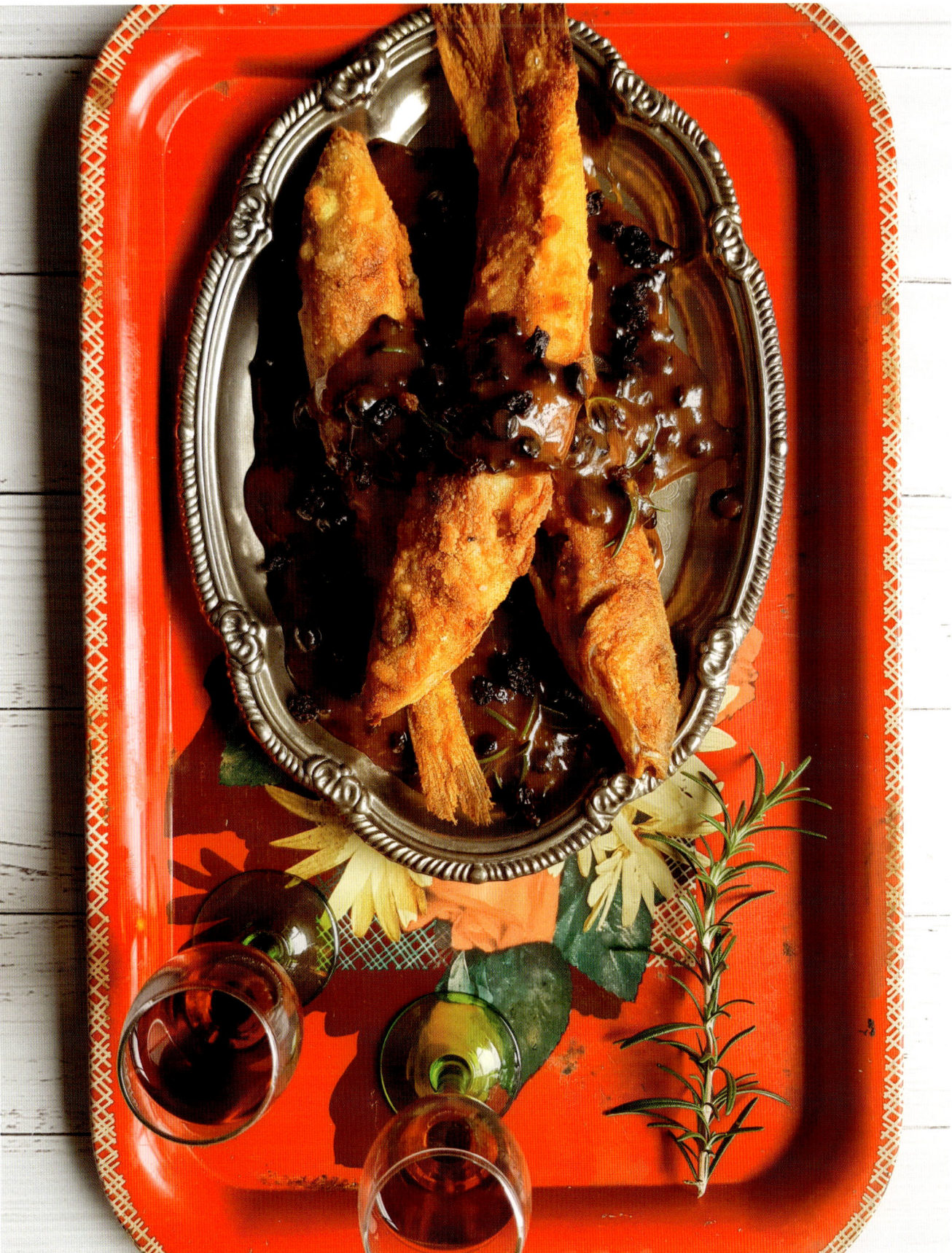

Μπακαλιάρος κοκκινιστός με πιπεριές
- COD STEW WITH CAPSICUMS -

This stew is light in contrast to most hearty stews. Representative of Corfiot cuisine, this stew is more Italian in its influence than Greek due to the centuries of Venetian rule. It is simple to prepare with few ingredients, yet it boasts big flavors. It can be served with rice or baked potatoes. If cod fish is not available, use any other white filleted fish.

Serves: 4 · 30–45 minutes · GLUTEN FREE

½ cup olive oil

1 small onion, diced

2 garlic cloves, minced

2 large red bell peppers, sliced 1cm (0.4 in.) thickness*

½ cup tomato purée

½ cup red or white wine

1 teaspoon castor (superfine) sugar

Salt and pepper, to taste

1 tablespoon parsley, chopped

1 kg desalted cod (35.2 oz.) or any choice of white flesh fillets, cut into serving pieces

TO SERVE

2 tablespoons mint, chopped

Heat oil in a large saucepan. Add the onion and garlic, sautéing until soft. Add the bell peppers, purée, wine, sugar, salt, pepper, and parsley. Cover, lower heat, and cook for 15 minutes or until sauce has thickened slightly. Now place the fish fillets on top of the sauce and add ½ cup water. Cover and cook for 8–10 minutes or until fish is cooked through.

Scatter chopped mint over the top and serve the fish immediately, ensuring you add a spoonful of the sauce to each serving.

*You could substitute brined capsicums for a further depth of flavor.

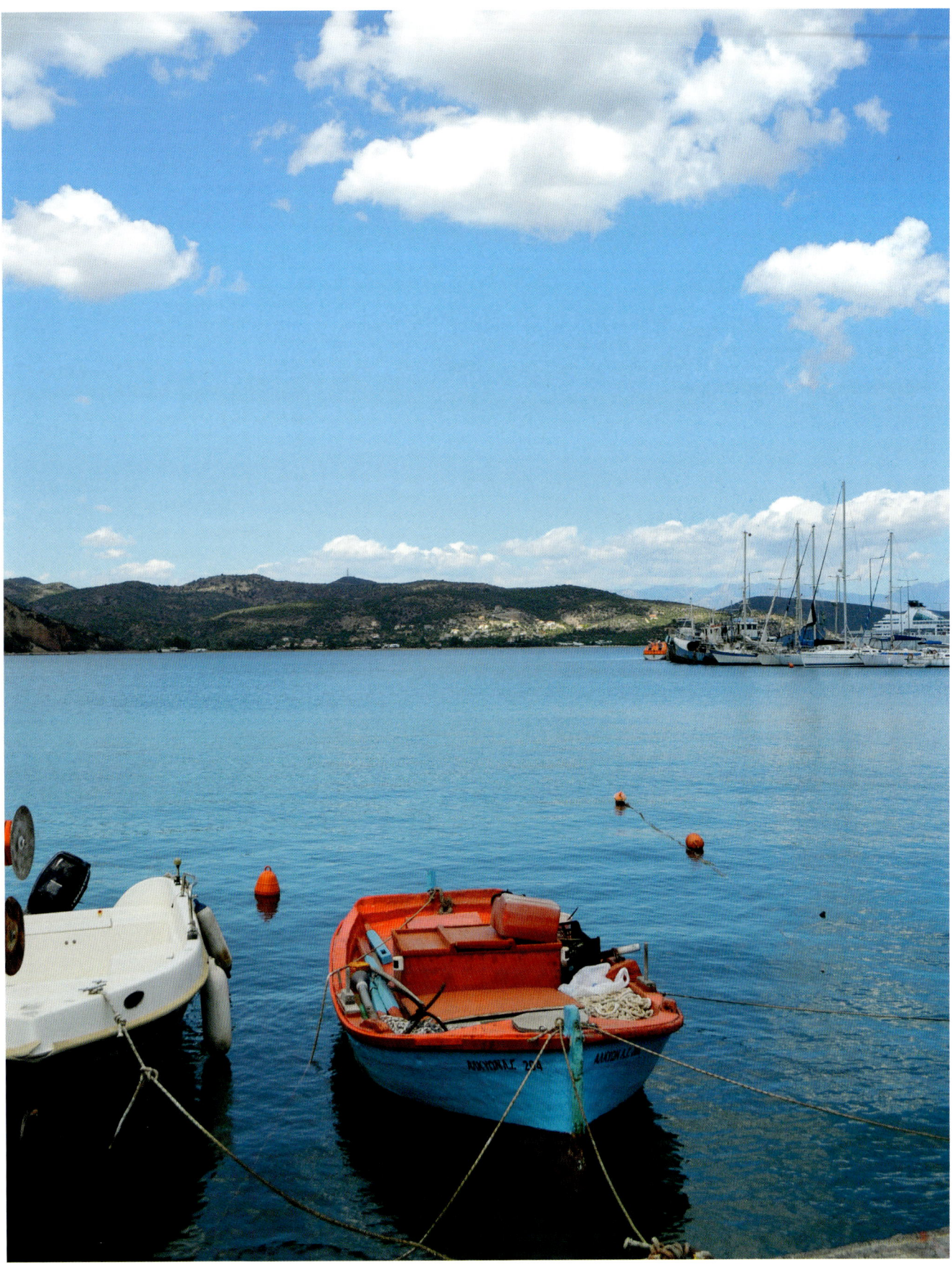

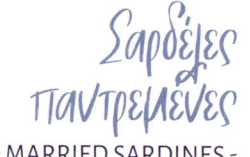

Σαρδέλες Παντρεμένες
- MARRIED SARDINES -

¼ cup parsley, chopped finely

¼ cup spring onions, chopped

½ cup breadcrumbs*

1 garlic clove, minced

Salt and pepper, to taste

Zest of one lemon

¼ cup olive oil, divided

1 large onion, sliced

18 sardines, filleted

2 lemons, juiced

Greeks love eating the humble sardine! They are full of protein and loaded with omega-3 fatty acids, vitamin D, phosphorus, calcium, vitamin B12, and selenium. You can cook them whole, filleted, fried, baked, and barbequed. This is a remarkably simple recipe common throughout Greece, and it is literally translated "married sardines"! It's a super cute name for two fillets that get sandwiched together.

Serves: 9 · 40 minutes · GLUTEN FREE

Preheat oven to 200° C/390° F.

Place the parsley, spring onion, breadcrumbs, garlic, salt, pepper, lemon zest, and one tablespoon olive oil in a small bowl. Mix and set aside.

Place the onion slices over the base of a baking dish. Place 9 cleaned and butterflied sardines skin side down. Sprinkle salt over each one, and then place a teaspoon of the filling on top of the fillet. Top with the remaining sardines. Pour the remaining olive oil and lemon juice over the fish, sprinkling with some additional salt over the top.

Bake for 20 minutes or until the sardines are cooked through.

Serve immediately with a side salad and a squeeze of lemon juice.

*For a gluten-free option, use gluten-free breadcrumbs.

TIP: Filleting sardines is not hard, but it is tedious. To speed things up, you can request your fishmonger to do it for you or purchase them already cleaned.

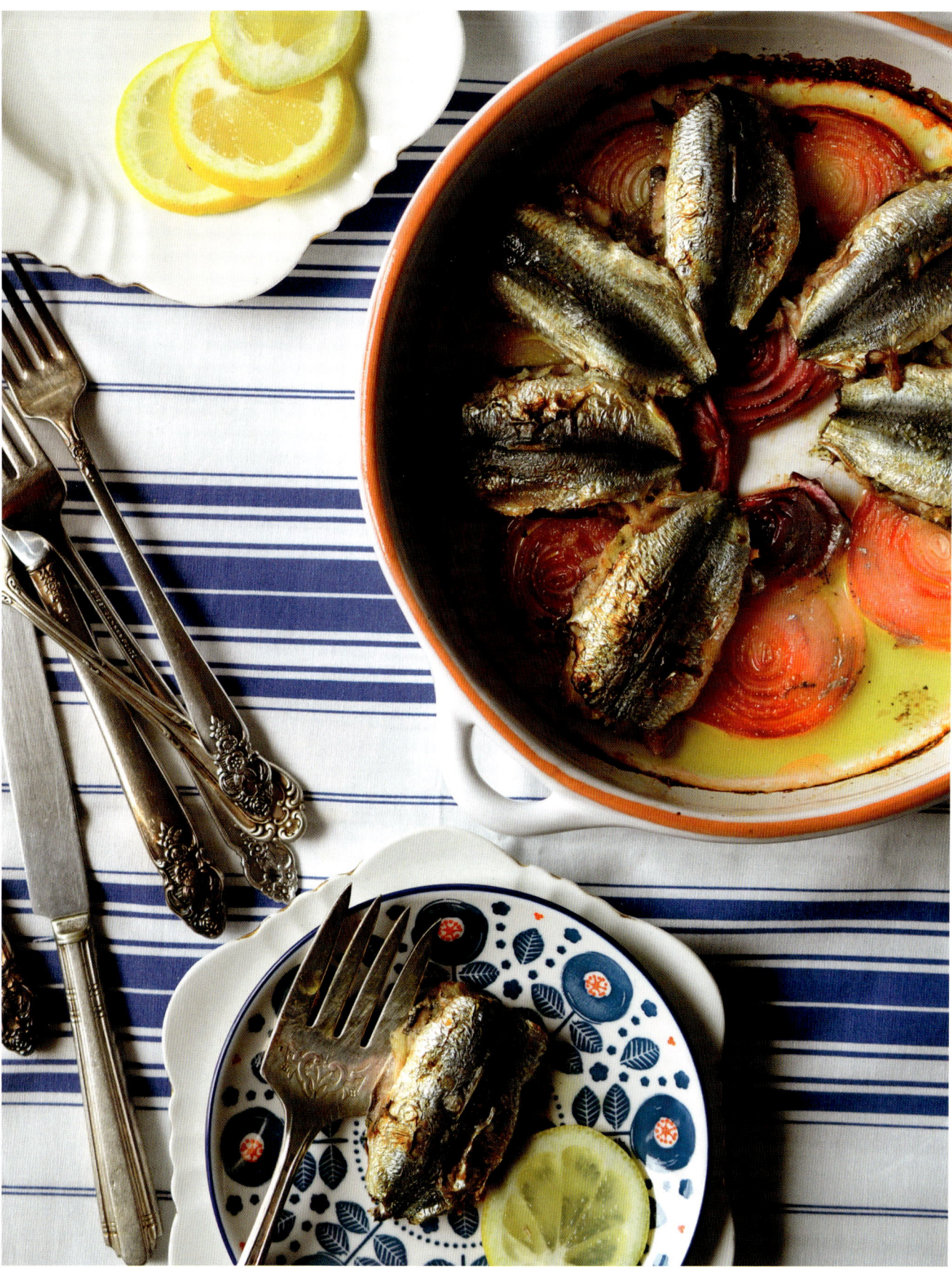

Τραγανές σαρδέλες φούρνου
- CRISPY BAKED SARDINE ROLLS -

3 teaspoons parsley, finely chopped

1½ cups breadcrumbs (preferably panko breadcrumbs)

2 garlic cloves, minced (optional)

Salt and pepper

½ teaspoon chili flakes, optional

1 lemon, zest and juice

1 cup olive oil, divided

16 sardines (250 g. or 8.8 oz.), filleted

3 tablespoons olive oil, extra

TO SERVE

Caper mash (recipe on page 78)

Lemon, wedge

These sardine rolls are a great meze served with a squeeze of lemon juice. They are crispy and slightly spicy. Double the amount—trust me, you will love them!

Serves: 4 · 35 minutes

Preheat oven to 200° C/390° F.

Place the parsley, breadcrumbs, garlic, salt, pepper, chili flakes, zest, and ¼ cup oil in a bowl. Mix to combine. Set aside.

In another bowl, add ¼ cup olive oil with a teaspoon of salt. Add sardines and coat with the oil.

Dip each sardine fillet into the breadcrumb mixture (both sides) so that the mixture sticks to the fillet. Roll each fillet tightly and secure with a toothpick. Place on a baking tray. Pour over the lemon juice and remaining olive oil. Bake for 20–30 minutes or until sardines are cooked through and crunchy.

Serve with a squeeze of lemon juice alongside the caper mash.

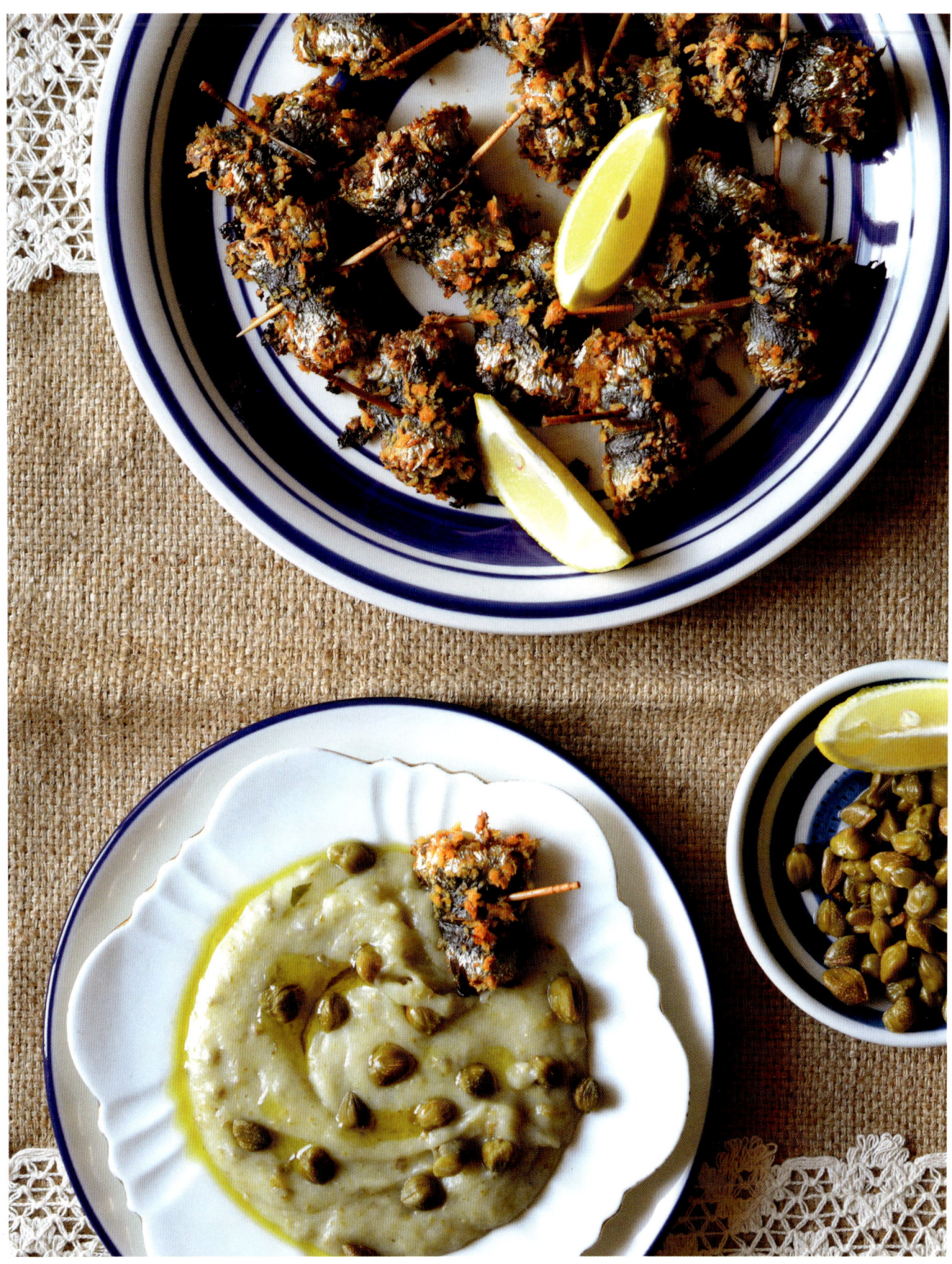

Χταπόδι στιφάδο

- OCTOPUS STIFADO -

1 kg (35.2 oz.) octopus, cleaned and beak removed

1 kg (35.2 oz.) pickling onions, whole

¾ cup olive oil

2 tablespoons tomato paste

10 peppercorns

4 pimento, whole

5 garlic cloves, whole

1 cup tomato purée

1 cup red wine

½ cup red wine vinegar

1 orange rind

1 cinnamon stick

5 cloves, whole

1 tablespoon honey

Salt, to taste

TO SERVE

Fried potatoes (recipe on page 89)
Crusty bread

Stifado literally means "stewed" (*stufado*) in Italian. It is a dish brought to Greece by the Venetians in the thirteenth century after the fall of Constantinople. Small pickling onions are stewed on a low and slow heat either with beef or rabbit, spices, and wine (see the recipe for rabbit *stifado* in my book *Hellenic Kanella*). However, Greeks also have a vegetarian and pescatarian version, like this recipe. Baby octopus is my preference as I like the thin tentacles amid the softened onions. It is lean, low in calories, and high in protein. It is best made a day ahead to allow flavors to intensify. Refrigerate and reheat the next day.

Serves: 6 · 2 hours · GLUTEN FREE

Cut the cleaned octopus into bite-size pieces and place in a large saucepan with the lid on. Cook on medium heat for 20 minutes. Do not add any liquid as it will release its own juices. Add all the remaining ingredients except the salt (this will toughen the octopus).

Cover and simmer on low for 1 hour and 30 minutes or until onions are cooked through, the liquid has evaporated by half, and oil risen to the top. Season with salt to taste.

Serve with fried potatoes and crusty bread to mop up the juices.

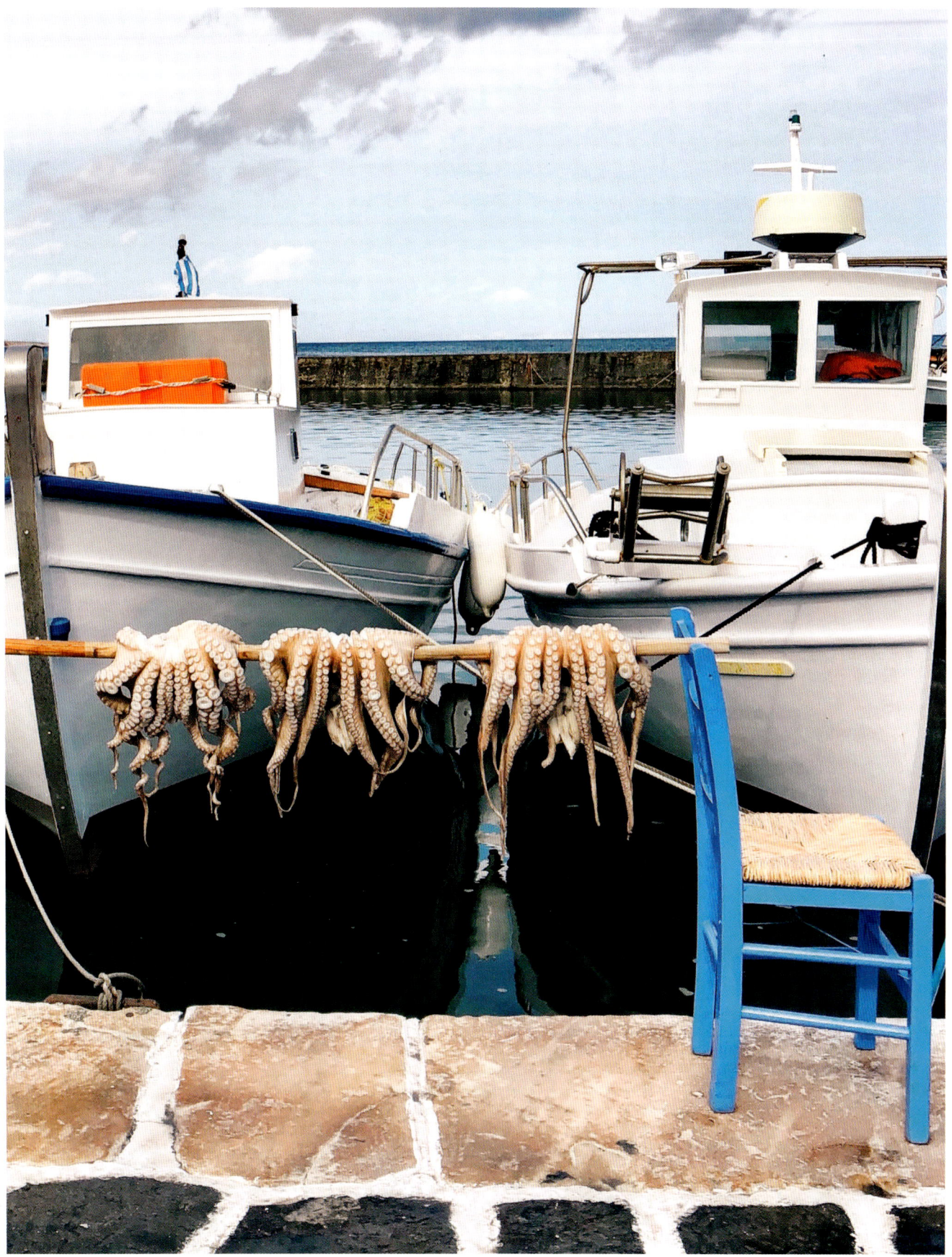

Αγιορείτικες μπάμιες με ψάρι στο φούρνο
- BAKED FISH WITH OKRA -

¾ cup olive oil

1 large onion, sliced

2–3 garlic cloves, sliced

700 g (24.6 oz.) okra, fresh or frozen

2 tablespoons balsamic vinegar

1 cup tomato purée

1 teaspoon castor (superfine) sugar

2 bay leaves

½ teaspoon cumin powder

½ teaspoon cinnamon powder

Salt and pepper, to taste

2 tablespoons parsley, chopped

1 whole snapper (1 kg. or 35.2 oz.) cleaned and gutted, head and tail intact*

TO SERVE

Lemon wedge

Parsley, chopped

Crusty bread

Many vegetarian recipes come from the monasteries in Greece. Monks fast from meat most of the year and therefore have developed tasty and healthy vegetarian meals. They eat from their own produce, which has exceptional flavor as they are grown on mountainous and nutrient-filled fields. Okra is one of those vegetables. If okra is not cooked correctly, it can release sliminess, which can be off putting. To avoid this, some acid needs to be added to the cooking of the okra. Balsamic vinegar is added in this recipe, which aids in that and elevates the flavor of the whole dish.

Serves: 4 · 1 hour · GLUTEN FREE

Heat olive oil in a wide saucepan. Add the onion and garlic and sauté until soft and translucent. Add okra and vinegar and cook for 3–5 minutes. Add the tomato purée, sugar, bay leaves, cumin, and cinnamon powders and season well with salt and pepper. Cook for 15 minutes, and then remove from heat.

Take a large baking tray and place the fish in the center. Pour the onion and okra mixture over the fish and scatter the parsley on top. Add 1½ cups of water to the pan, sprinkle some salt and pepper over the fish, and bake for 35–40 minutes at 200° C/390° F or until okra and fish are cooked, the sauce has thickened, and oil has risen to the top.

Serve with a wedge of lemon, some fresh chopped parsley, and some crusty bread.

TIP: You can add 3 potatoes quartered to the baking dish if desired.

*Fillets can be substituted rather than a whole fish.

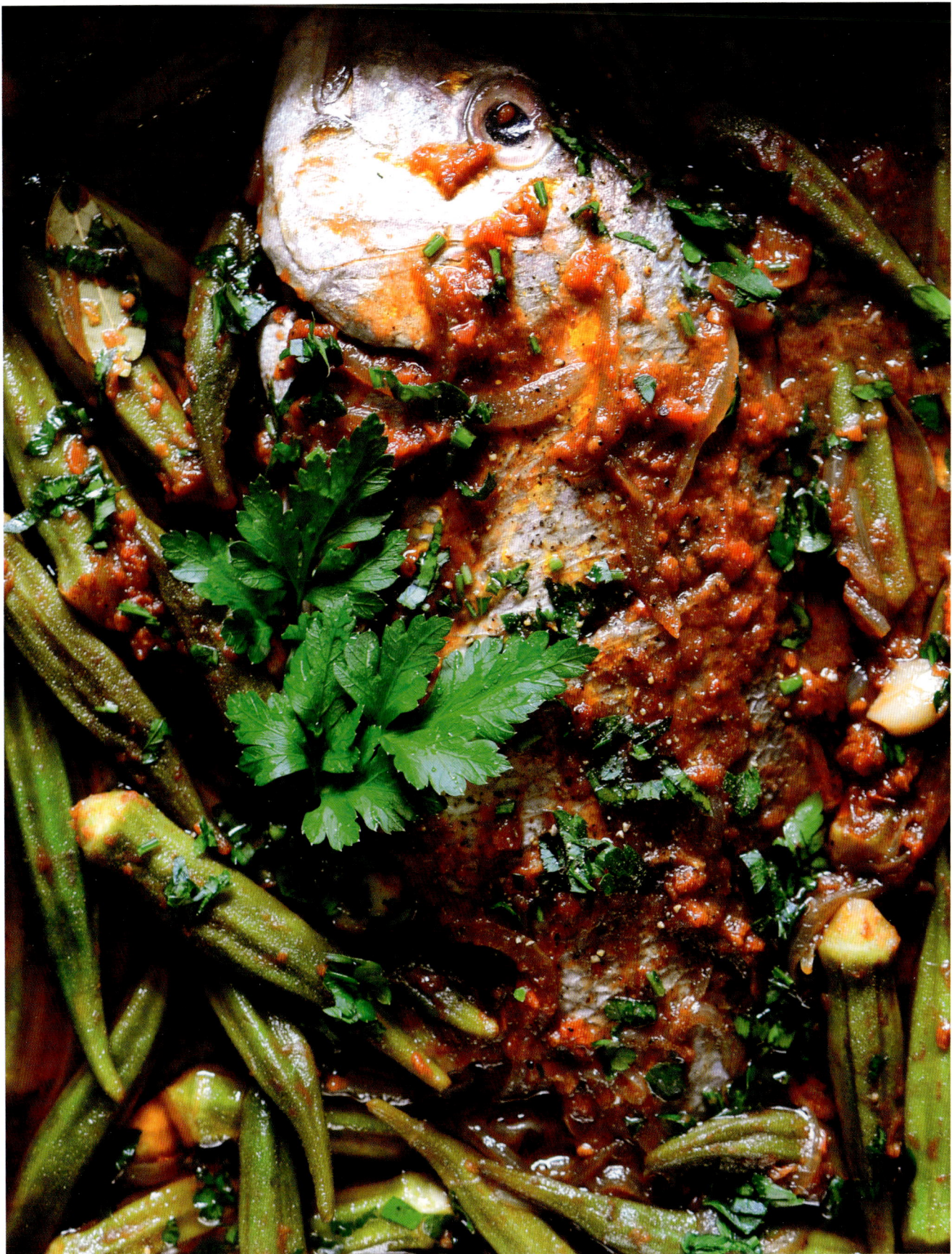

Μπακαλιάρος Τσιλαδιά
- BAKED COD WITH FRIED POTATO, ZUCCHINI, AND RAISIN SALSA -

2 cups olive oil, divided

1 large onion, diced

1 cup tomato purée

½ cup water

2 teaspoons castor (superfine) sugar

Salt and pepper, to taste

¾ cup Peloponnese raisins*

3 medium potatoes, peeled and sliced into scallops

3 medium zucchinis, sliced into scallops

500 g (17.6 oz.) salt cod, rockling, or any white-fleshed fish of choice*

¾ cup all-purpose flour

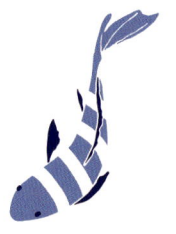

This recipe is cooked throughout different regions in Greece, mostly known by the name *plaki* (πλακί). However, in Messinia, a region of the Peloponnese, a similar dish called Μπακαλιάρος Τσιλαδιά with the addition of raisins is made (also known as Corinthian currants). Raisins are a small superfood loaded with vitamins, micronutrients, and minerals. Rich in natural sugars and a great source of fiber, these raisins are used to sweeten the dish and simultaneously provide many health benefits. This dish can be a little tedious as there are a few steps, but I can assure you it is well worth the effort. Traditionally, salt cod is used, but feel free to use any white-fleshed fish. I use two large frying pans simultaneously to speed up the process. Any raisins can be used if Corinthian variety cannot be purchased in your local area.

Serves: 4 · 1.5 hours

Place two large frying pans on the stove top. Use one for the sauce and the other for frying the fish.

In one pan, heat ½ cup olive oil together with the chopped onions and sauté until incredibly soft. Add tomato purée, water, sugar, salt, and pepper, and continue to cook on low heat for 10 minutes. Add the raisins and cook for a further 5 minutes or until the sauce has thickened slightly.

While the sauce is cooking, take the other frying pan and heat 1½ cups oil. Add the potatoes and fry on both sides until golden and cooked through. Drain on a paper towel and sprinkle with some salt. Do the same with the zucchinis, and then set aside. Now dust the fish fillets with flour, ensuring they are covered well, and fry in the same pan until golden and crispy. Place on paper towel to drain any excess oil.

Take a large baking tray and pour in the tomato and raisin mixture. Top with the potatoes and zucchinis. Mix gently so that vegetables are coated in the sauce. Now place the fish on top (do not mix).

Bake at 190° C/370° F for 15–20 minutes or until the fish starts to further golden and the juices in the pan have evaporated by half.

*Peloponnese raisins can be purchased from European grocers. Alternatively, any other raisins will do.

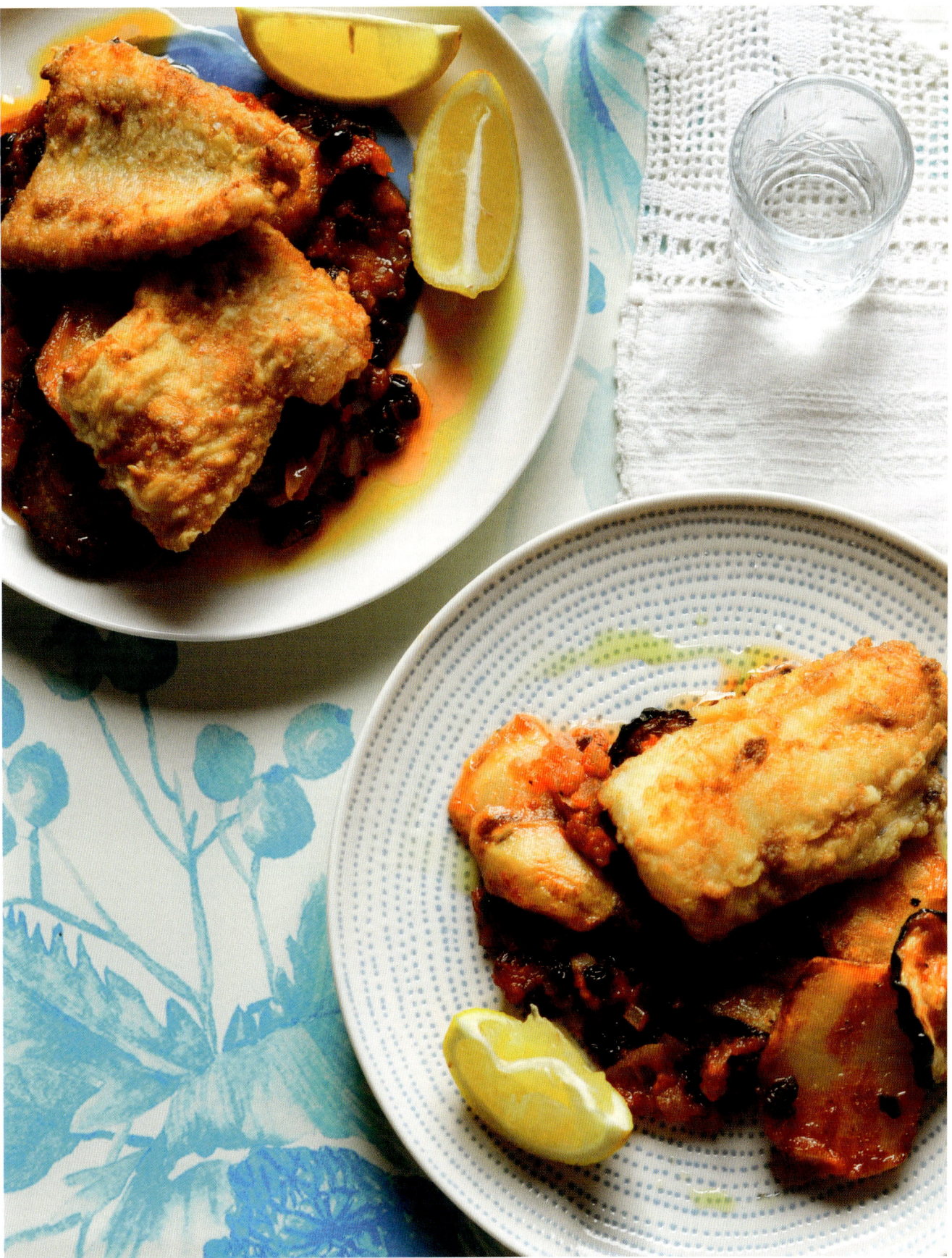

Γαρίδες σαγανάκι με λεμόνι, μάραθο και τυρί φέτα

- PRAWN *SAGANAKI* WITH LEMON, FENNEL, AND FETA CHEESE -

Prawn *saganaki* is a quintessential dish found in most tavernas around Greece. Sautéed prawns are cooked in a rich, flavorsome tomato sauce, a good helping of feta cheese is placed on top, and then they are grilled. My recipe has lemon juice and ground fennel, which intensifies the flavor of this dish. Serve with a glass of iced ouzo.

Serves: 4 • 35 minutes • GLUTEN FREE

¼ cup olive oil

1 small onion, finely chopped

2 garlic cloves, minced

2 teaspoons fennel seeds, ground

1 cup tomato purée

2 bay leaves

1 teaspoon sweet paprika powder

Salt and pepper, to taste

1 teaspoon chili flakes, optional

1 teaspoon castor (superfine) sugar

½ cup white wine

450 g (15.8 oz.) large uncooked prawns*

½ cup feta cheese, crumbled

TO SERVE

2 tablespoons parsley, chopped

2 tablespoons lemon juice

Heat olive oil in a large ovenproof pan. Sauté the onion and garlic until soft but not browned. Add the fennel and cook for 30 seconds. Add the tomato purée, bay, paprika, salt, pepper, chili flakes, sugar, and wine. Simmer for 10–15 minutes on a medium heat. Stir in the prawns and mix to coat with the sauce. Cover and simmer on low heat for a further 10 minutes or until the prawns have turned pink and are cooked through.

Taste the sauce and adjust seasoning if needed. Scatter the crumbled feta cheese over the top and place under a hot grill to brown and for the cheese to melt slightly.

Garnish with chopped parsley and lemon juice and serve with crusty bread.

*I use half cleaned prawns and the other half with skins on.

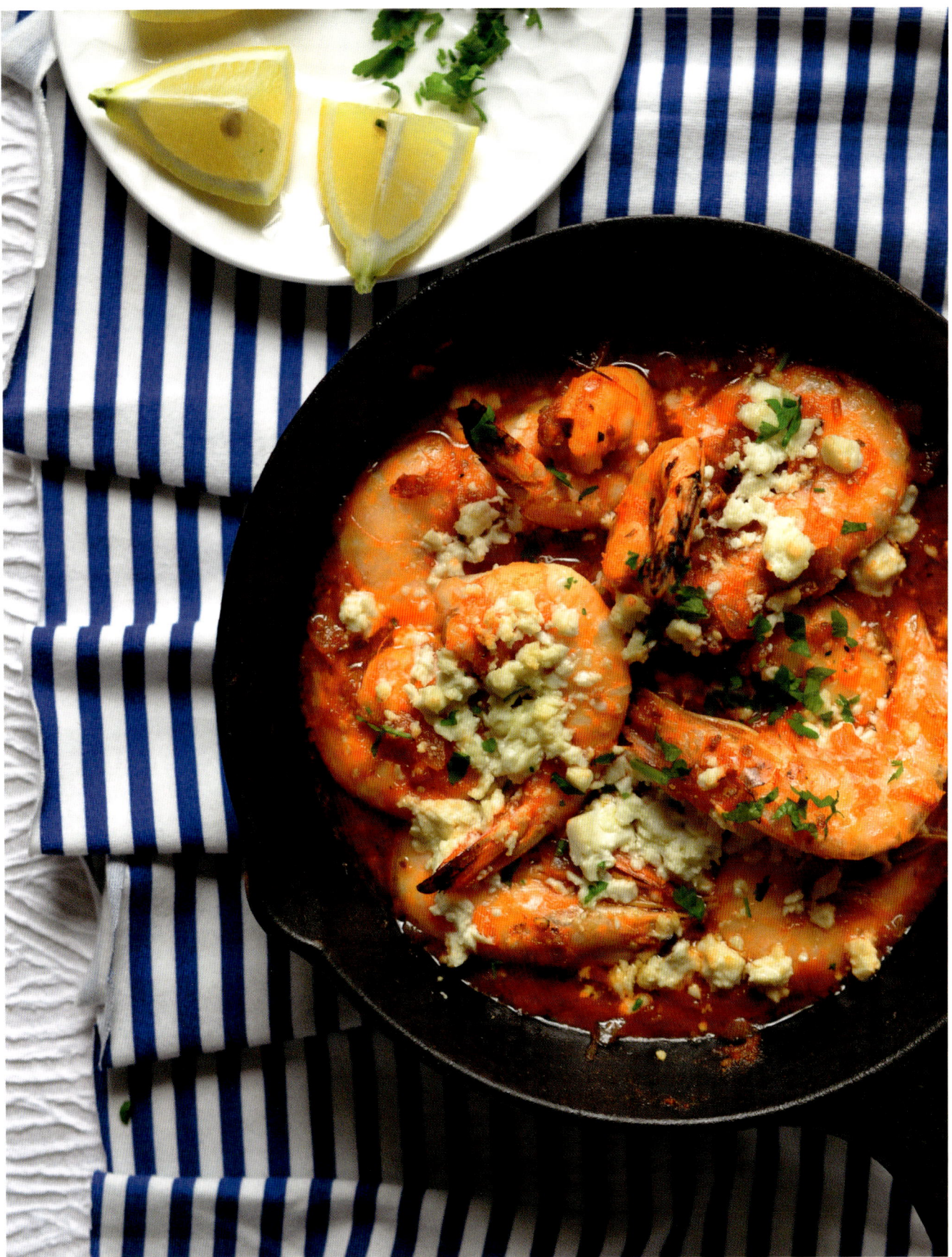

Γεμιστές Σαρδέλες σε αμπελόφυλλα
- STUFFED SARDINES WRAPPED IN VINE LEAVES -

This is a recipe quite commonly eaten in monasteries and on Greek islands. Grape leaves are a staple ingredient used in Greek cooking. Leaves are generally picked in late spring and early summer while they are tender and plentiful. They are used immediately in recipes such as this or preserved for the winter months.

Makes: 25 pieces · 1 hour · GLUTEN FREE

In a bowl, mix together the marinade ingredients. Add the sardines, turning them over to ensure both sides are coated well. Set aside to marinate for 15 minutes.

In another bowl, add the filling ingredients. Mix to combine.

Place a leaf stem side up on your workbench. Place one sardine fillet on top, and then add one teaspoon of the stuffing onto the sardine and gently roll away from you, bringing in the sides and enclosing the fillet. Place onto a baking tray and repeat with all the sardines.

Drizzle the additional 3 tablespoons olive oil over the vine leaves.

Bake at 190º C/374º F for 30–40 minutes or until sardines are cooked through and slightly crispy.

Serve with a dollop of yogurt or caper mash.

*Brined vine leaves must be rinsed with water and then drained to remove excess salt. If using fresh leaves, blanch in boiling water for 1 minute. Allow to cool.

*May be substituted with gluten-free breadcrumbs.

MARINADE

¼ cup olive oil

2 garlic cloves, minced

1 lemon, juiced

25 sardines, filleted

FILLING

1 cup breadcrumbs (preferably panko breadcrumbs)*

3 tablespoons mint, chopped

2 tablespoons parsley, chopped

1 teaspoon salt

½ teaspoon pepper

3 tablespoons olive oil

1 lemon, juice and zest

25 vine leaves, fresh or brined*

Additional 3 tablespoons olive oil

TO SERVE

Caper mash (recipe on page 78)

Yogurt

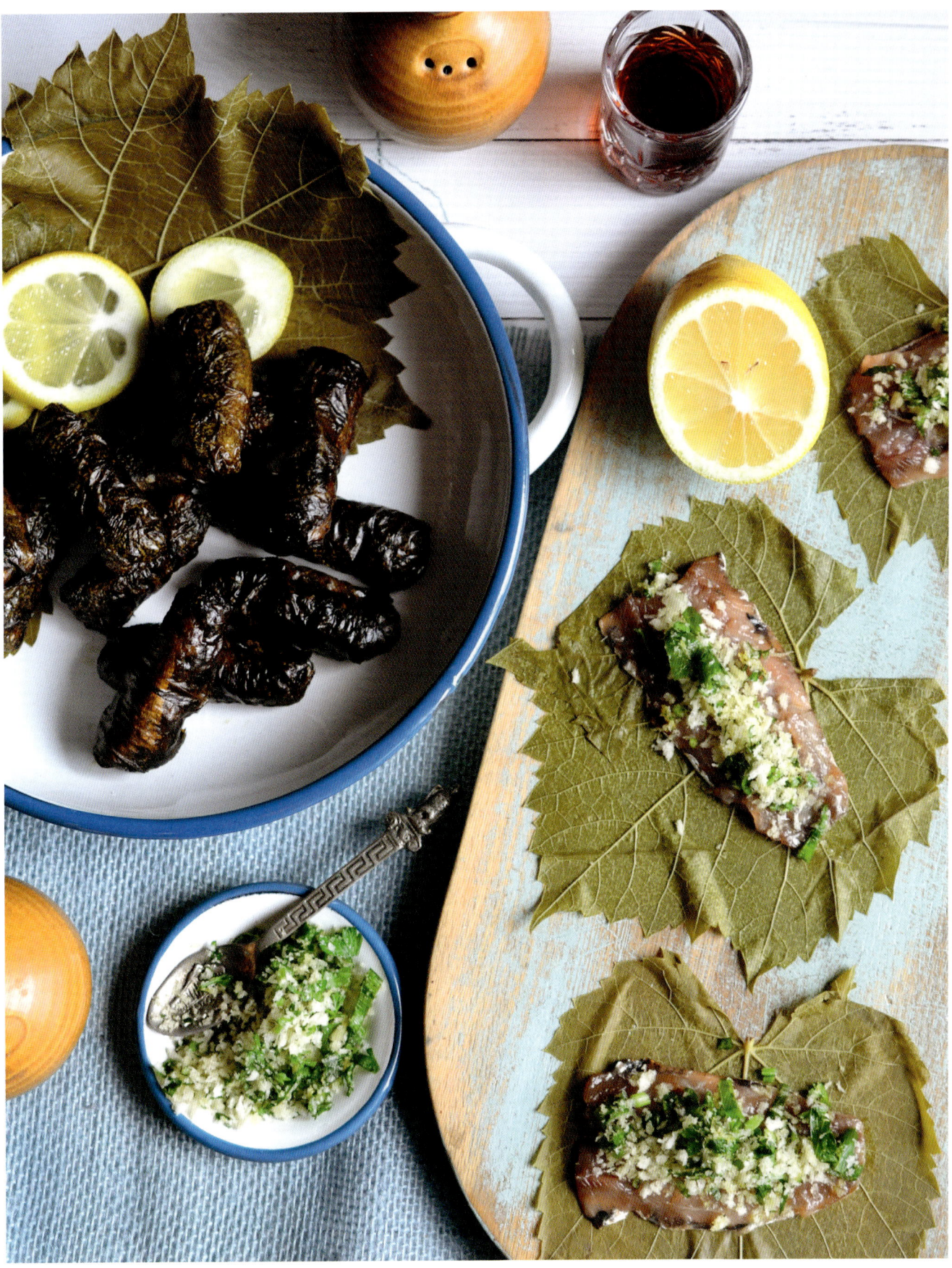

Σκορδαλιά με χταπόδι και μέλι
- ROASTED GARLIC MASH AND HONEY OCTOPUS -

Skordalia is a potato mash made with garlic that is commonly served alongside fish such as cod. However, in Corfu it is also served with octopus that has been cooked and marinated in a honey, orange, and balsamic dressing. It is both sweet and sour and pairs wonderfully well with the creamy potato and garlic mash.

Serves: 4-6 • 1.5 hours • GLUTEN FREE

---

1 kg (35.2 oz.) octopus, cleaned and beak removed

¼ cup olive oil

2 bay leaves

DRESSING

¼ cup olive oil

2 tablespoons balsamic vinegar

2 tablespoons orange marmalade

2 tablespoons runny honey

1-2 tablespoons water

Salt and pepper, to taste

GARLIC MASH

10 garlic cloves, skin on

2 tablespoons olive oil

6 medium potatoes, quartered

1 tablespoon salt

¼ cup olive oil

1 lemon, juiced, or to taste

Place the octopus in a pot with bay leaves and olive oil. Cover and simmer on low heat for approximately 45 minutes. Do not add any liquid as it will release its own juices. Octopus should be fork tender; if not, keep cooking for a further 20 minutes. Remove from the pot. Allow it to cool slightly, and then cut into bite-size pieces and set aside.

Place all dressing ingredients into a bowl, whisking to combine. Taste and adjust seasoning if needed. Pour marinade over the cooked octopus and allow to marinate for 35 minutes or until the potato mash is ready. Keep warm.

To make the mash, place the garlic cloves onto a baking tray. Drizzle the olive oil over them and sprinkle with some salt. Bake at 180º C/356º F for 30 minutes or until soft. Remove, allow to cool, and then peel the skins.

In a pot of water, add the potatoes and salt. Bring to a boil and simmer until potatoes are fork tender. Immediately place the potatoes into a blender together with the garlic, ¼ cup oil, and the lemon juice. Blend until a smooth mash is achieved. Taste and adjust seasoning if needed.

To serve, place the potato mash onto a plate or platter, and then add the octopus with some marinade over the top. Octopus is best served at room temperature, but it can be heated slightly if you prefer it warmer.

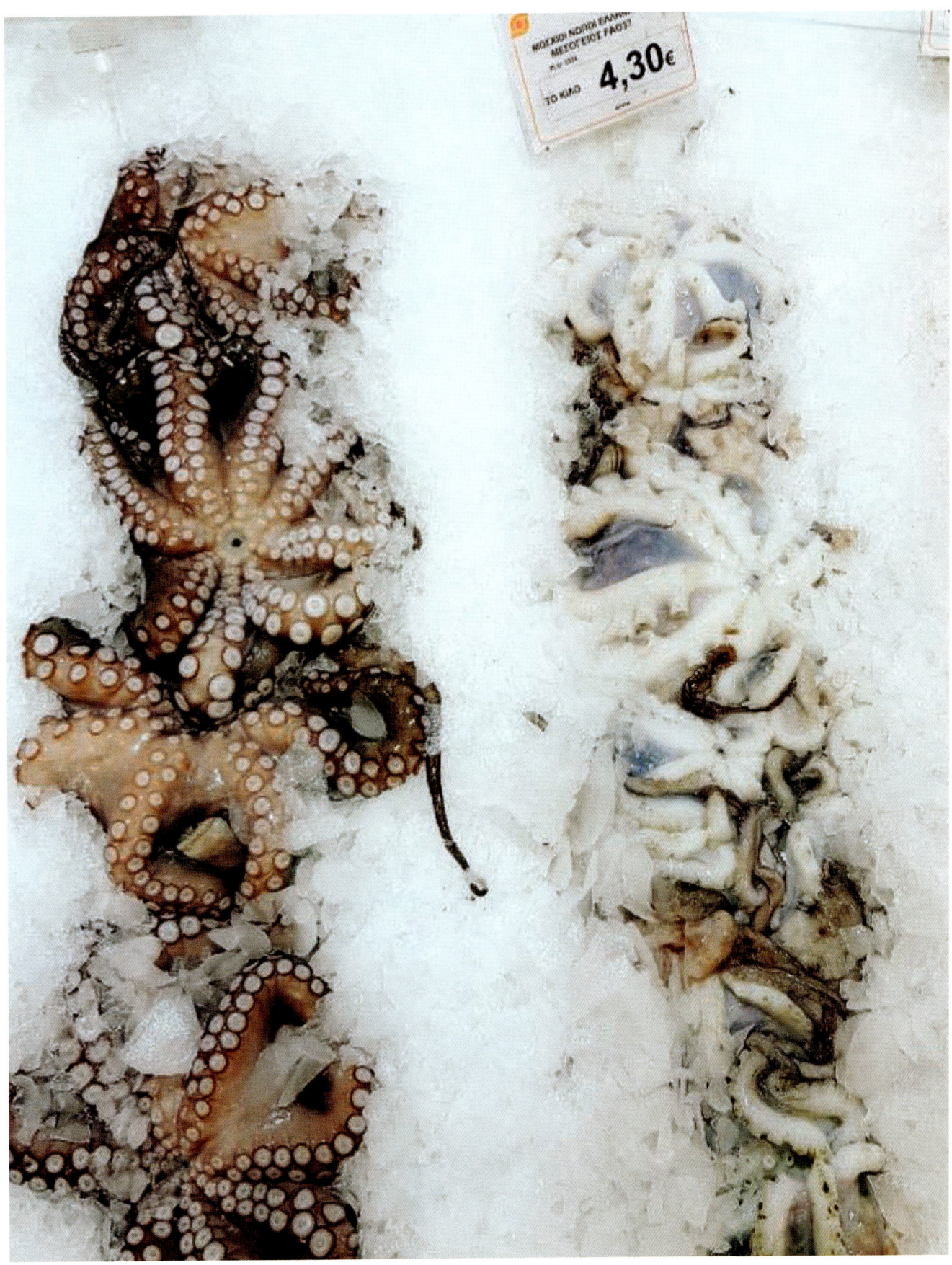

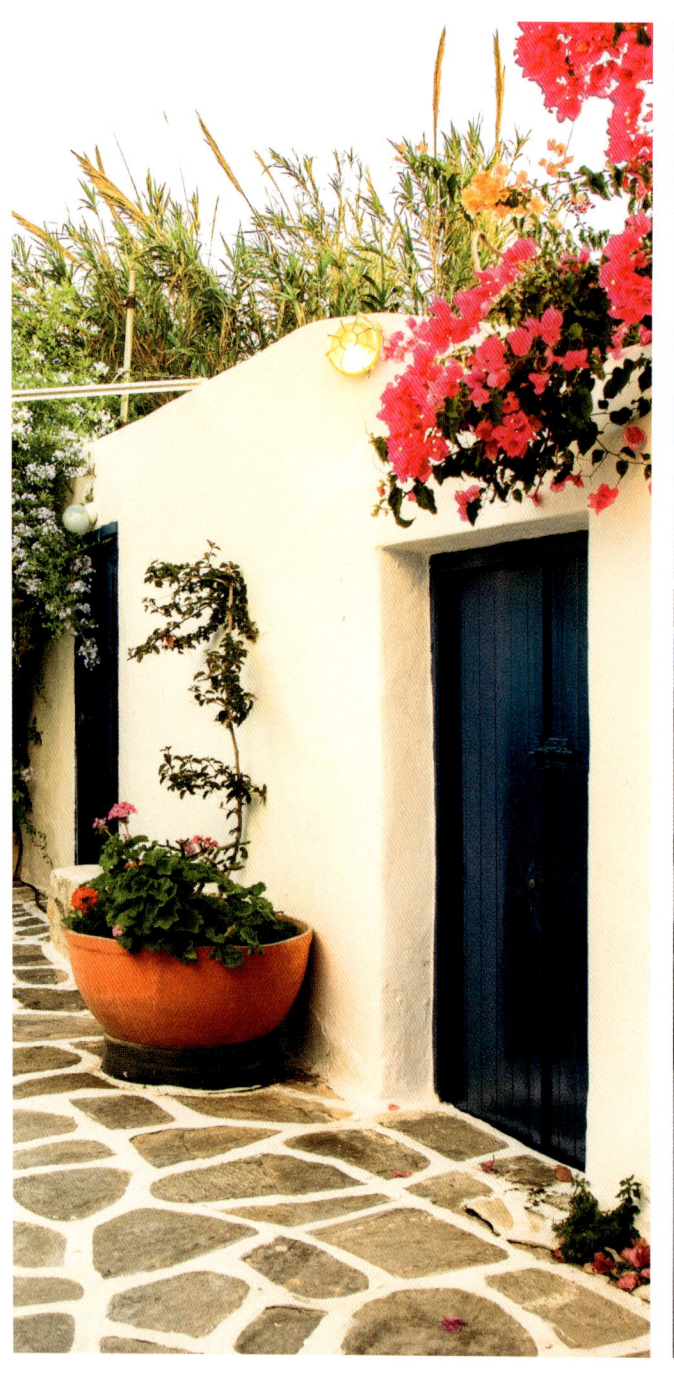
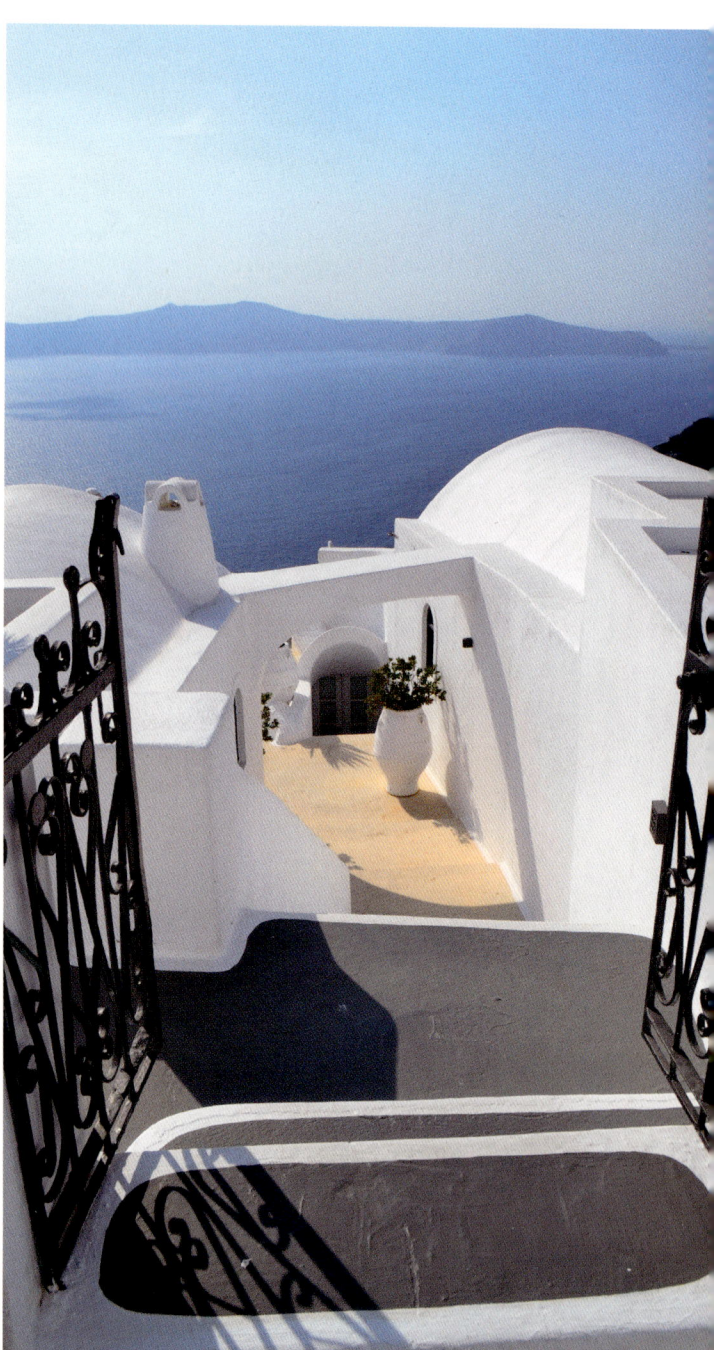

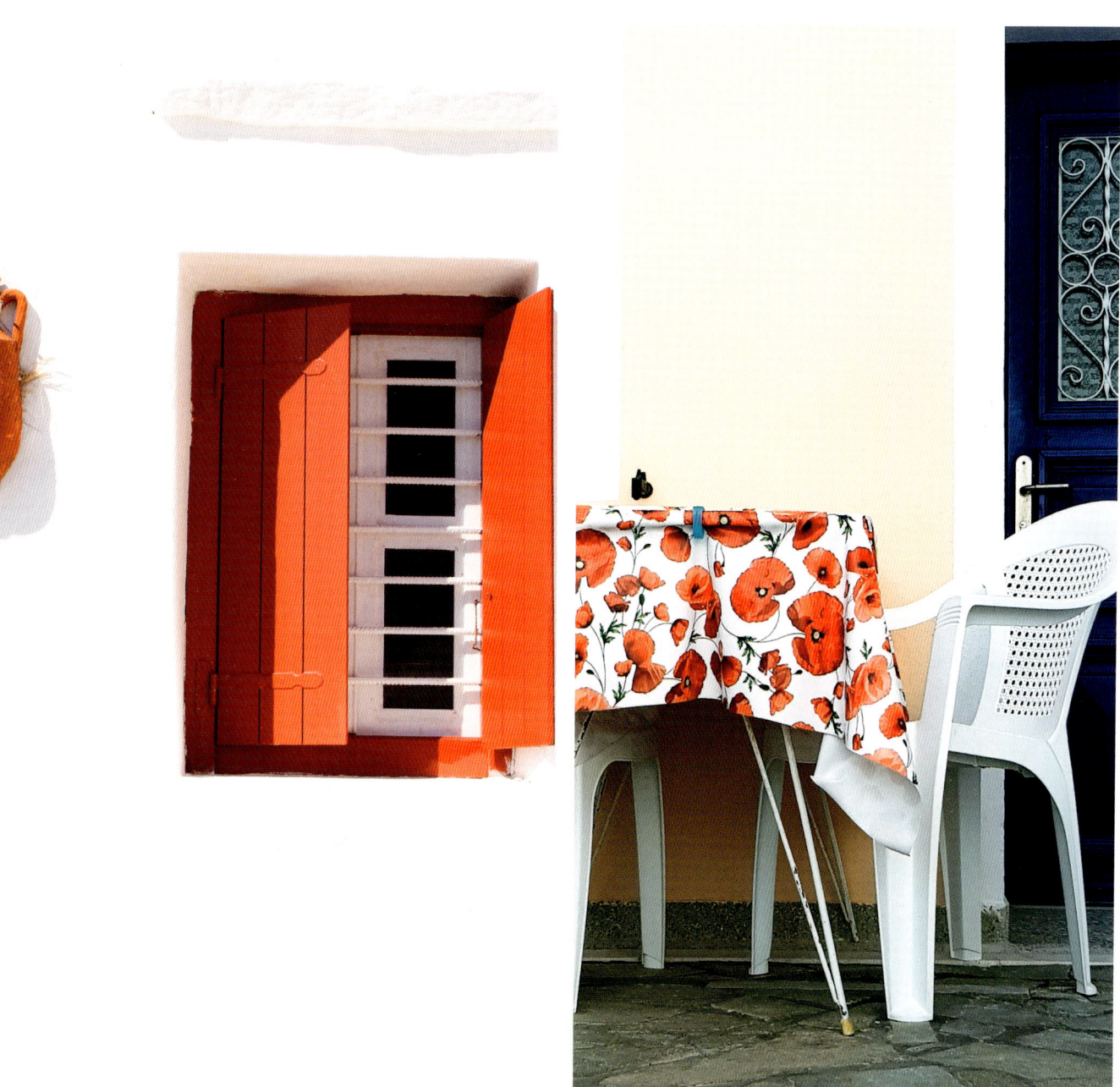

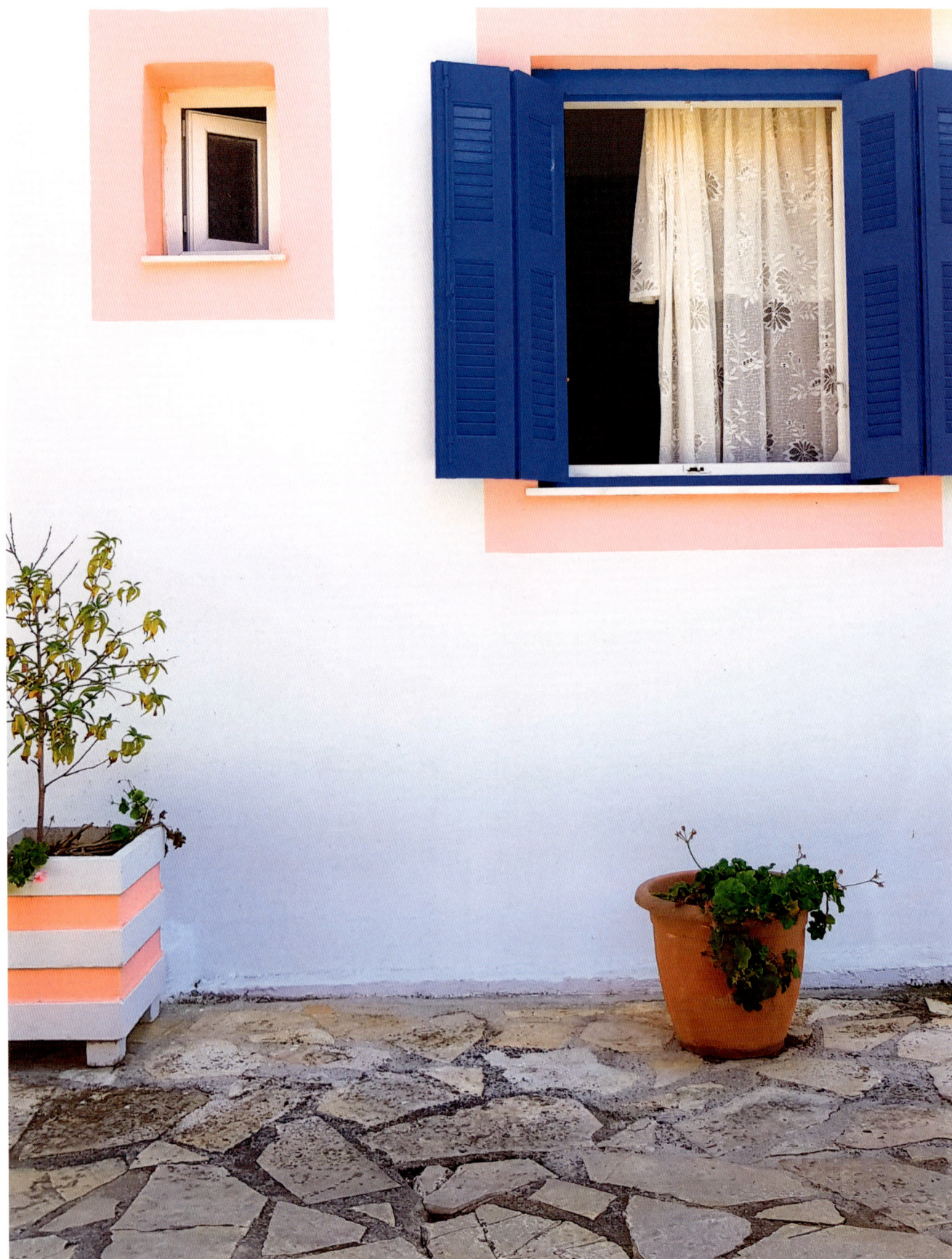

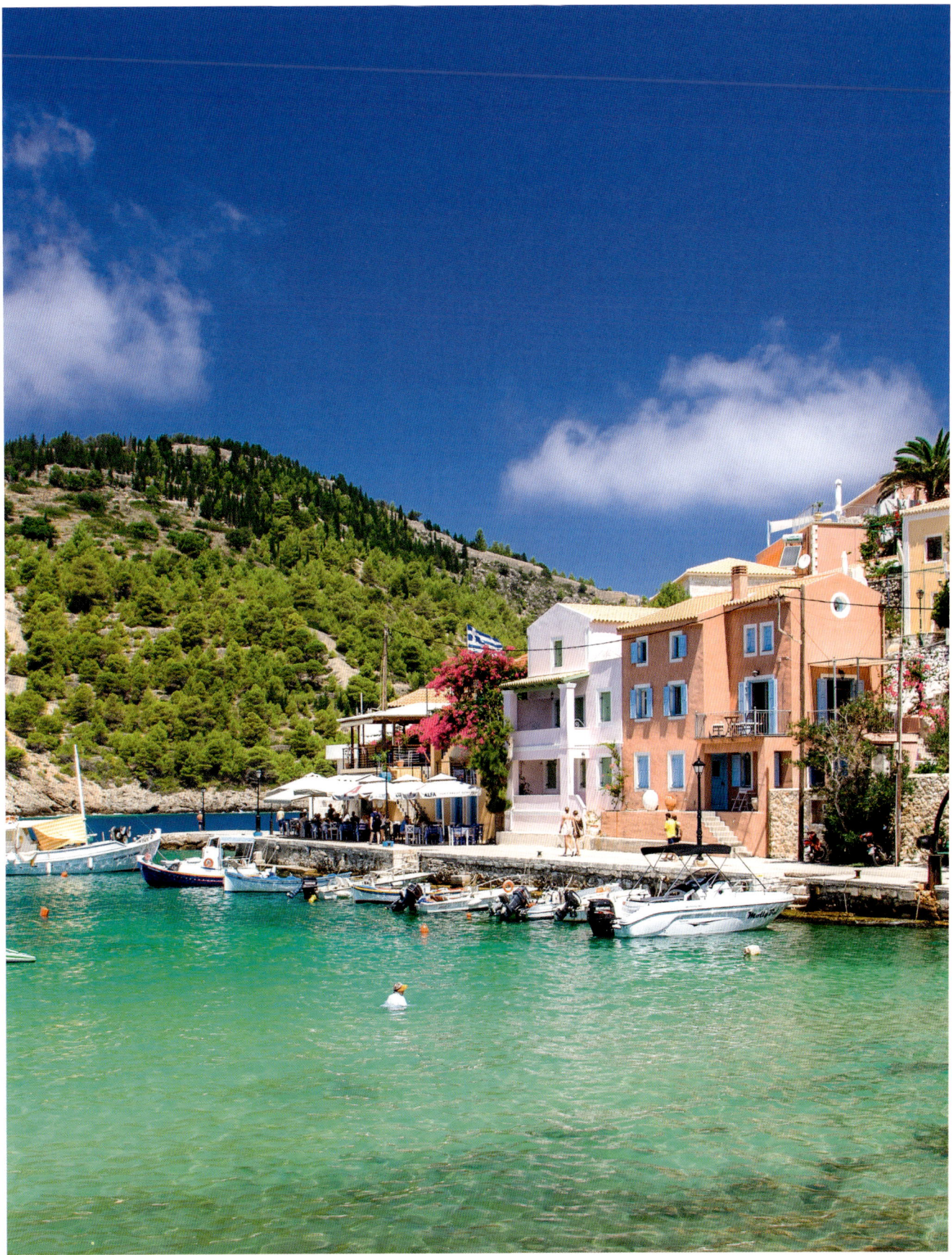

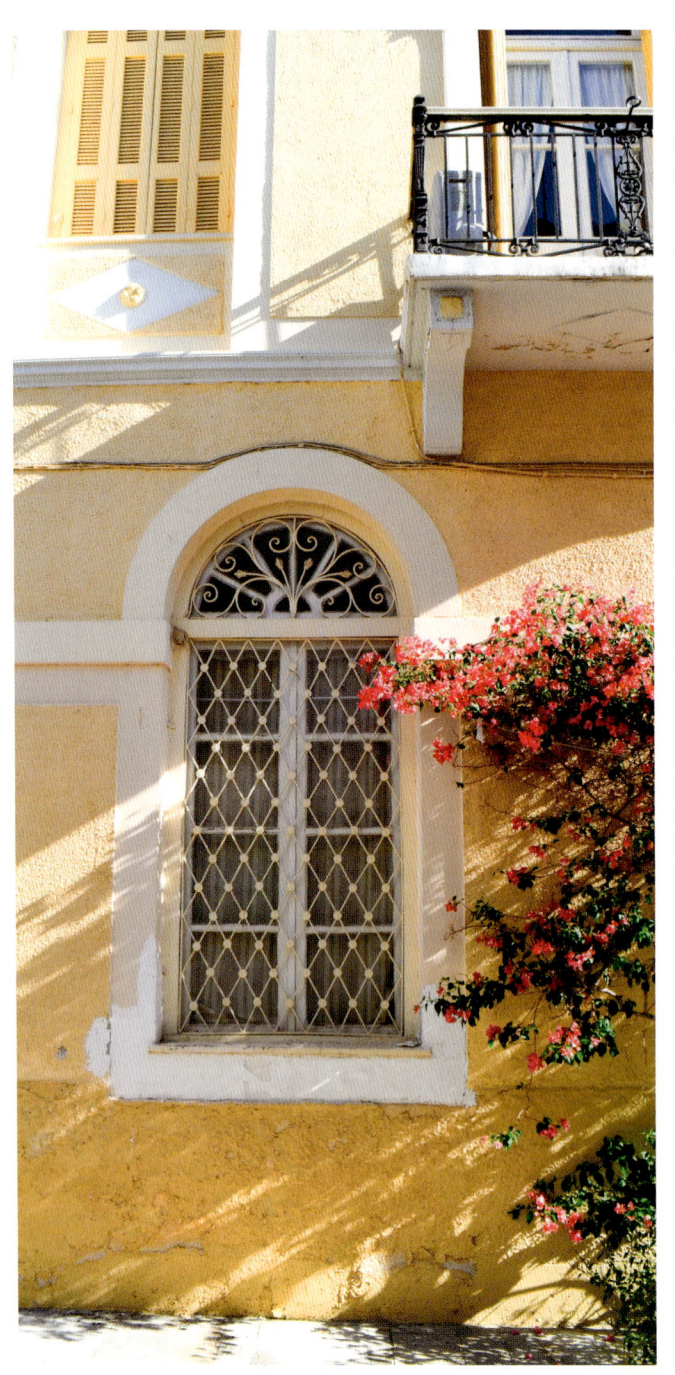
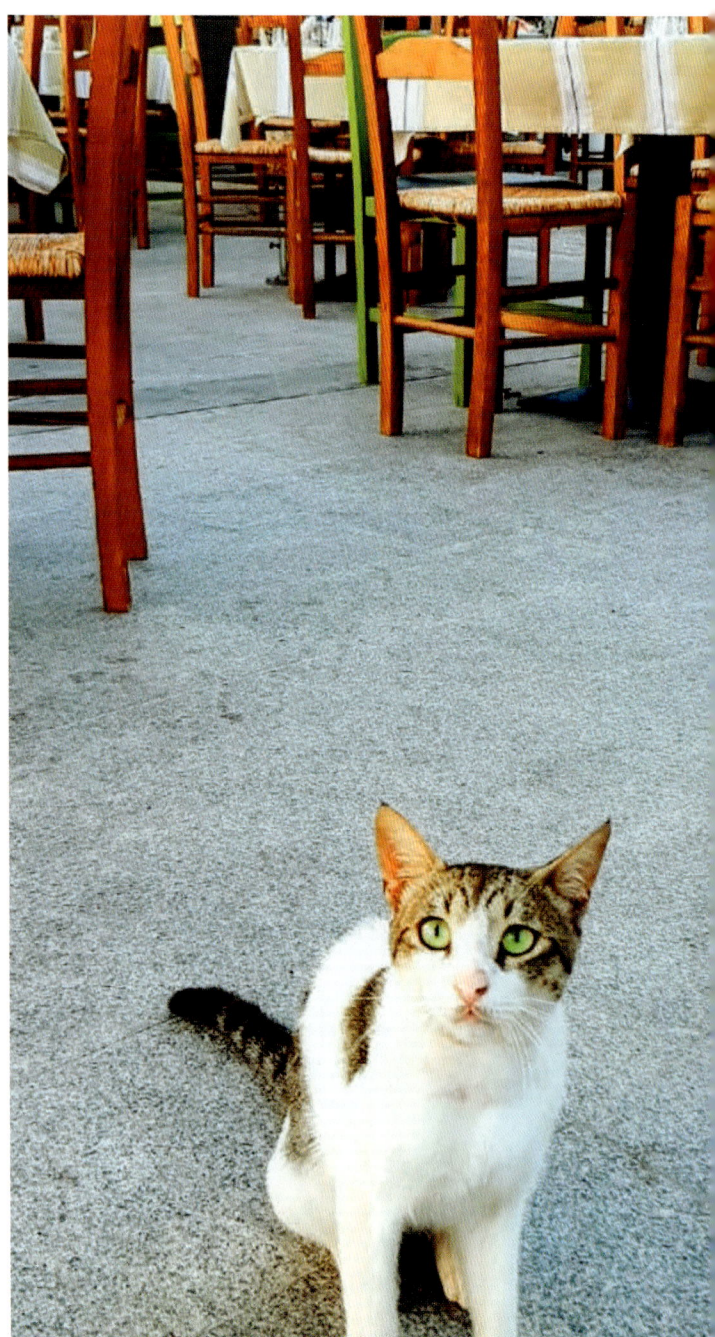

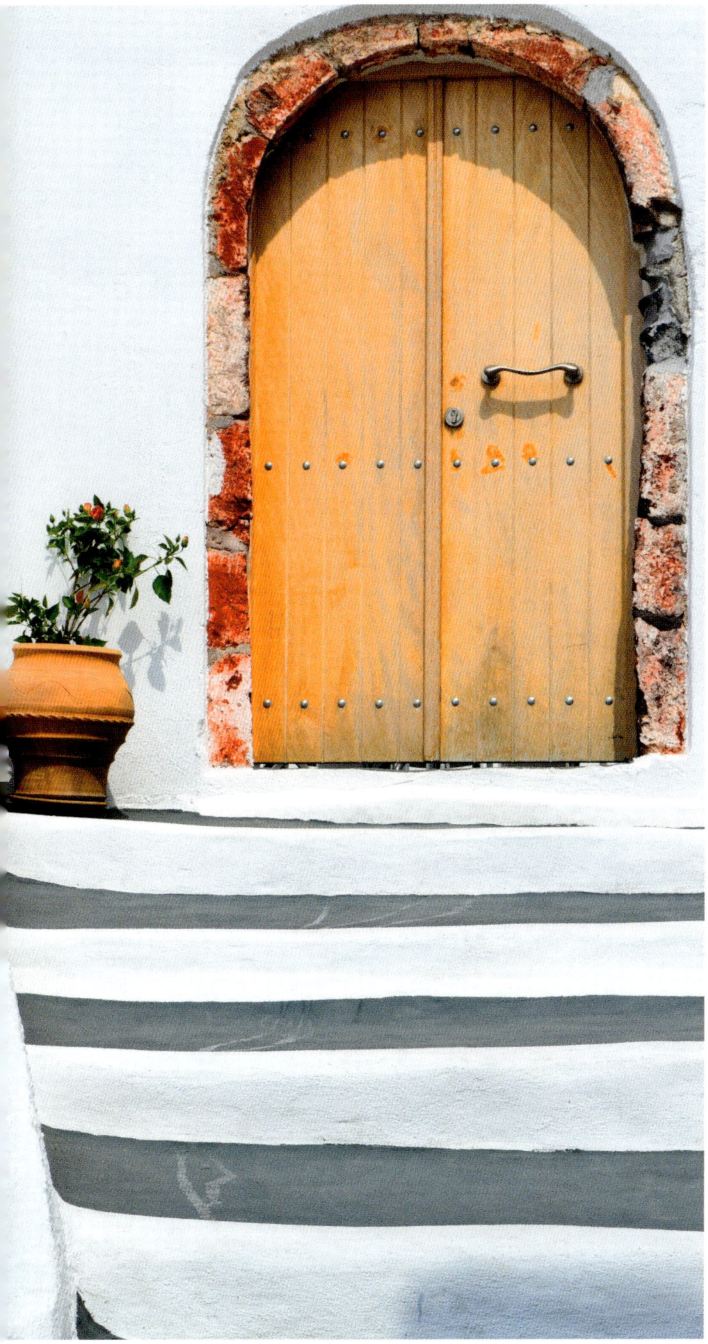

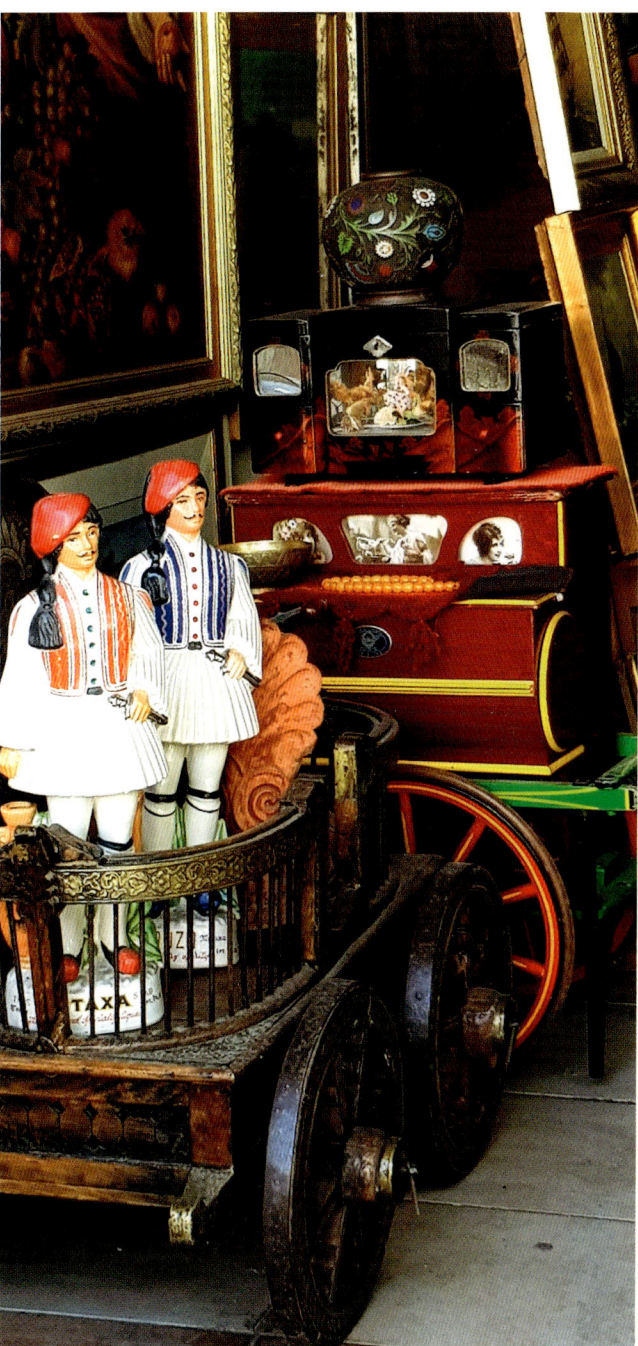

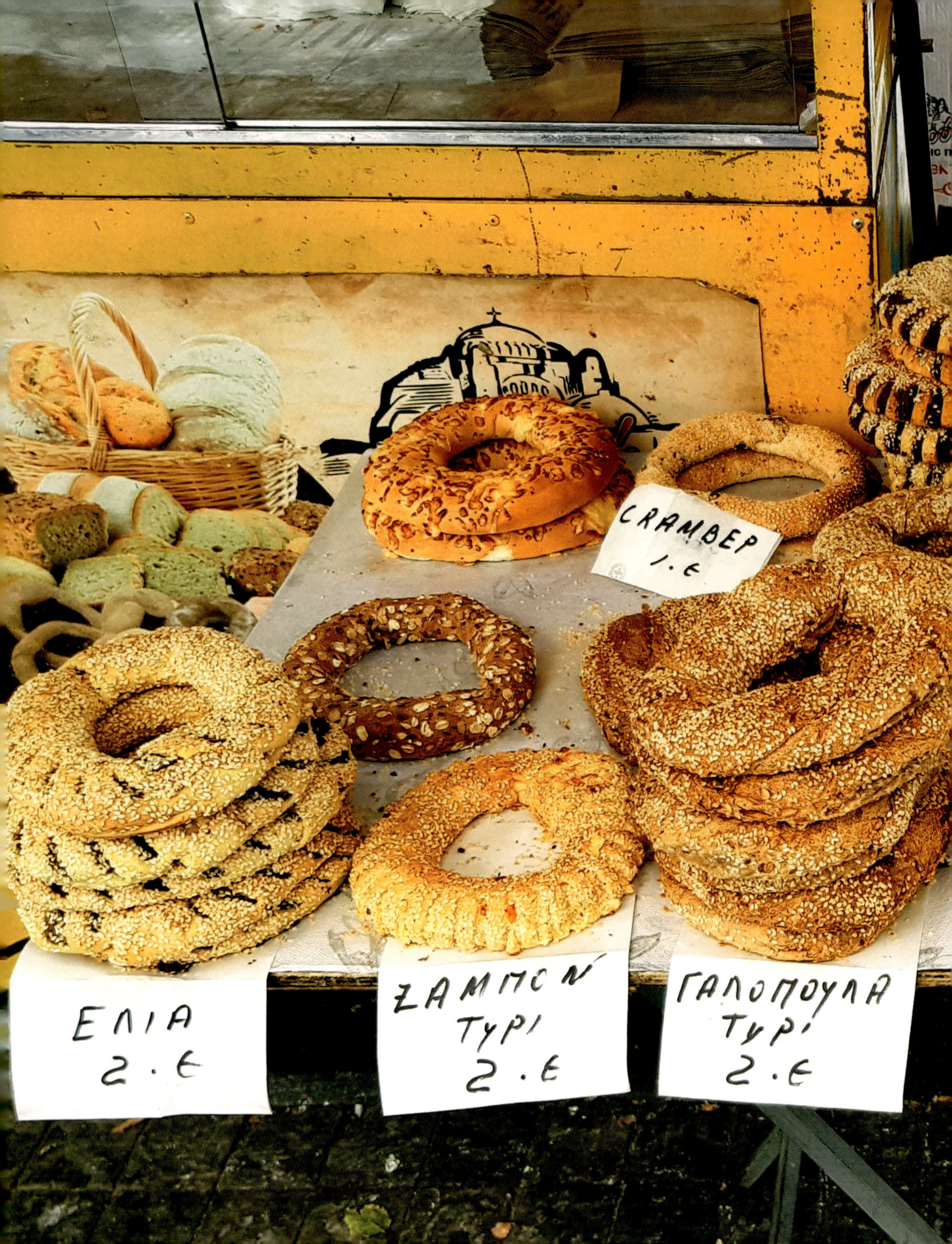

Ο ΦΟΥΡΝΑΡΗΣ
THE BAKER

ΤΟ ΦΥΛΛΟ ΣΤΗΝ ΠΑΡΑΔΟΣΗ
TRADITION

In the village.

She rises early, occasionally before the sun exposes its first light. She considers the day ahead; she will be required to provide food for her household. She does not have supplies in abundance. She must think and create.

She has freshly milled flour from the grain fields cultivated by her husband. She gathers fresh eggs that have been laid by her free-ranging chickens, and then she forages through her vast land for fresh herbs and vegetables. It looks like simple roughage, yet unbeknownst to her is that it is fueled with vitamins and nutrients. She fills her apron pockets and then wipes her sharp knife now covered in soil.

She takes a large bowl and starts to combine the ingredients for the dough: milled flour, cold-pressed extra-virgin olive oil, and salt. She swirls it around with her fingertips and then slowly pours in exactly enough water. She continues to mix with her hands. Experience has taught her the magic of touch and feel, knowing when enough water is absorbed. She stops pouring. She knows it is enough; she is precise. She removes the dough from her bowl and places it onto a low bench. She crouches, overexposing her now hunched back—evidence of hard work. She pushes the dough with her palm outward, stretching and repeating until a silky soft, pliable dough is achieved. She puts it aside to rest, covered by a cotton tea towel.

This is the beginning.

She proceeds to prepare the filling. Today it is a greens pie. She fills her kitchen trough with water and submerges all her soiled greens. She carefully and meticulously washes each one, removing any insects or dirt attached to the leaves. It is a wonderous assortment, a variety of spinach, silverbeet, leeks, and wild greens. She cuts and places them into another bowl. She does not forget to add the abundance of herbs: evergreen parsley, perfumed mint leaves, and long spring onions. She finely chops these, and into the bowl of greens they are added.

She cracks a few fresh eggs, pours a generous amount of olive oil, and crumbles in a good helping of feta cheese. She mixes these well to combine and sets it aside.

ΗΝ ΠΑΡΑΔΟΣΗ

She separates the dough into small balls.

The dowel is now in her hands. Lightly flouring the surface of her bench, she places the dough in the center. Her dowel is placed on top, and with gentle motions, she presses down and forward until the ball starts to expand. She pulls the dough closer to her. She places the dowel on the one end, wrapping some dough over it and then rolling up all the dough. She gently presses the dough over the dowel, and the dough expands ever so slightly. With a quick flip, she loosens it and repeats until she has a large, thin pastry. She picks up speed, and before long, she has sheets upon sheets of thin pastry. She oils her aluminum baking tray. She rolls up one piece of pastry with her dowel and then places it over the tray. She gently loosens the pastry from side to side so it drops into the baking tray like a ruffled drape. It hangs over the edges. She oils the pastry and repeats with a few more sheets. She now scatters the filling over the pastry and proceeds to repeat the pastry layers, but this time she ensures no pastry is overhanging. It is layered into the tray. Her last layer is added, and she now brings in the outer pastry, gathering and twisting to create a thick rope edge. She scores the pie with her small knife. She pours oil into her palm and splatters it onto the top. The pie is ready to be baked.

Her husband has gathered wood and lit a blazing fire in their outdoor clay oven, which is a hollow dome-shaped structure with a chimney. Most meals are cooked here. She places her tray into the oven and with much strength pushes closed a heavy steel door to seal the heat in.

An hour later, she proceeds to remove the cooked pie from the oven using a thick towel so as to not burn her hands. The family gathers around the table. The hot baking tray is placed in the center. She takes a knife and begins to cut the pie. The pastry is crispy and crunchy. The only additional sounds to be heard are the expressions of deep hunger by the mouths ready to devour this humble pie.

A piece is given to all.

Groans of satisfaction are expressed and then the joyful silence of contentment.

Έβαλα την ζυγαριά μου
στην γωνία σήμερα.
και θα μείνει εκεί
μέχρι να ζητήσει συγνώμη

ΠΙΤΕΣ ΚΑΙ ΨΩΜΙΑ
THE SAVORY BAKER

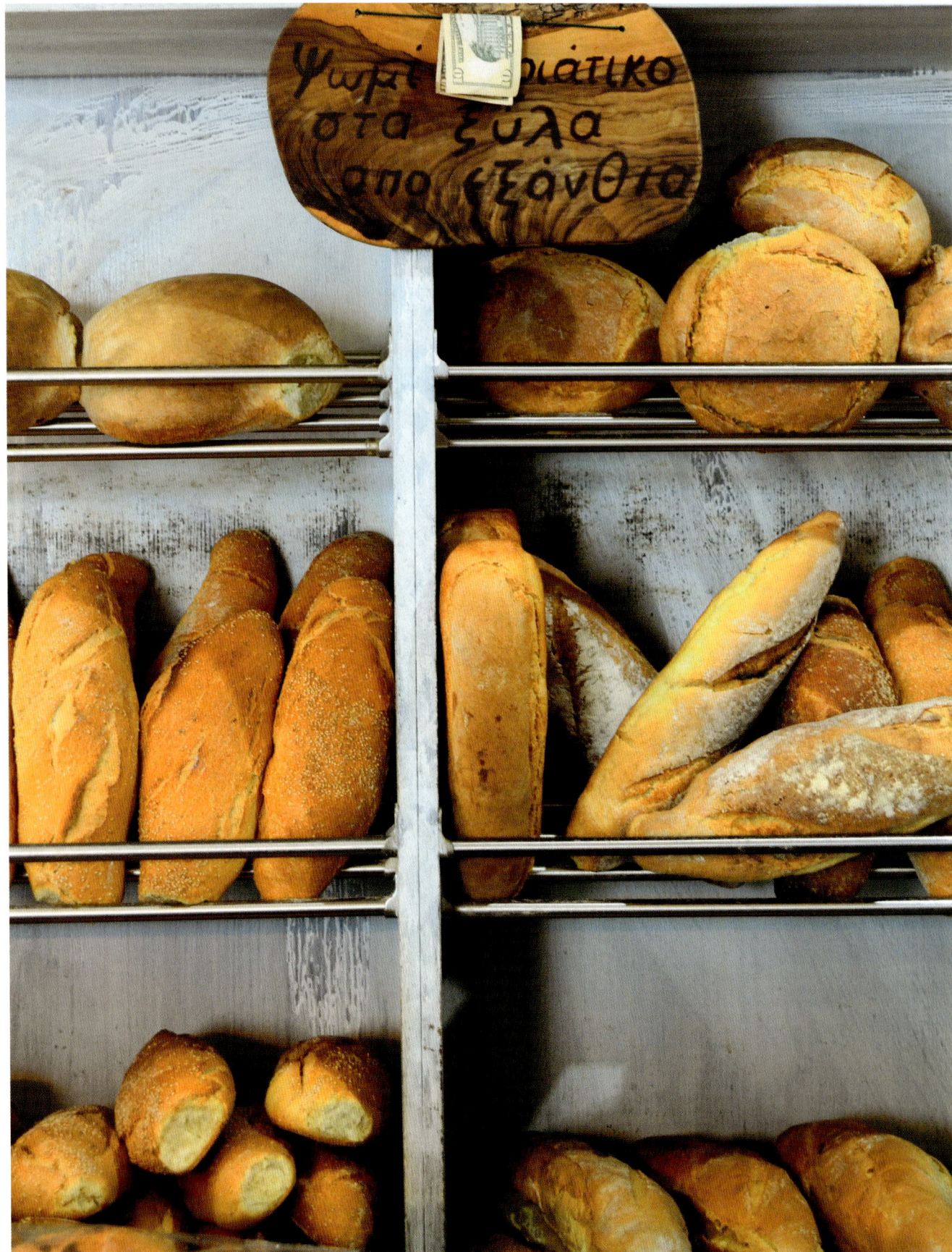

ΠΙΠΕΡΟΠΙΤΑ ΦΛΩΡΙΝΗΣ ΜΕ ΧΩΡΙΑΤΙΚΟ ΦΥΛΛΟ
143   CAPSICUM AND CHEESE PIE WITH VILLAGE PASTRY

ΤΥΡΟΠΙΤΑ ΜΕ ΦΥΛΛΟ ΑΠΟ ΓΙΑΟΥΡΤΙ ΚΑΙ ΓΑΛΑ
145   CHEESE PIE MADE WITH YOGURT AND MILK PASTRY

ΠΡΑΣΟΠΙΤΑ ΜΕ ΦΥΛΛΟ ΜΕΘΟΔΟΣ ΤΟΥ ΗΛΙΟΥ
146   LEEK PIE—"SUNRAY" PHYLLO PASTRY

ΠΑΤΑΤΟΠΙΤΑ ΜΕ ΕΛΙΑ ΚΑΙ ΔΕΝΤΡΟΛΙΒΑΝΟ ΜΕ ΧΩΡΙΑΤΙΚΟ ΦΥΛΛΟ
159   POTATO, OLIVE, AND ROSEMARY PIE WITH VILLAGE PASTRY

ΤΙΓΑΝΟΠΙΤΕΣ ΜΕ ΧΩΡΙΑΤΙΚΟ ΦΥΛΛΟ
152   STOVE TOP FRIED CHEESE PIES WITH VILLAGE PASTRY

ΞΕΣΚΕΠΑΣΤΗ ΣΠΑΝΑΚΟΤΥΡΟΠΙΤΑ
154   SPINACH, CHEESE, AND TOMATO OPEN PIE

ΤΥΡΟΠΙΤΑ ΣΤΟ ΠΙ ΚΑΙ ΦΙ ΜΕ ΕΤΟΙΜΟ ΦΥΛΛΟ
157   CHEESE PIE IN A FLASH WITH STORE-BOUGHT PASTRY

ΚΑΣΕΡΟΠΙΤΑ ΜΕ ΧΩΡΙΑΤΙΚΟ ΦΥΛΛΟ
158   *KASEROPITA* WITH VILLAGE PASTRY

ΚΟΛΟΚΥΘΟΤΥΡΟΠΙΤΑ ΜΕ ΧΩΡΙΑΤΙΚΟ ΛΕΠΤΟ ΦΥΛΛΟ ΣΤΡΙΦΤΗ ΣΕ ΛΑΔΙ
159   PUMPKIN CHEESE PIES WITH VILLAGE PASTRY IN OIL

ΛΑΔΕΝΙΑ ΚΙΜΩΛΟΥ
163   *LADENIA* FROM KIMOLOS

ΕΛΙΟΨΩΜΟ ΧΩΡΙΣ ΖΥΜΩΜΑ
165   NO-KNEAD OLIVE CIABATTA

ΠΕΪΝΙΡΛΙ
167   *PEINIRLI*

ΚΥΠΡΙΑΚΗ ΦΛΑΟΥΝΟΠΙΤΑ
169   CYPRIOT *FLAOUNOPITA*

ΤΥΡΟΚΟΥΛΟΥΡΑ ΜΕ ΓΛΥΚΑΝΙΣΟ
170   FETA CHEESE AND FENNEL KOULOURI

ΠΙΤΕΣ ΚΑΙ ΨΩΜΙΑ

THE SAVORY BAKER

What would a Greek do without bread of some sort to dip into oil-based ladera (λαδερά) dishes, or the bread ring koulouri (κουλούρι), which is enjoyed for breakfast with a strong Greek coffee, or the most popular snack of spinach and cheese pies at every corner store and bakery around Greece? Basically, one of the most popular things at every table is bread or a pie in some form, generally homemade by the home cook. The truth is, bread ties a meal together and is the heart of hospitality. Bread, a bowl of olives, cheese, and a good wine is always at the meal table and is a gesture of invitation. Know well that a Greek will only cry out hungry if they are without bread! Bread is the basis and a staple in Greek cuisine.

All Greeks have grown up eating a myriad selection of Greek pies and pastries. Developed and derived from absolute necessity due to scarcity of ingredients, these pies are an absolute treat and delight to eat. Many home cooks are vigilant in wanting to continue the tradition of making pastry from scratch and ensuring this tradition does not end with this generation.

Flour, water, salt, oil, a few filling ingredients, hands willing to knead, and the use of a dowel (a thin rolling pin) creates a meal substantial enough to feed a crowd and please the fussiest of eaters. Traditional Greek pies have many variances. They range from thin (phyllo) sheets to thicker (puff) pastries, some oiled, some buttered, some with dairy and eggs, and some without. Fillings also are endless. The most widespread traditional Greek pie is the cheese pie (τυρόπιτα), clearly because feta cheese is the most popular cheese product in Greece. Cheese is also added to other pies such as spinach, leek, various greens, pumpkin, peppers, eggplant, and the list goes on. My other two cookbooks have many other pies differing from the selection in this book. The recipes in this chapter are a mixture of other bread-like recipes eaten in Greece that extend beyond phyllo pastries.

Homemakers dating back to antiquity would make what was needed to provide a year's worth of dried pasta, *trahana* (a wheat and sour yogurt product), *hilopites* (a small square pasta), and other pastas, ensuring they had plenty of flour to make bread daily to provide for their families. For some, there was nothing else to eat but bread, fruit, and vegetables gathered from the wild and seafood if they were close to water. The life of the poor and middle class was not easy. It was survival with what was reared on one's land, and thus the amazing plethora of breads and pies were created.

Bread was available not only for consumption, but also for religious purposes. Symbolism on breads and some Christian imagery stamped on celebratory breads are still made today. Various symbols such as eggs inserted in Easter breads (*τσουρέκι*), and coins in the New Year's cake (*βασιλόπιτα*), breads with the cross representing Christ and his death, and engagement and wedding breads (made a certain way to aid for wedding peace) are all a key part of the importance of bread to the Greek. Though I am Greek, I do not follow any form of superstition, nor do I think that bread has any given function as depicted by the tradition of Greek culture (such as bread eaten on behalf of the dead). I eat and make them for the joy and pleasure of eating and enjoying all things. As it is written, "Man shall not live by bread alone, but by every word that proceeds out of the mouth of God" (Matthew 4:4, ESV).

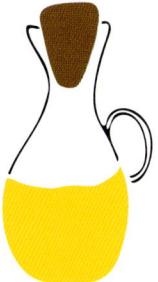

η τέχνη της πίτας
TIPS AND TRICKS FOR MAKING PASTRY

1 ΕΝΑ
Use a plain flour known as pastry, cake, or unbleached flour. This is a low-protein flour designed to make pastries lighter and more delicate than those made with all-purpose flour.

2 ΔΥΟ
Always add salt to the dough. This helps stabilize the gluten in the flour and helps the dough to retain moisture and not dry out.

3 ΤΡΙΑ
For a crispier pie, add vinegar and or lemon juice to the dough. This also helps the pastry to rise.

4 ΤΕΣΣΕΡΑ
Always have a cup of spare flour and water next to your bowl to add if required.

5 ΠΕΝΤΕ
Water is added slowly to the flour (or vice versa) so that it gets absorbed appropriately.

6 ΕΞΙ
Water must be room or lukewarm in temperature.

7 ΕΠΤΑ
To help keep pastry thin and stretchy, do not use any leavening agents.

8 ΟΚΤΩ
Allow the dough to rest for a minimum of 1 hour. This allows the gluten to relax, creating a more tender pastry. During the resting time, the water in the dough spreads out, resulting in even hydration and a more consistent result.

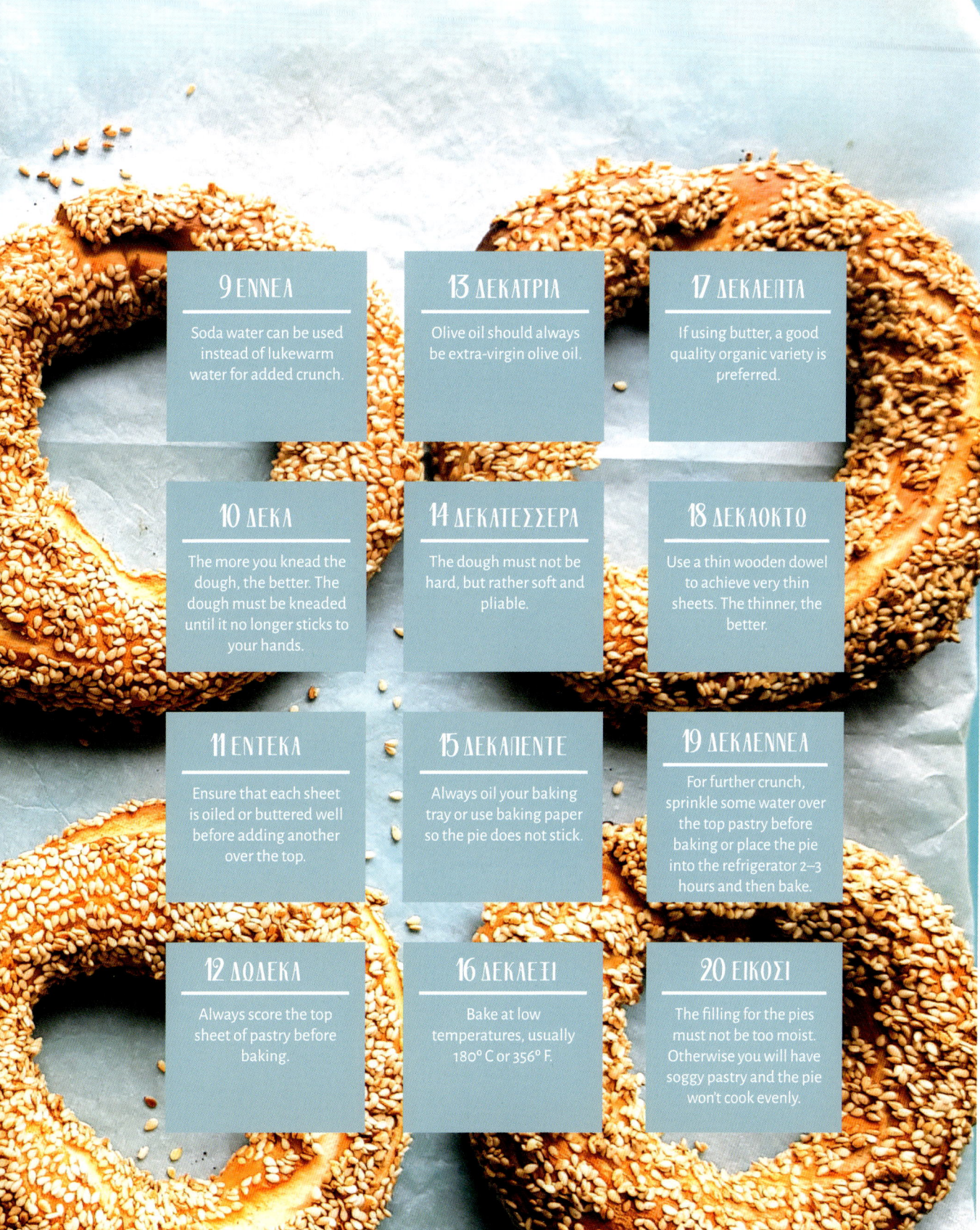

9 ΕΝΝΕΑ
Soda water can be used instead of lukewarm water for added crunch.

10 ΔΕΚΑ
The more you knead the dough, the better. The dough must be kneaded until it no longer sticks to your hands.

11 ΕΝΤΕΚΑ
Ensure that each sheet is oiled or buttered well before adding another over the top.

12 ΔΩΔΕΚΑ
Always score the top sheet of pastry before baking.

13 ΔΕΚΑΤΡΙΑ
Olive oil should always be extra-virgin olive oil.

14 ΔΕΚΑΤΕΣΣΕΡΑ
The dough must not be hard, but rather soft and pliable.

15 ΔΕΚΑΠΕΝΤΕ
Always oil your baking tray or use baking paper so the pie does not stick.

16 ΔΕΚΑΕΞΙ
Bake at low temperatures, usually 180º C or 356º F.

17 ΔΕΚΑΕΠΤΑ
If using butter, a good quality organic variety is preferred.

18 ΔΕΚΑΟΚΤΟ
Use a thin wooden dowel to achieve very thin sheets. The thinner, the better.

19 ΔΕΚΑΕΝΝΕΑ
For further crunch, sprinkle some water over the top pastry before baking or place the pie into the refrigerator 2–3 hours and then bake.

20 ΕΙΚΟΣΙ
The filling for the pies must not be too moist. Otherwise you will have soggy pastry and the pie won't cook evenly.

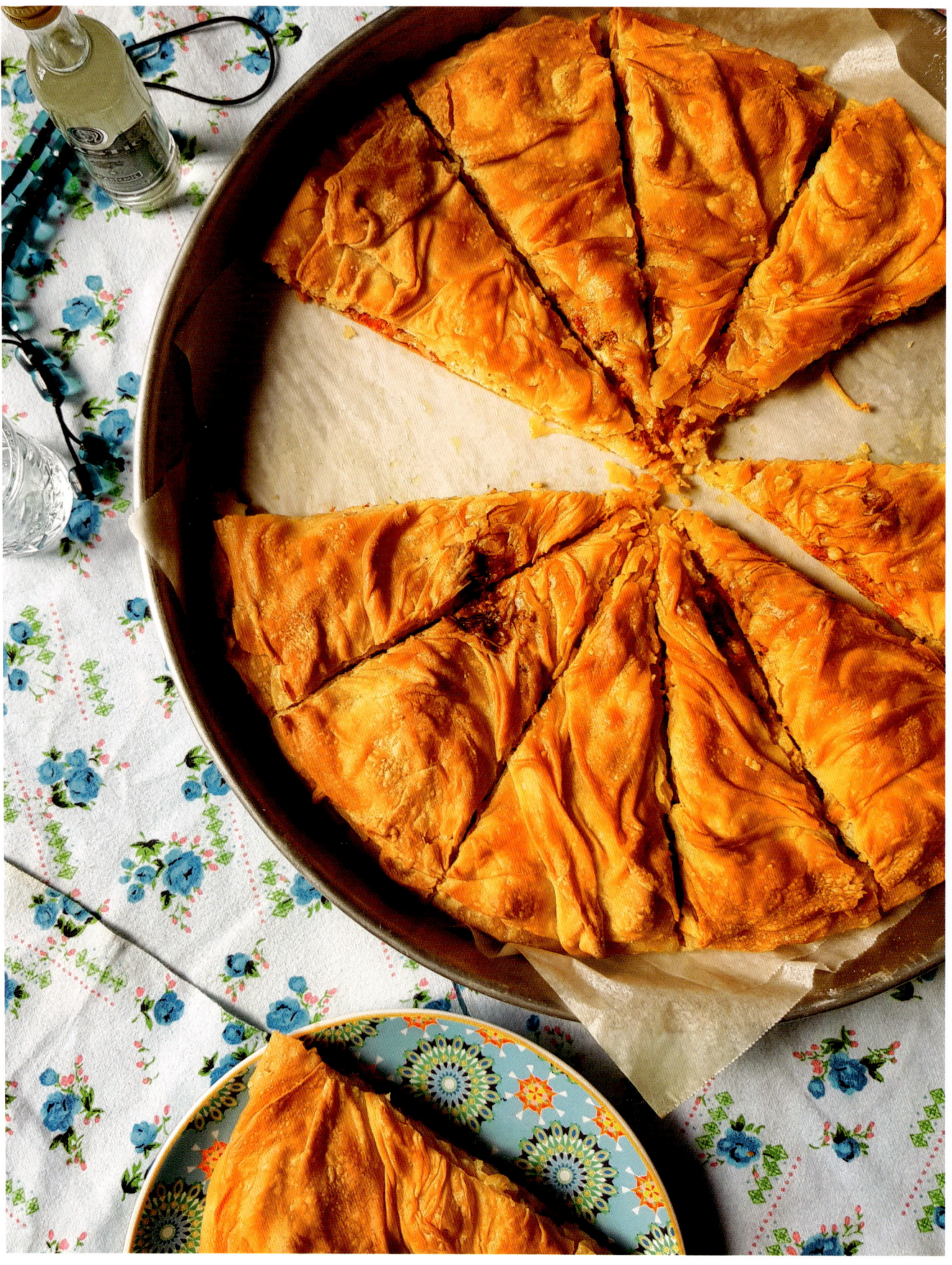

The name of this pie comes from a specific variety of peppers used from the region of Florina. For this recipe, I have used bell peppers as they are more readily available. This pie is very appetizing and tastes a lot like a stuffed pizza. The dough used for this recipe is a simple olive oil dough known as village pastry (χωριάτικη). It has two sheets on the bottom and two on the top. It is extremely easy to make.

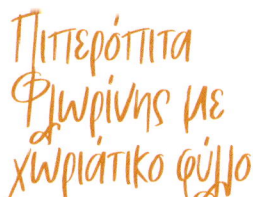

– CAPSICUM AND CHEESE PIE WITH VILLAGE PASTRY –

Makes: 12 large pieces • 2 hours

Prepare pastry: Place all the ingredients into a large bowl. Bring together with a wooden spoon, and then tip onto a floured benchtop and knead until soft and smooth. Add more flour if needed, or water if it is too dry. This should take a few minutes. Cover and rest for a minimum of 1 hour.

To prepare peppers, place them whole onto a baking tray and roast at 200° C/395° F until soft and slightly blackened. Remove from oven, and when they are cool enough to handle, remove the tops and gently peel off the outer skins. They should come away easily. Set aside.

Place the feta cheese and eggs into a bowl. Mix and set aside.

Take the dough and divide into four pieces. Dust a workbench with corn flour and place one piece of dough on the bench. Dust more corn flour on top, and with a rolling pin (or thin wooden dowel), start to roll out the dough into a very large sheet. Ensure the pastry is rolled out a little larger than the tray you use. It must have an overhang. In this case, I used a size 37 cm (14.56 in.) circular tray.

Line the baking tray with parchment paper and put in the first piece of pastry. Drizzle some olive oil on top and repeat with the second sheet of pastry.

Place the cheese filling onto the pastry, and then place the peppers over the top in one layer over the cheese. Fold over the overhang to enclose the filling and keep it from seeping out. Roll out the third sheet of pastry and place it on top, scrunching all the extra overlay on the top to create a ruffled effect. Drizzle oil on top and repeat with the last sheet of dough. Drizzle olive oil on top and score with a sharp knife into desired squares or slices.

Bake at 180° C/350° F for 35 minutes or until golden. Serve warm or at room temperature.

Best eaten the day it is made. Do not cover, otherwise the dough will soften and lose its crispiness.

PASTRY

2 cups all-purpose plain flour

2 tablespoons olive oil

1 tablespoon salt

1 teaspoon white or red wine vinegar

1 cup warm water

TO ROLL OUT

Corn flour (starch) to roll out dough

½ cup olive oil for brushing pastry layers and top

FILLING

5–6 long red peppers

300 g (10.5 oz.) feta cheese, crumbled

2 whole eggs, whisked

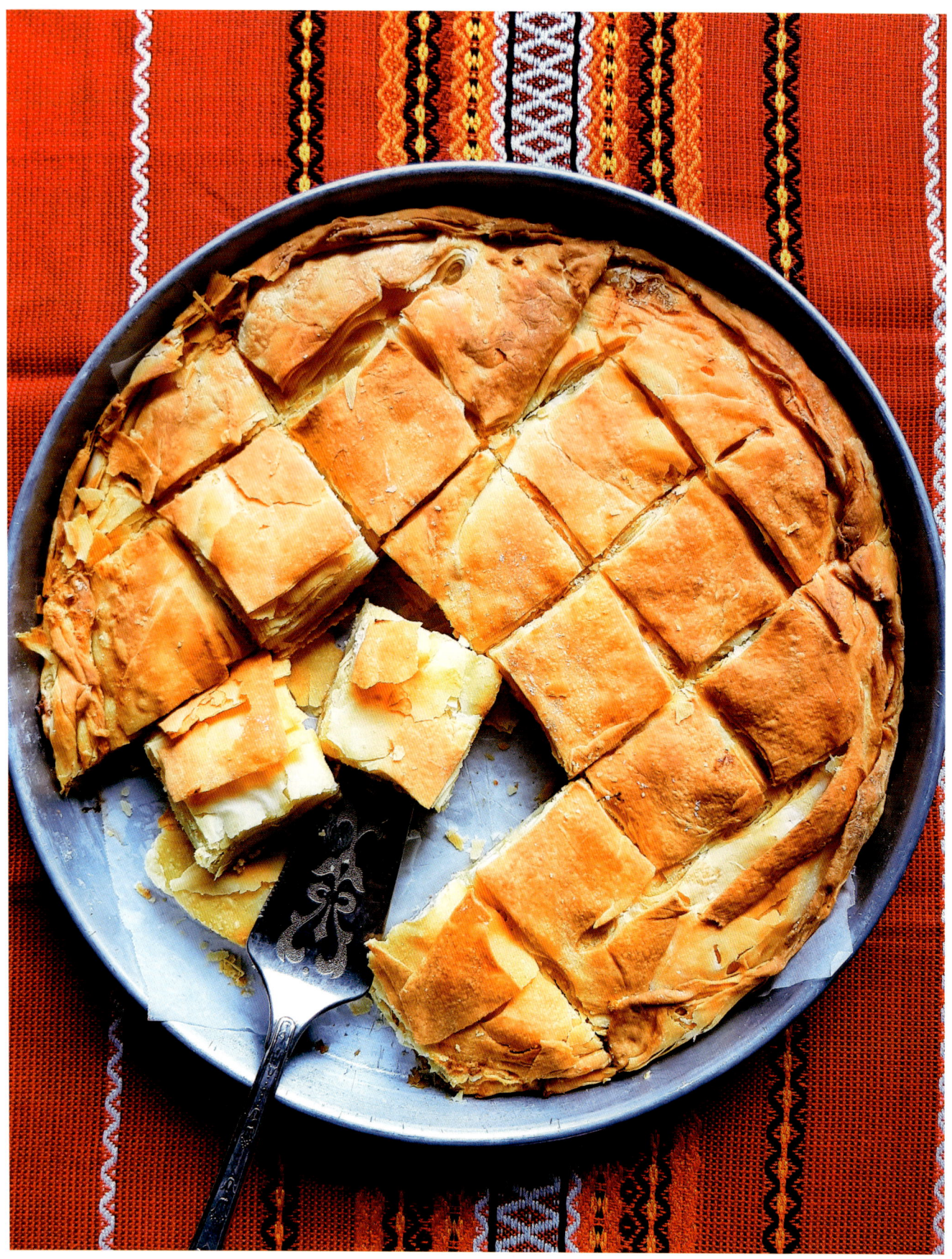

This pastry is made with yogurt, milk, and eggs instead of the usual vinegar and oil. It has a softer texture than most other doughs and is not supposed to be very crispy. The dough comes together very easily. This recipe is a little more tedious as 14 sheets need to rolled out one by one, but it is well worth the effort.

Makes: 20 pieces · 2 hours

In a large bowl, whisk to combine the yogurt, milk, oil, eggs, baking powder, and salt. Slowly incorporate the flour little by little, stirring with a wooden spoon, and then use your hands to bring it all together. Knead until a smooth dough is achieved that does not stick to your hands. Add additional flour if needed. Cover with a towel and set aside to rest 20–30 minutes.

Prepare the filling by adding all the ingredients into a bowl. Mix. Set aside.

Separate dough into 14 small even balls. Place a ball of dough between two pieces of parchment paper, and, using a rolling pin, roll each ball into the size of a large dessert plate. The parchment paper helps the dough not to stick to the rolling pin. Make 2 piles of 7 sheets, placing them on top of each other, liberally dusting each one with corn flour so they don't stick. They must have plenty of corn flour between each layer as this is what will help separate the sheets once baked.

Oil and line a baking tray (35 cm/14 in.) with parchment paper. Set aside. Preheat oven to 180° C/356° F.

Now using the same two sheets of parchment paper, place one pile (7 sheets) between the paper. Gently push down, being careful not to push too hard, and roll it out to create one large sheet of pastry (this will separate into 7 layers when baked). It should stretch easily. Carefully remove the paper from the top and bottom and place onto the baking tray. Add filling and repeat with the second pile of 7 sheets and place over the top. Bring in any overhanging pastry, neatening the edges. Score with a knife and drizzle a little more olive oil over the top. Bake for 40 minutes or until golden.

Τυρόπιτα με φύλλο από γιαούρτι και γάλα

- CHEESE PIE MADE WITH YOGURT AND MILK PASTRY -

PASTRY

½ cup yogurt

1 cup whole milk

1 cup olive oil

2 whole eggs, beaten

1 teaspoon baking powder

½ tablespoon salt

4½ cups all-purpose flour

TO DUST

Corn flour (starch) for dusting

Olive oil for additional brushing

FILLING

300 g (10.5 oz.) ricotta cheese

200 g (7.0 oz.) feta cheese, crumbled

¼ cup whole milk

½ teaspoon salt

½ teaspoon cracked pepper

1 teaspoon dried mint

1 whole egg, beaten

Πρασόπιτα με φύλλο μέθοδος του ήλιου

- LEEK PIE WITH "SUNRAY" PHYLLO PASTRY -

PASTRY

4 cups all-purpose flour

1 tablespoon olive oil

1 tablespoon vinegar

1 teaspoon salt

2–3 cups of warm water

TO DUST

Corn flour (starch) for dusting

30 g butter, melted

¼ cup olive oil plus a little more

FILLING

2 cups spinach, chopped

1 cup leeks, chopped

½ cup spring onions, chopped

¼ cup parsley, chopped

¼ cup mint, chopped

1 cup feta cheese, crumbled

1 whole egg, lightly whisked

½ teaspoon white pepper

3 tablespoons olive oil

This phyllo pastry is made using the "sunray technique." A large round sheet of pastry is made, oiled, and cut into what looks like sunrays. These rays are then placed on top of each other to create the layers of a delicious thin pastry without having to individually roll out many sheets. It is a great dough to freeze, thaw, and use as required. Flour and humidity play a role in how your pastry turns out, and therefore the amount of water used is crucial. Start by adding half the water, mixing it well into the flour, and adjusting as the water is absorbed by the flour. The pastry should be soft and pliable. If the dough is too crumbly or dry, add a little more water (just a few tablespoons at a time). If it is too wet, add a little more flour. You must knead it for a few minutes to assess what is needed.

Makes: 14 large pieces · 15 minutes (plus resting or freezing time)

Combine all the pastry ingredients in a large bowl (starting with half the water) and mix by hand until it comes together. Add the remaining flour, then more water, a little at a time, as needed to form a soft, pliable pastry. Place onto a floured surface and knead for 5–10 minutes. Cover and allow to rest for 1 hour. The resting time ensures that the pastry has softened and can be rolled out easily. Divide the pastry into two.

Dust a work surface with corn flour. Place one ball of pastry onto the floured surface and sprinkle a little more corn flour onto the pastry to prevent it from sticking to your rolling pin or surface. Roll out the pastry with a thin dowel, turning the pastry occasionally, until it becomes a very thin round sheet a little larger than the size of your baking tray (with an overhang).

Drizzle 4–5 tablespoons olive oil (combined with the melted butter) onto the pastry. Brush over the pastry to cover completely. Take a knife and cut a shape like a sun with rays. See picture on page 147.

Now place each section over the center to create a parcel. Cover with plastic wrap and place in the freezer for a minimum of 20 minutes (if using on the same day). The purpose of this is to allow the oil/butter to harden slightly. Repeat with the remaining dough.

Prepare the filling by placing all the ingredients into a bowl. Mix to combine and set aside.

To assemble the pie: Remove the pastry from the freezer and place onto a lightly floured surface. I use corn flour rather than regular flour. Allow it to thaw slightly if it has frozen (it should not take long). It is best to be cold and not very soft to handle. Add some corn flour over the top, and with a rolling pin (or thin dowel), gently press down and out to roll pastry into a large sheet. Oil may ooze out of the pastry, but that's okay. Add a little more corn flour if it is too sticky, being careful not to add too much so it becomes dry and floury. The size of the sheet should be larger than the baking tray so that it has an overhang once assembled. This recipe is for a 35 cm/14 in. diameter tray.

Lift and place pastry onto the baking dish. Add the filling. Repeat with the top phyllo. When placing the top layer onto the pie, place all the pastry inside (with no overhang) ruffling it to fit into the tray.

Score with a knife and drizzle olive oil over the top. Sprinkle 1 tablespoon over the top and bake at 180° C/356° F for 40 minutes or until golden both on the top and bottom.

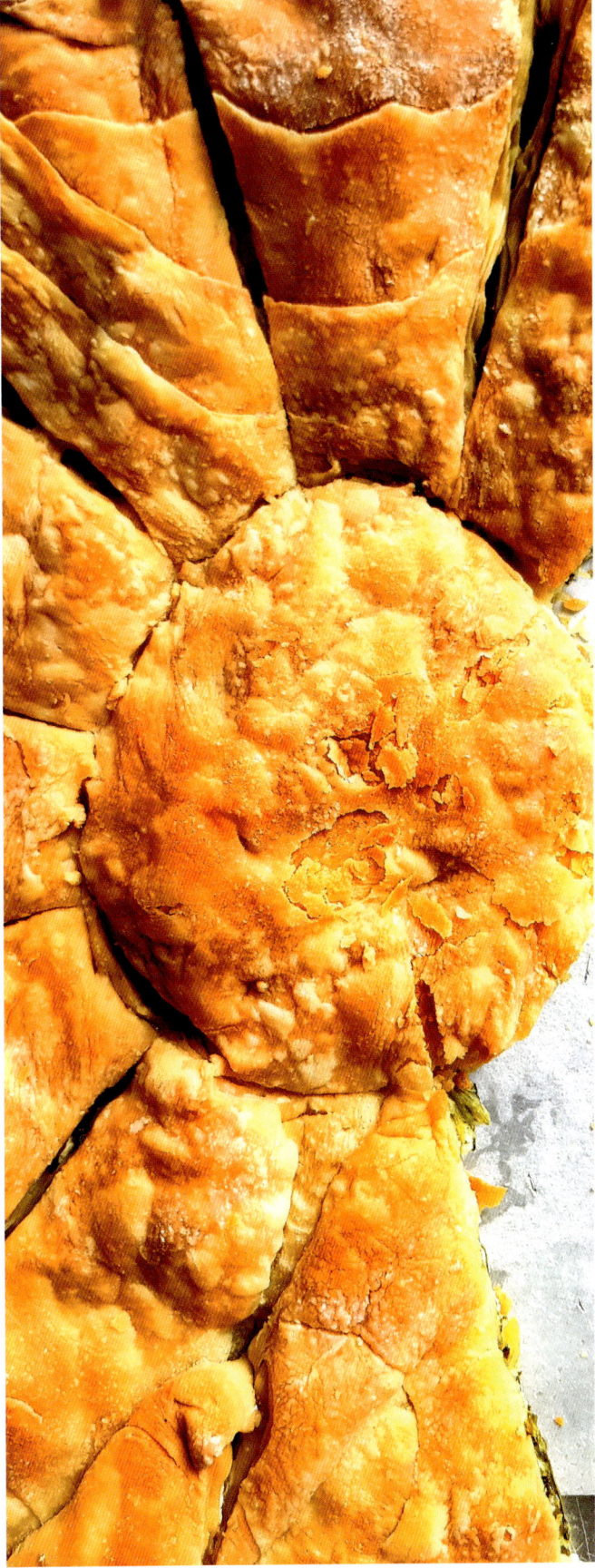

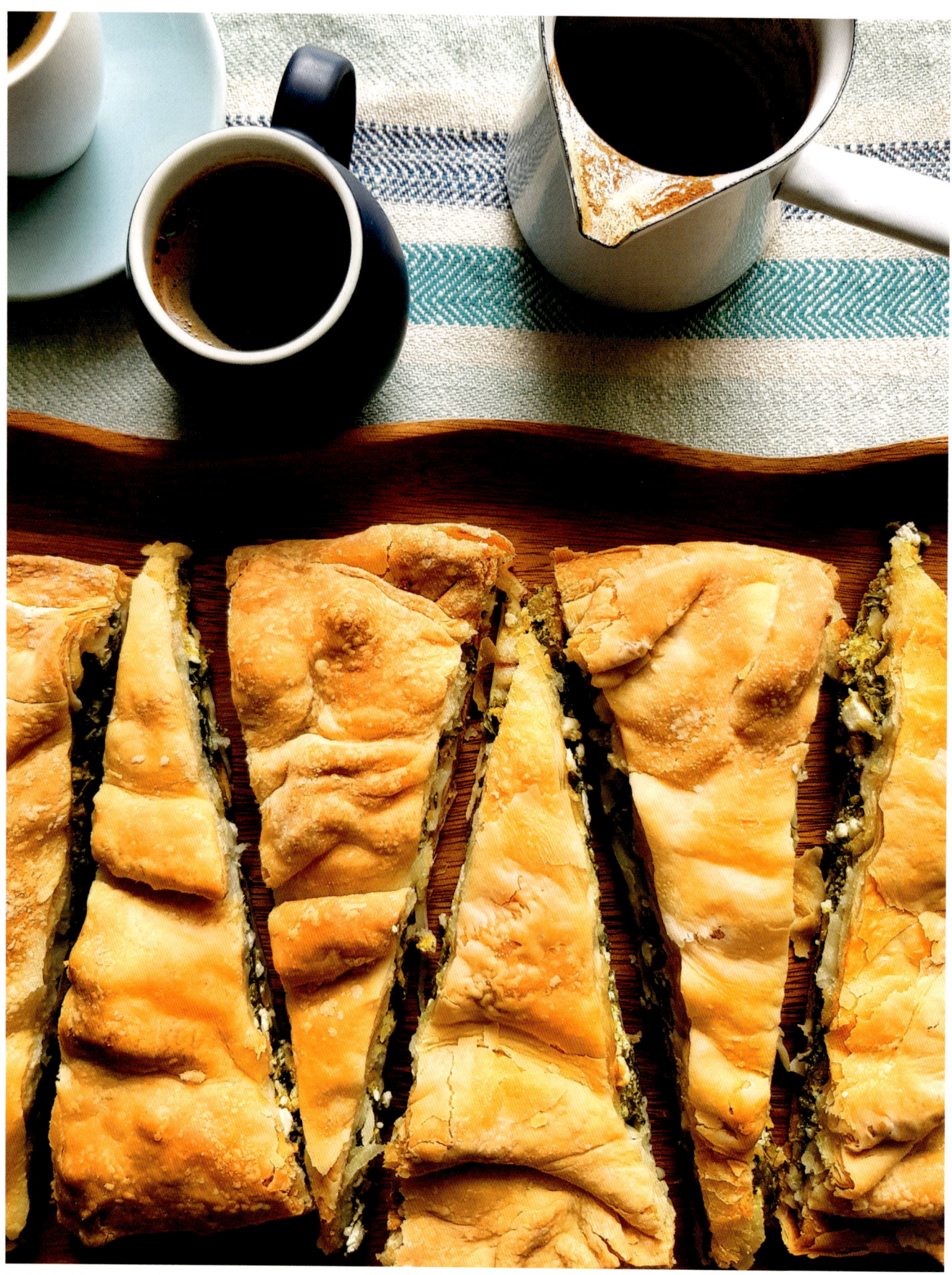

Leek Pie with "Sunray" Phyllo Pastry, page 146-147.

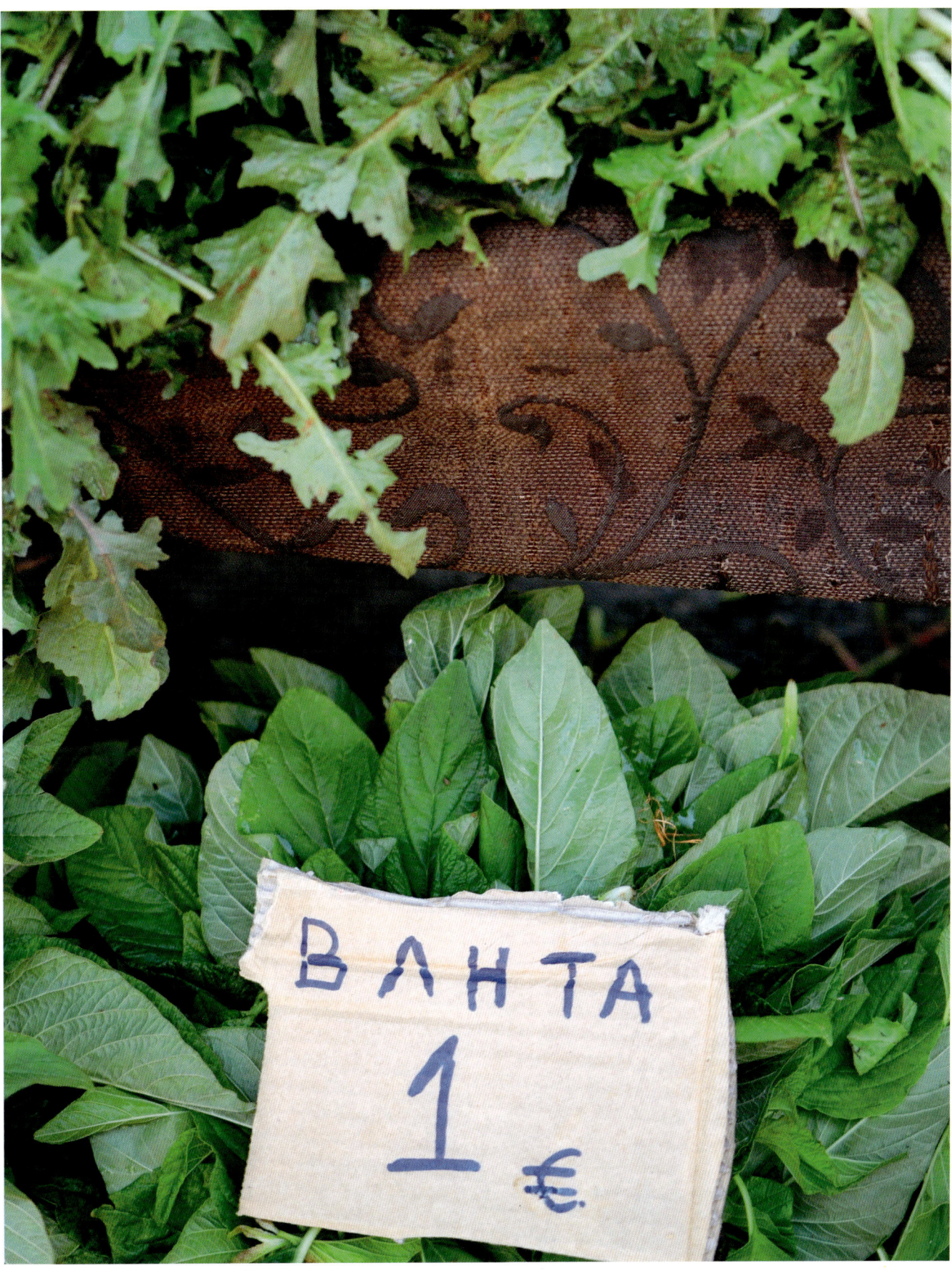

Πατατόπιτα με ελιά και δεντρολίβανο με χωριάτικο φύλλο
- POTATO, OLIVE, AND ROSEMARY PIE WITH VILLAGE PASTRY -

This recipe is from Metsovo (a village in the northwestern part of Greece). It is a potato pie flavored with cheeses, rosemary, and olives. The phyllo dough for this recipe is a very thin dough also known as a village pastry (as with the previous recipe); however, due to the method of preparing, the sheets are much thinner, and the result is even crispier and crunchier. Use kitchen scales to weigh the dough for this recipe. Once the dough is made, it is divided into balls roughly 90 g each (3.1 oz.), dusted with cornflour and left to rest for 30 minutes. You can leave the floured balls covered and refrigerated overnight to be rolled out the next day. Ensure they are not placed too close together as they do expand a little if left to prove for longer.

Makes: 16–20 pieces · Time: 2 hours

PASTRY
- 350 ml lukewarm water
- 1 tablespoon vinegar
- 2 tablespoon olive oil
- 1½ teaspoons salt
- 600 g (21.1 oz.) all-purpose flour

TO ROLL OUT
- Corn flour (starch) to roll out pastry
- Olive oil, additional for brushing

FILLING
- 800 g (28.2 oz., roughly 7–8 medium size) potatoes, boiled and roughly mashed
- Salt and pepper
- 1 tablespoon oregano, dried
- 80 g (2.8 oz.) Kalamata olives, pitted and sliced
- 1 tablespoon rosemary, chopped
- ¼ cup spring onion, chopped finely
- ½ cup feta cheese, crumbled
- ½ cup kefalograviera* or other yellow hard cheese, grated

Prepare pastry.

Put the water, vinegar, oil, salt and half the flour in a bowl. Using a wooden spoon, mix together, adding the remaining flour little by little until a soft, pliable dough is formed. You may not require all the flour. If it is too sticky, keep adding flour. If it is too dry, add 1–2 tablespoons water.

Place the pastry onto a floured workbench and knead by hand for a further 5–10 minutes. Weigh the dough. The key here is that each ball is roughly 90–100 g (3.1 oz.) each. You should have anywhere from 8–10 balls. Dip each ball into corn flour. Place on a tray and set side covered with plastic wrap for 30 minutes.

To prepare the filling, peel, cut, and boil potatoes in water until very soft. Drain and place into a bowl. Allow to cool completely. With a fork, break up the potatoes until they are mashed, and then add all the filling ingredients and mix to combine well. Set aside.

Preheat oven to 170° C/340° F.

To prepare the pastry sheets, take one ball at a time and place on a floured workbench. Using a thin dowel (or rolling pin), gently roll out into a large circle or square a little larger than the baking dish. This pastry is incredibly soft, so be gentle when pressing down on the pastry with the dowel. Sprinkle extra corn flour to help the pastry not to stick onto the bench or the dowel. You will use half the balls for the bottom and half for the top.

To assemble: Line a baking tray 37 cm (14.56 in.) with parchment paper and place the first piece of pastry.

Drizzle 2 tablespoons olive oil on top, and then repeat with half the sheets, oiling between each one. Place the filling onto the pastry and fold over the overhang to hold the filling and keep it from seeping out.

Roll out the next sheet of pastry and place it on top, scrunching all the extra overlay on the top to create a ruffled effect. Drizzle 2 tablespoons oil on top and repeat with the remaining sheets of dough, oiling each layer.

Drizzle olive oil on top and score with a sharp knife into desired squares or slices.

Bake for 35 minutes or until golden. Serve warm or at room temperature. Best eaten the day it is made.

*Kefalograviera cheese can be purchased at European grocers. Parmesan cheese can be used as a substitute or any other hard yellow cheese.

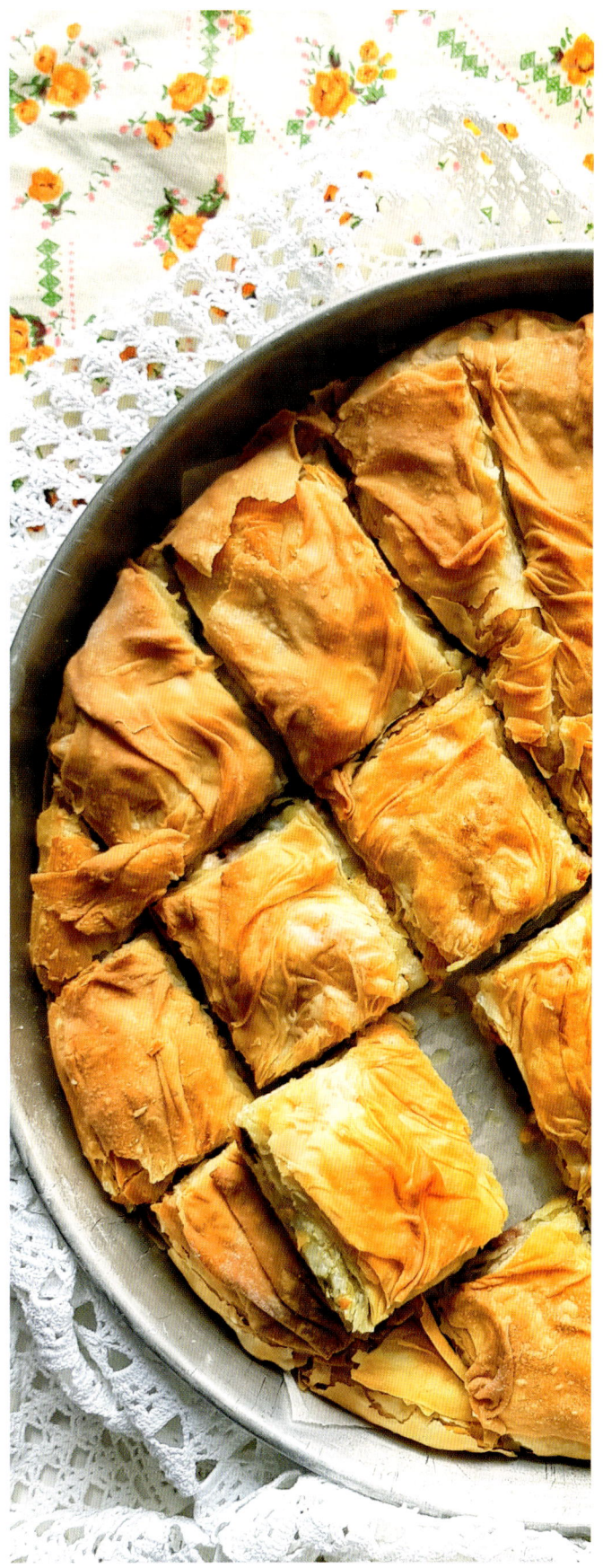

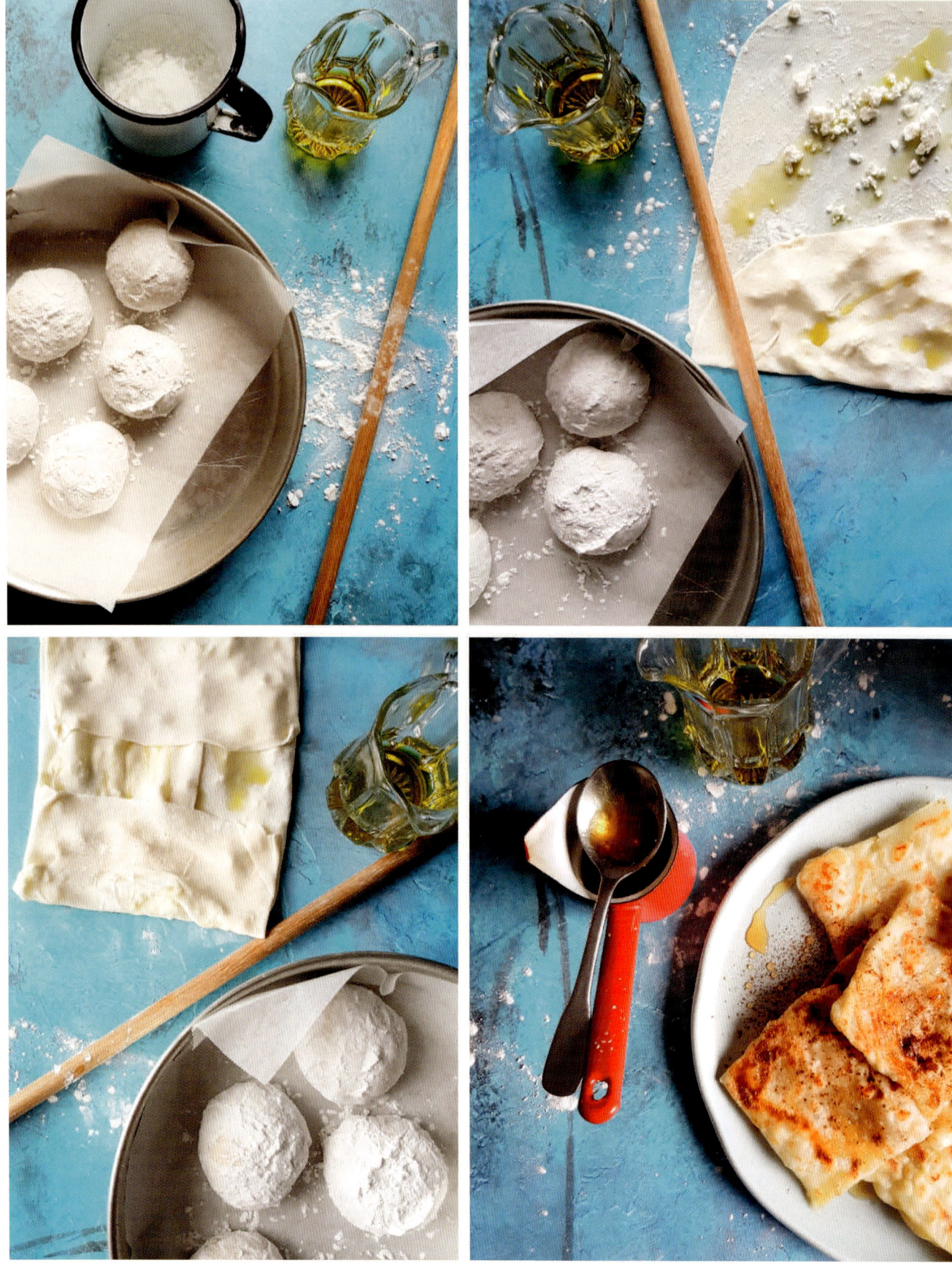

These pies are super quick and easy to make for a last-minute snack or craving. The pastry is the same dough as the potato and rosemary recipe on page 150. These pies are very shallow fried in oil for approximately 4–5 minutes on each side. They can be eaten hot or cold. I always like to drizzle runny honey and sprinkle cinnamon over the top. I recommend doubling the recipe—five are just not enough.

Makes: 5 parcels · 40 minutes

In a bowl, place the water, vinegar, oil, salt, and half the flour. Using a wooden spoon, mix adding the remaining flour little by little until a soft, pliable dough is formed. You may not require all the flour. If it is too sticky, keep adding flour. If it is too dry, add 1–2 tablespoons water. Place the dough onto a floured workbench and knead by hand for a further 5–10 minutes. Divide the dough into 5 pieces (roughly 80–100 g. or 3.52 oz. or 0.22 lb.) each. Dip each ball into corn flour, place on a tray, and set side covered with plastic wrap for 30 minutes.

Take one ball at a time, dust a workbench with corn flour, and, using a thin dowel, gently roll out into a large circle. Use extra corn flour to help the dough not to stick onto the bench or the dowel. Once you have a large thin sheet, sprinkle 2 tablespoons of feta cheese (or more if you like it cheesy) over the pastry. Sprinkle 2 tablespoons olive oil over the top. Fold the pastry halfway, and then bring the other half over the top. Sprinkle a little more oil, and then overlap the ends to create a parcel.

Heat a nonstick pan with 2 tablespoons oil. Add the parcel and cook for 4–5 minutes on each side. You can add more oil if you desire. Remove from pan and repeat with all the remaining dough.

Serve immediately with a drizzle of runny honey and a sprinkle of cinnamon.

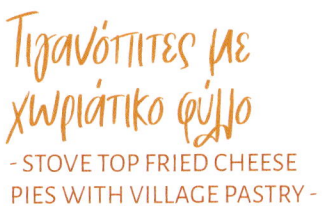

Τιγανόπιτες με χωριάτικο φύλλο
- STOVE TOP FRIED CHEESE PIES WITH VILLAGE PASTRY -

PASTRY

175 ml lukewarm water

½ tablespoon vinegar

1 tablespoon olive oil

1 teaspoons salt

300 g (10.5 oz.) all-purpose flour

TO ROLL OUT

Corn flour (starch) to roll out dough

Olive oil, additional for brushing

FILLING

1–2 cups feta cheese, crumbled

¼ cup olive oil, divided

TO SERVE

Runny honey

Cinnamon powder

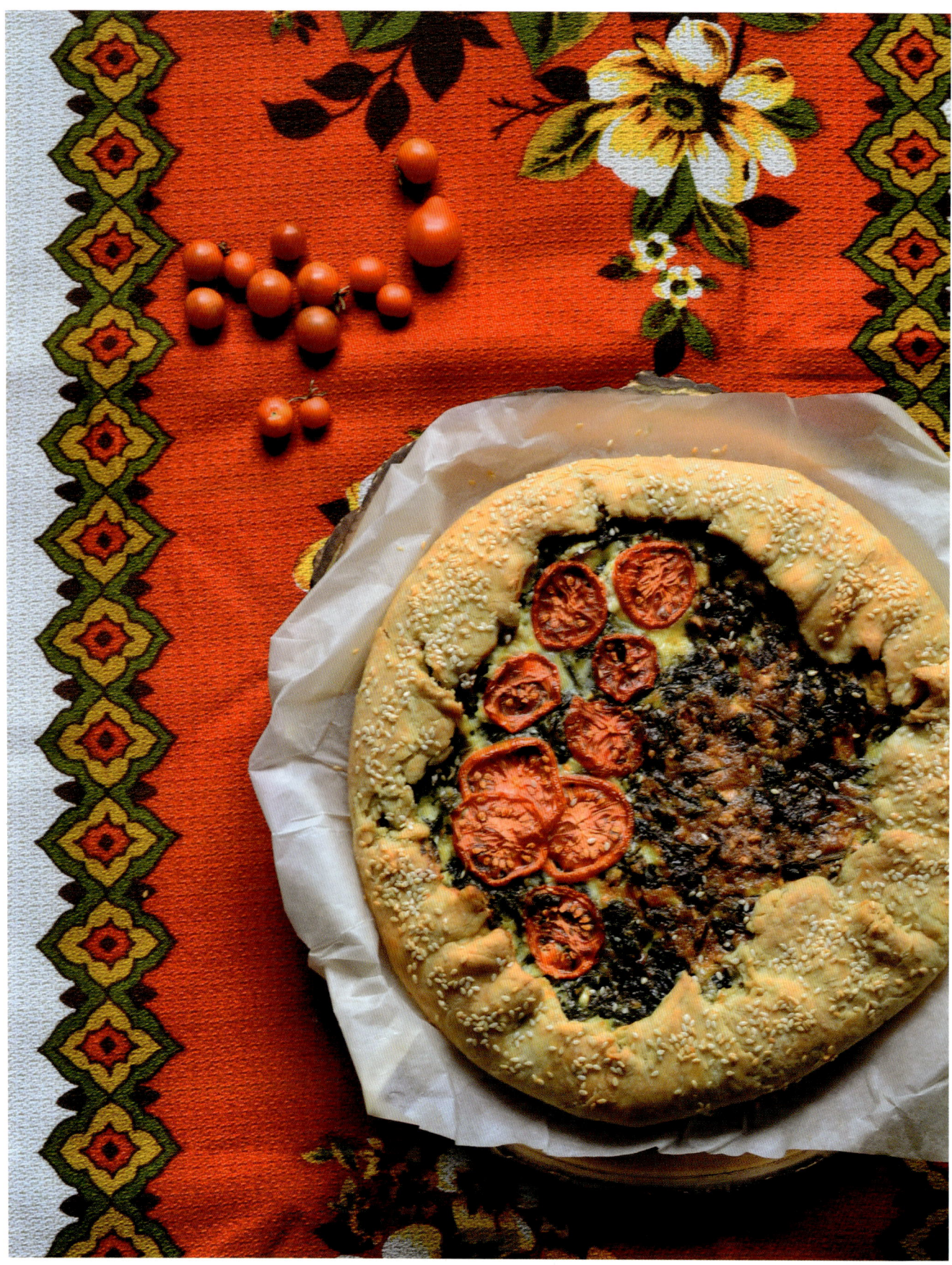

This recipe is for an open pie, using a crumbly olive oil pastry that comes together very easily. There is no need to rest the dough, which speeds up the process. Any greens will do nicely. I have added tomatoes over the top to retain moisture and so that the spinach mixture does not burn while baking. You can see the difference in the photo. This is a great pie served for lunch, snack, or even a main meal accompanied with a crispy salad.

Serves: 4 · 1.5 hours

Ξεσκέπαστη σπανακοτυρόπιτα
- SPINACH, CHEESE, AND TOMATO OPEN PIE -

PASTRY

2 cups all-purpose flour

¾ cup (150 ml) olive oil

⅓ cup chilled water

1 teaspoon salt

FILLING

¼ cup olive oil

5 cups spinach, chopped

¼ cup mint, chopped

¼ cup spring onions, chopped

Salt and pepper

⅓ cup kefalograviera cheese*

¾ cup feta cheese, crumbled

1 whole egg, whisked

2–3 tomatoes, sliced

2 tablespoons sesame seeds, raw

To make the pastry, add the flour, oil, water, and salt in a bowl. Using a wooden spoon, mix to form a dough. Place onto a work surface knead very lightly then wrap the dough in plastic wrap until the filling is ready. It should be slightly crumbly but still retain its shape.

To prepare the filling, heat oil in a fry pan. Add the spinach, mint, onions, salt, and pepper and sauté until just wilted (do not overcook). Remove and drain any excess liquid and place in a bowl. Allow to cool slightly, and then add the cheeses and beaten egg. Mix.

Preheat oven to 180° C/350° F.

To assemble, place the pastry between two sheets of parchment paper. Using a rolling pin, roll out pastry a little larger than the baking tray (30 cm/11.8 in. diameter). The thinner, the better. Remove the top sheet of parchment paper and place the pastry with the bottom paper onto the baking tray. There should be excess pastry overhanging.

Add filling over the base of the pastry, ensuring it is totally covered. Slice tomatoes and place on top. Fold in the excess pastry so that it covers around the ends, leaving the center exposed. Brush the pastry with some more olive oil and sprinkle sesame seeds over it.

Bake for 45 minutes or until golden. Serve warm or at room temperature.

*Kefalograviera cheese can be substituted with Parmesan cheese.

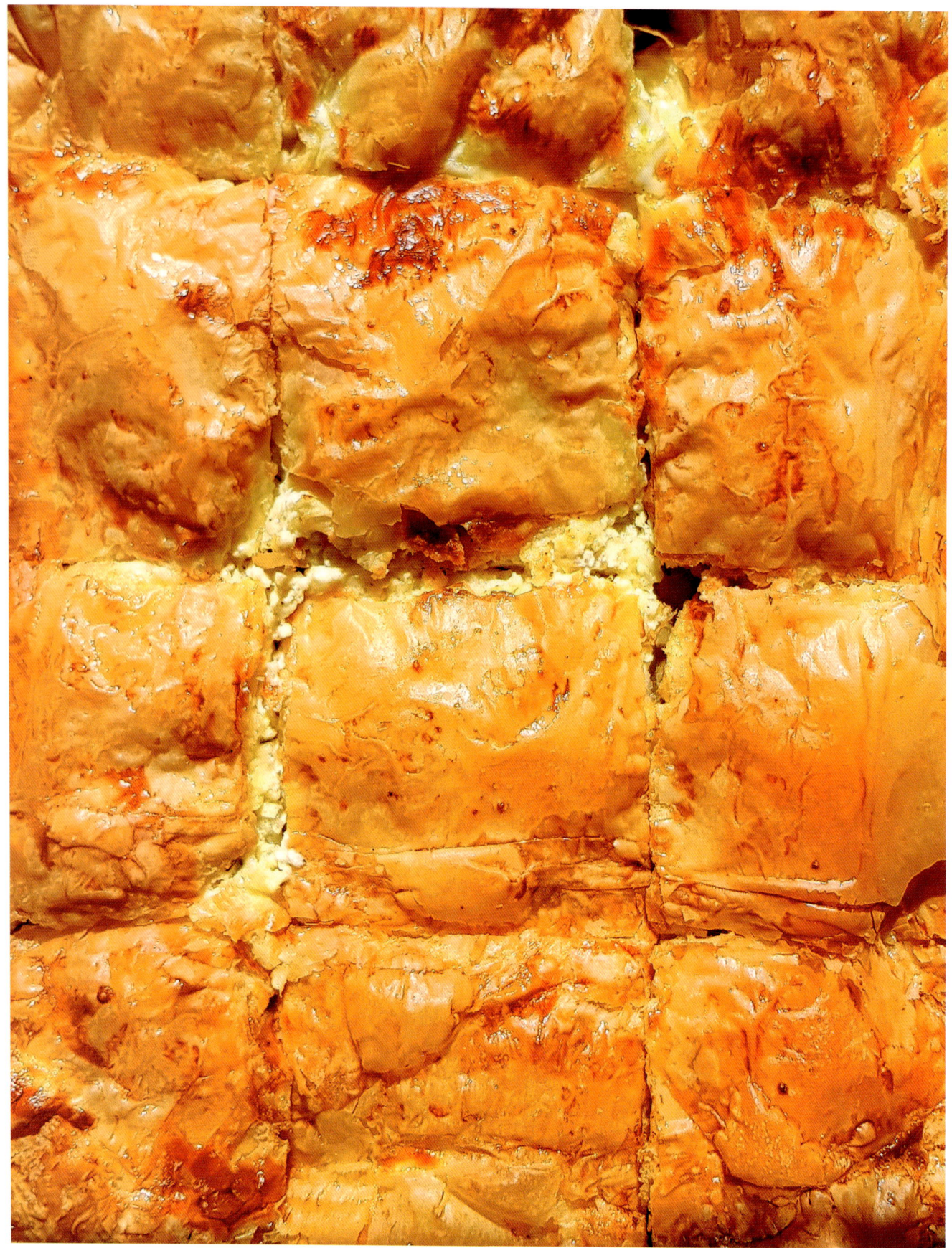

Though both of my other publications have various cheese pie recipes, I could not think of writing another Greek book without at least another using store-bought pastry to speed up the process and give a variance to homemade pastry. We all have a box stored in our refrigerator. This recipe is super moist and creamy as it has milk and eggs that get poured over the top before baking. This technique gives the pie a crispy exterior and soft interior.

Τυρόπιτα στο πι και φι με έτοιμο φύλλο
- CHEESE PIE IN A FLASH WITH STORE-BOUGHT PASTRY -

Makes: 24 pieces · 1.5 hours

Preheat oven to 180° C/350° F.

Place filling ingredients into a bowl, mix, and set aside.

Oil a baking tray (30x40 cm/11.8x15.7 in.). Place two sheets of phyllo pastry to cover the base of the baking tray, leaving a slight overhang. Drizzle with some oil (do not brush directly onto the pastry). Repeat with 3 more sheets of pastry but with no overhang. Instead ruffle and layer each sheet to fit into the pan, oiling each layer. Pour ¼ of the cheese mixture over the top, and then continue to place 3 more ruffled sheets of pastry (oiling each layer) into the tray. Pour another ¼ of cheese mixture. Repeat the same process with another 3 sheets of pastry. Add the remaining cheese and layer another 4 sheets of pastry, oiling each layer as you go.

Gently push in the overhang so it is nicely folded into the pan. Drizzle the remaining oil over the top. Score the pie as desired. Whisk together the eggs and milk and pour over the pie. Lift baking tray and tilt so that the egg mixture distributes evenly through the pie. Sprinkle sesame seeds over the top.

Bake for 45 minutes or until golden. Allow to cool slightly, and then serve.

*Parmesan or graviera cheese are available at European delicatessens.

FILLING

250 g (8.8 oz.) feta cheese, crumbled

50 g (1.7 oz.) semihard yellow cheese, grated (Parmesan or graviera cheese)*

1 teaspoon dried mint (optional)

15 sheets of store-bought phyllo pastry

½ cup olive oil

---

2 whole eggs, lightly whisked

250 ml whole milk

2 tablespoons sesame seeds, optional

Κασερόπιτα με χωριάτικο φύλλο
- KASEROPITA WITH VILLAGE PASTRY -

This is the cheese pie my husband always opts to eat first when in Greece. He loves the intense saltiness from the specific cheeses. Its name is a compound word from "kasseri" (the specific cheese) and "pita," for pie. It is a great breakfast pie to help kickstart your day. It is crispy and salty all in one. In this recipe, there are also some chopped tomatoes and some feta cheese to balance the saltiness from the cheeses.

Makes: 30 pieces • 1.5 hours

PASTRY

- 2 cups all-purpose plain flour
- 2 tablespoons olive oil
- 1 tablespoon salt
- 1 teaspoon white or red wine vinegar
- 1 cup warm water

TO ROLL OUT

- Corn flour (starch) to roll out dough
- ½ cup olive oil for brushing pastry layers

FILLING

- 1 cup kasseri cheese, grated*
- 1 cup kefalograviera cheese, grated*
- Pinch of salt and pepper
- 1 cup feta cheese, crumbled
- 1 cup tomatoes, chopped into small pieces
- 1 tablespoon dried oregano

Prepare pastry. Place all the ingredients into a large bowl. Bring together with a wooden spoon, and then place onto a floured workbench and knead until soft and smooth. Add more flour if needed, or water if it is too dry. This should take a few minutes. Cover and rest for a minimum of 25 minutes.

Preheat oven to 190° C/374° F. Place all the filling ingredients into a bowl, mixing to combine. Set aside.

Take the dough and divide into four pieces. Dust workbench with corn flour and place one piece of dough onto bench. Dust more cornflour on top, and with a thin wooden dowel (or rolling pin), start to roll out the dough into a large circle slightly bigger than the baking dish so that it has an overhang. I used a 37 cm/14.56 in. circular baking tray.

Line baking tray with parchment paper and place the first piece of pastry. Drizzle with a few tablespoons olive oil and repeat with the second sheet. Pour in the filling, spreading it out to cover the pastry. Fold the overhang onto the filling to keep it from seeping out.

Roll out the third sheet of pastry and place it on top, scrunching all the extra overlay on the top to create a ruffled effect. Drizzle oil on top and repeat with the last sheet of pastry. Score with a sharp knife into desired squares or slices, and then drizzle a few more tablespoons of oil over the top.

Bake for 35 minutes or until golden. Serve warm or at room temperature.

*Kasseri and kefalograviera cheese are available at European delicatessens. A mixture of Parmesan cheese and another semihard yellow cheese can be used as a substitute.

Here is a simple and absolute foolproof pie that can be made into a large spiral pie or as small individual spirals. I have opted for the latter to give variance to this chapter. The dough is left to rest in olive oil. This is helpful in ensuring the pastry stretches out very thinly to give a crispy, wafer-thin result. Surprisingly, the pastry is not oily when baked, and, in fact, it needs a drizzle of olive oil before baking.
See page 160 - 161 for images.

Κολοκυθοτυρόπιτα με χωριάτικο λεπτό φύλλο στριφτή σε λάδι
- PUMPKIN CHEESE PIES WITH VILLAGE PASTRY IN OIL -

Makes: 6 pieces · 2.5 hours

PASTRY

- 2 cups all-purpose flour
- 1 teaspoon salt
- 2 tablespoons olive oil
- 1 cup warm water

TO SOAK

- 1¼ cups light olive oil, for soaking
- Additional olive oil, for drizzling
- 4 tablespoons sesame seeds

FILLING

- 300 g (10.6 oz.) pumpkin, grated
- ¼ teaspoon nutmeg, ground
- ¼ teaspoon each salt and pepper
- 2 cups feta cheese, crumbled

Place the flour, salt, 2 tablespoons of olive oil, and water into a bowl. Mix with a wooden spoon, and then, using your hands, knead onto a floured workbench until you have a soft, pliable dough. It must not be stiff. Add a little more water if it is too dry or flour if it is too wet. It is a matter of feel and touch.

Place the 1¼ cups light olive oil into a bowl and set aside.

Divide the dough into 6 pieces. Roll into balls, flatten, and then, using a rolling pin, roll them out into 10 cm (4 in.) discs. Place the discs in the oil, turning to coat both sides. Repeat with all the dough, placing them on top of each other in the oil. Allow to rest for a minimum of one hour.

Prepare filling by placing all ingredients into a bowl. Mix well and set aside.

Place a tablecloth that you do not mind getting oily on a workbench. Remove one piece of dough from the oil, allowing any excess oil to drip back into the bowl. Place the dough onto the tablecloth and gently start to pull the dough outwards, stretching as much as possible until it is paper-thin. If it rips slightly, do not worry; it will get rolled up.

Divide the filling into 6 portions. Scatter 1/6 of it over the dough. Gently lift the side of the tablecloth closest to you and pull up and forward, rolling the dough into a long cylinder. Coil into a spiral shape with the seam side down and place onto a lined baking tray. Lightly brush with some olive oil and scatter some sesame seeds over it. Repeat with the remaining dough.

Bake at 190° C/375° F for 25 minutes or until golden.

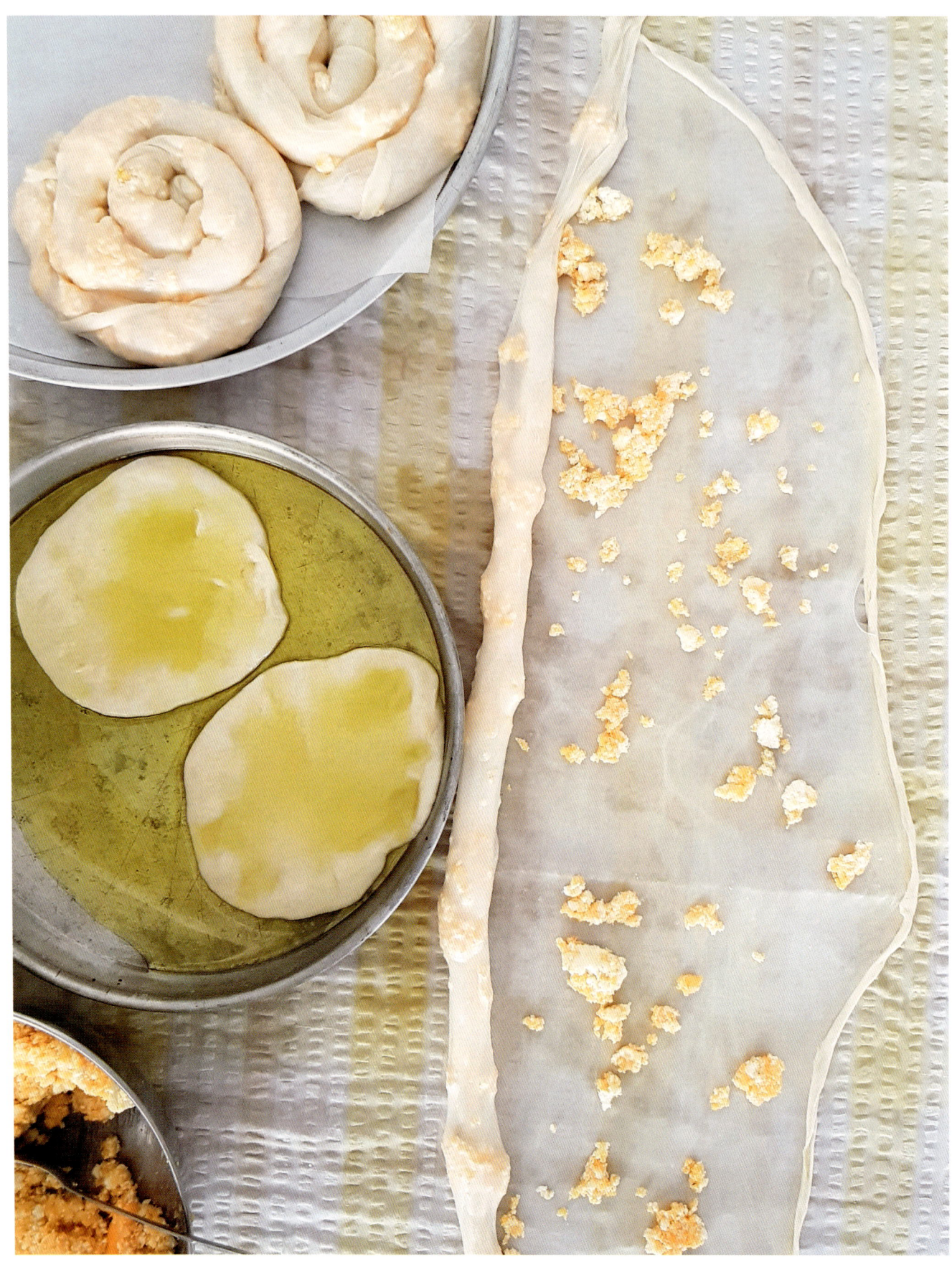

Pumpkin Cheese Pies with Village Pastry in Oil, page 159.

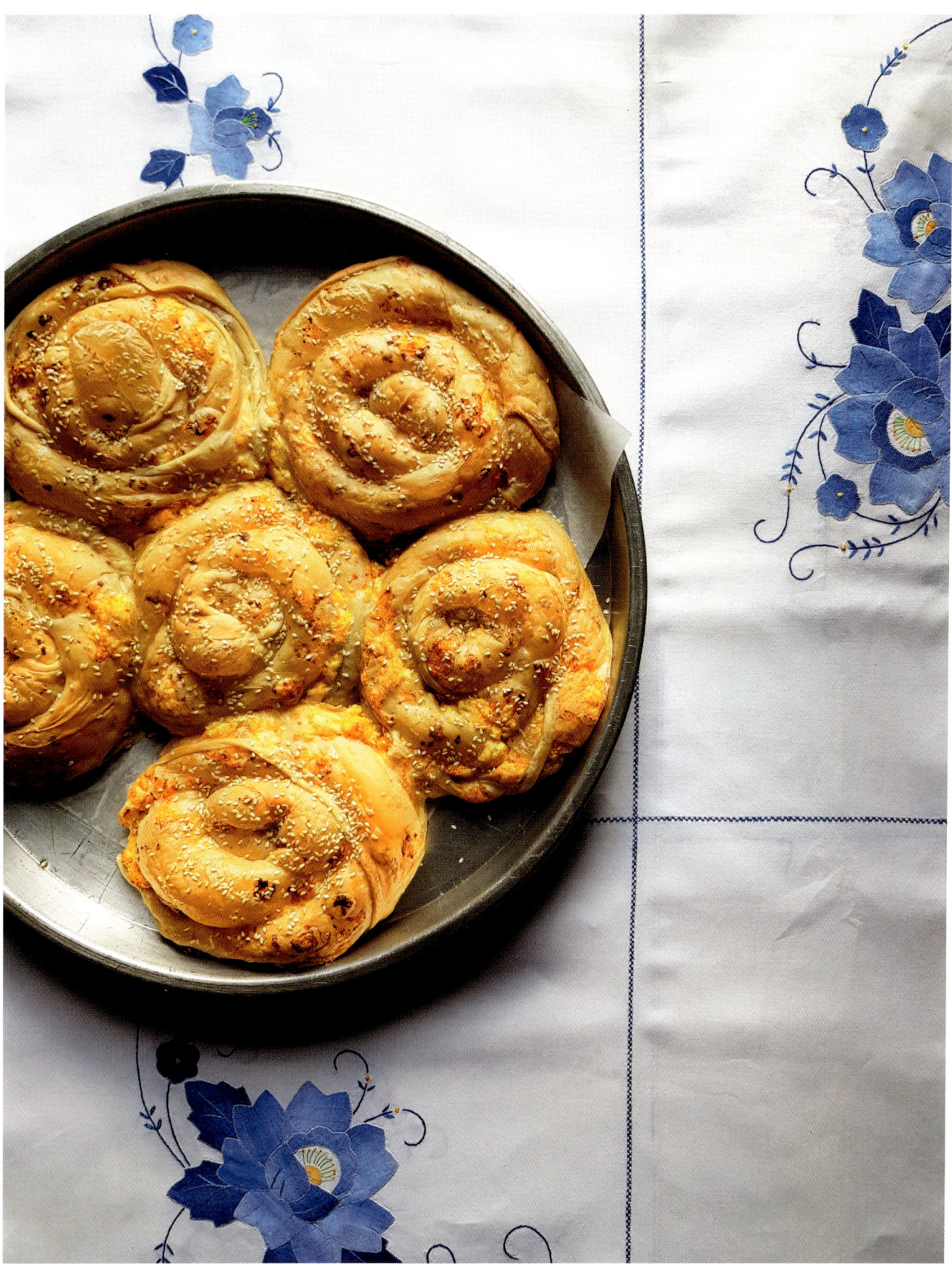

Pumpkin Cheese Pies with Village Pastry in Oil, page 159.

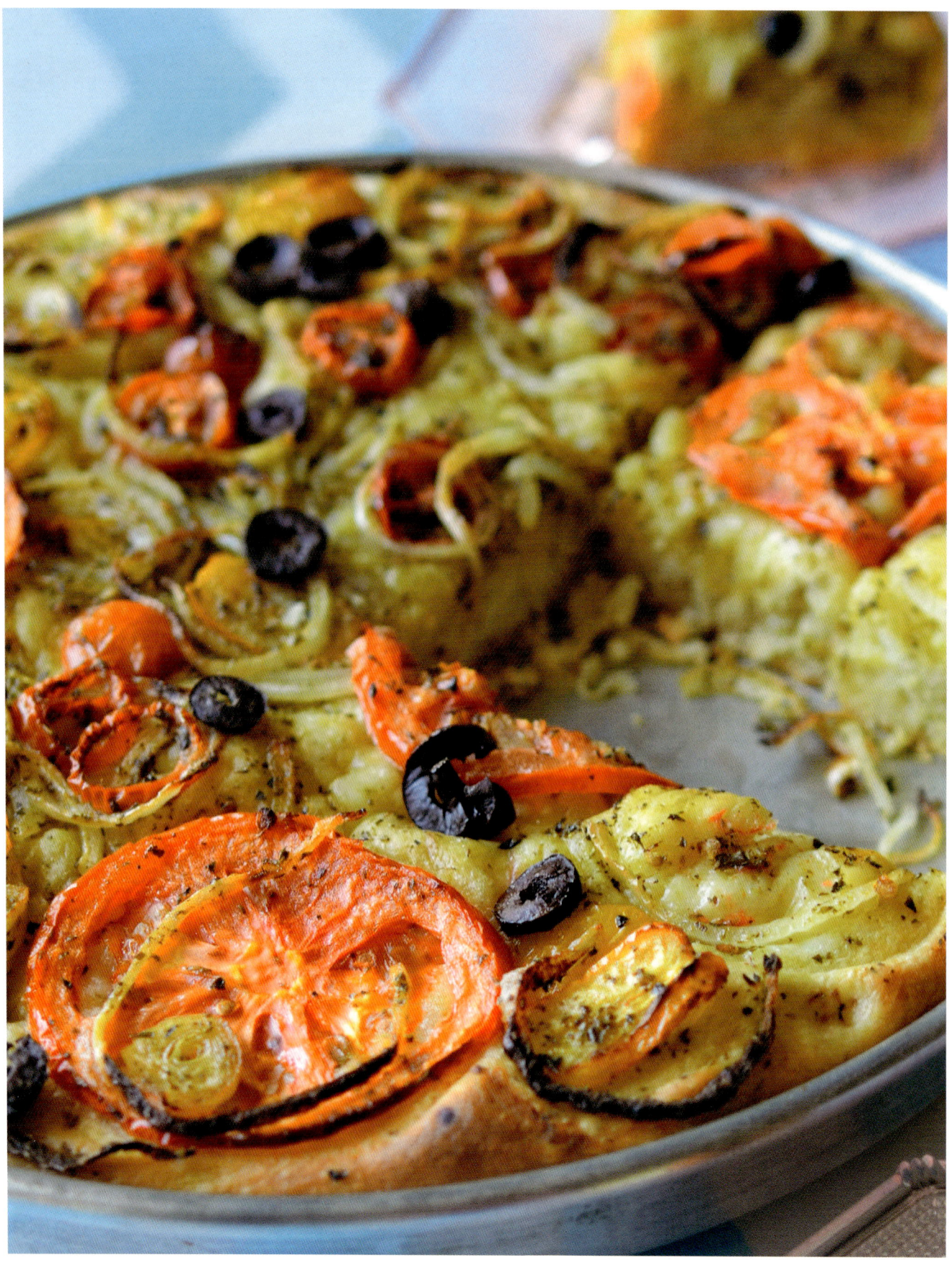

Λαδένια (*ladenia*) is not to be confused with λαγάνα (*lagana*). *Ladenia* is a traditional open-faced tomato and onion style bread from the Cyclades region of Greece. The latter is a Greek flatbread traditionally eaten to break the Lenten fast. *Ladenia* from Kimolos is a bread traditionally topped with onions, tomato, olive oil, and oregano. I have also added some olives to add a little more saltiness. It is obvious that this has come from the Venetian influence on the island as it has similarities to an Italian pizza

Makes: 15 pieces · 1.5 hours

In a large bowl, combine yeast, sugar, and warm water. Set aside for 5 minutes or until the yeast starts to bubble. Add flour, oil, and salt and, with a wooden spoon, mix the ingredients to form a soft, pliable dough. If the dough is too dry, add a little more water, and if it is too wet, add a little flour.

Oil a baking tray (30 cm/11.81 in. in diameter). Place the dough onto it, pushing down and out and stretching the dough to cover the entire base (like a focaccia). Set aside, covered with a tea towel, and allow it to rise for 30 minutes. In the meantime, place all the filling ingredients into a bowl. Mix to coat with the oil, being careful not to break up the tomatoes.

Preheat oven to 200° C/390° F.

After 30 minutes, press down on the dough with your fingertips to make indentations. Spread the filling mixture over the dough to distribute evenly.

Bake for 30–40 minutes or until the base is cooked and the top is golden.

Remove from oven, cut into pieces, and serve warm or at room temperature.

Λαδένια Κιμώλου
- LADENIA FROM KIMOLOS -

1 tablespoon instant yeast

1 teaspoon castor (superfine) sugar

1½ cups lukewarm water

2½ cups all-purpose flour

¼ cup olive oil

1 teaspoon salt

TOPPING

1 large tomato, sliced thinly

6 cherry tomatoes, sliced thinly

1 medium onion, sliced thinly

1 tablespoon oregano, ground

½ cup olive oil, divided

½ cup Kalamata olives, pitted and sliced (optional)

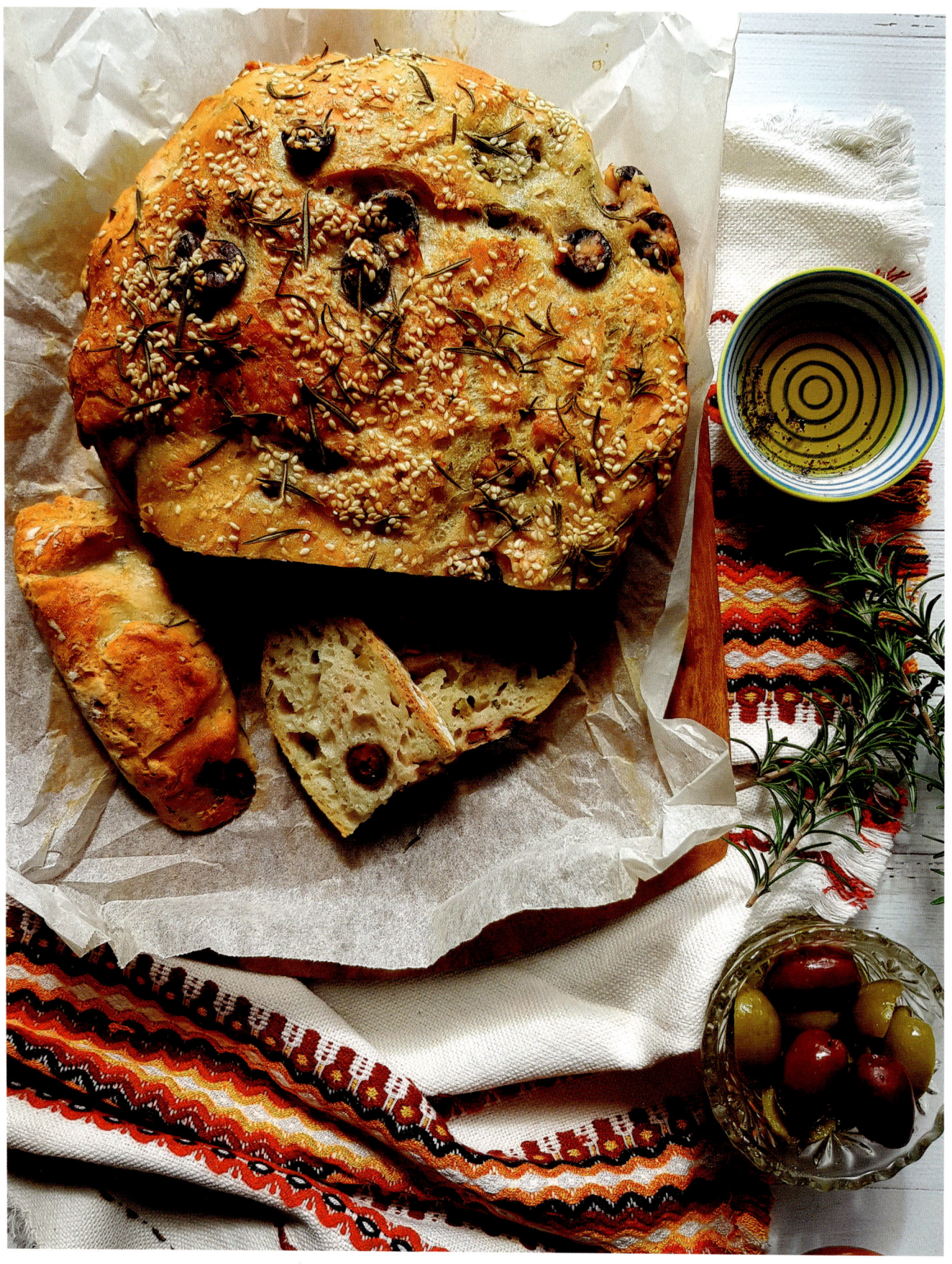

There is nothing quite like the smell and taste of freshly baked bread, a staple food never absent from the dinner table. There are many methods for baking breads, but here I have gone with a remarkably simple no-knead recipe. It is a very forgiving recipe that you really cannot get wrong. Feel free to play around with the flavorings. I have added olives and rosemary, which work wonderfully well for dipping in olive oil and can be enjoyed with some feta cheese. Start this recipe the night before or early in the morning, and then cook it for dinner.

Ψιόψωμο χωρίς ζύμωμα
- NO-KNEAD OLIVE CIABATTA -

Makes: 1 loaf · 1 hour (plus overnight proving)

In a bowl, place the flour, yeast, salt, rosemary, and olives and mix. Pour in the lukewarm water. Using a wooden spoon, gently stir until you have a wet, sticky dough, about 30 seconds. It should be lumpy and not totally combined.

Take a clean bowl and grease it with 2 tablespoons oil. Place the lumpy dough into the bowl, cover with cling wrap, and let it stand for a minimum of 7 hours or overnight. The dough will double in size and become very airy and bubbly.

Preheat oven to 200° C/390° F.

Place a cast-iron pot with lid (or other ovenproof pot) in the oven to heat for 20 minutes.

Generously dust a piece of parchment paper (30 cm/11.8 in. diameter) with flour. Gently tip out the from the bowl. Dust the top lightly with more flour. Gently pull the ends over the top, folding it onto itself to create an oval shape.

Remove the hot pot with lid from the oven (use mittens as it will be extremely hot). Pick up the edges of the parchment paper and place the dough into the pot together with the paper. Sprinkle the top with sesame seeds and extra chopped rosemary.

Place the lid back on and bake for 40 minutes at 200° C/390° F. Remove the lid and continue to bake another 20 minutes or until the top is golden brown. Remove from oven and place onto a cooling rack to cool completely.

3 cups (360 g or 12.6 oz.) all-purpose flour

2 teaspoons active dry yeast

1 teaspoon salt

1 teaspoon fresh rosemary, chopped finely

1 cup Kalamata olives (or mixture of green and black olives), chopped

2 cups lukewarm water

2 tablespoons olive oil

Sesame seeds

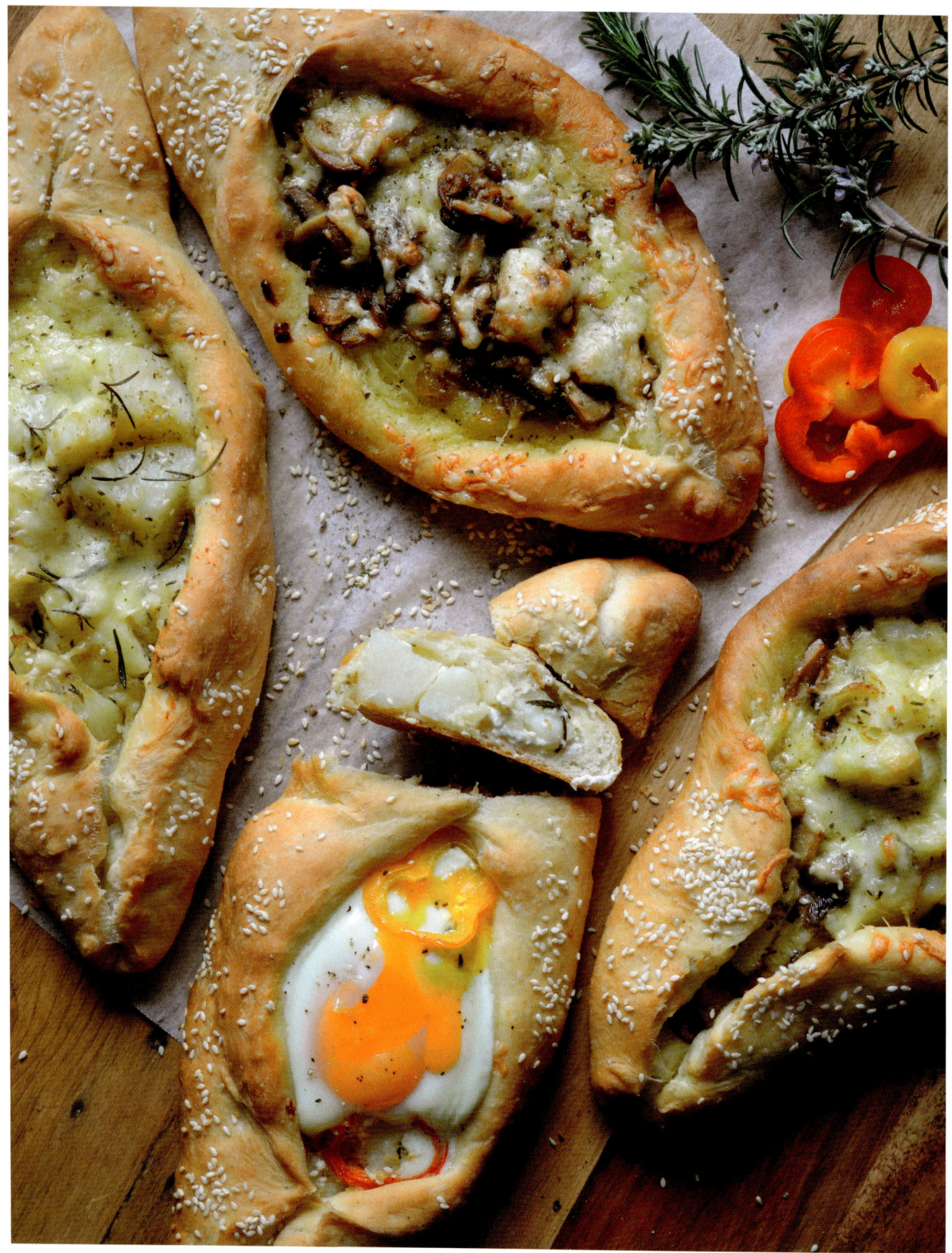

No doubt *peinirli* made its way into Greece via the Turks. They are mostly seen in food stores outside Thessaloniki. The name in Turkish means "with cheese." Greek cheeses such as feta cheese or kasseri work wonderfully well. Essentially, they are individual pizza boats. You can substitute the fillings to your liking but always ensure there is plenty of cheese. It can be prepared a few hours ahead of time and then baked when desired. You can always add capsicum or crack an egg into each boat 3 minutes before removing from the oven for a lovely breakfast/brunch alternative.

Serves: 4 · 2 hours

Prepare the dough: Place the flour, salt, yeast, sugar, olive oil, and water in a large bowl. Mix with a wooden spoon until a dough is formed. Sprinkle a little flour onto a workbench and knead dough until soft and not sticky. You can add a little more flour if needed. Do not add too much; otherwise it will become stiff. Roll into a ball and place into an oiled bowl. Cover with a cloth for a minimum of 1 hour to double in size. In the meantime, prepare the fillings.

Make the mushroom filling: Sauté the onion in the olive oil, and then add the mushrooms, oregano, salt, and pepper. Cook for 5–10 minutes or until mushrooms are cooked and slightly golden. Add 1–2 tablespoons additional olive oil if it is too dry. Remove from heat and add the lemon juice. Taste and adjust seasoning if needed. Set aside to cool.

Make the potato filling: Place potatoes into a saucepan of cold water. Add salt and boil until very soft. Drain. In a sauté pan, add olive oil and cook onion until it is soft and translucent. Add the rosemary, salt, pepper, and the boiled potatoes. Mix well and cook until the potatoes are coated in the oil and onion mixture and they are starting to brown. Remove from heat and add olives (if using).

Preheat oven to 200° C/390° F.

On a lightly floured bench, place the dough and knead again until smooth. Divide the dough into 4 parts and, with a rolling pin, make 4 oval shapes. Place the fillings along the center, leaving the edges empty. Add the cheeses on top of each (kasseri cheese for the mushroom and feta cheese for the potato). Fold and pinch the edges together so that the middle is exposed. Brush with olive oil and sprinkle sesame seeds onto the dough. Bake for 20 minutes or until golden.

*Kasseri cheese can be substituted with mozzarella cheese.

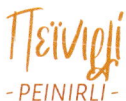

Πεϊνιρλί
- PEINIRLI -

DOUGH

400 g (14.1 oz.) all-purpose flour

½ teaspoon salt

2 teaspoons active yeast

1 teaspoon castor (superfine) sugar

3 tablespoons olive oil

350 ml warm water

FILLING

¼ cup olive oil

1 large onion, diced

3 cups mushrooms, sliced

2 tablespoons dried oregano or fresh thyme leaves

Salt and pepper, to taste

4 tablespoons lemon juice

½ cup kasseri cheese*

POTATO, ROSEMARY, AND FETA CHEESE

¼ cup olive oil

4 medium potatoes, cut into bite-size pieces

1 medium white onion, sliced

1 tablespoon fresh rosemary, chopped

Salt and pepper, to taste

½ cup feta cheese, crumbled

1 tablespoon sliced olives, optional

TO SERVE

Raw sesame seeds

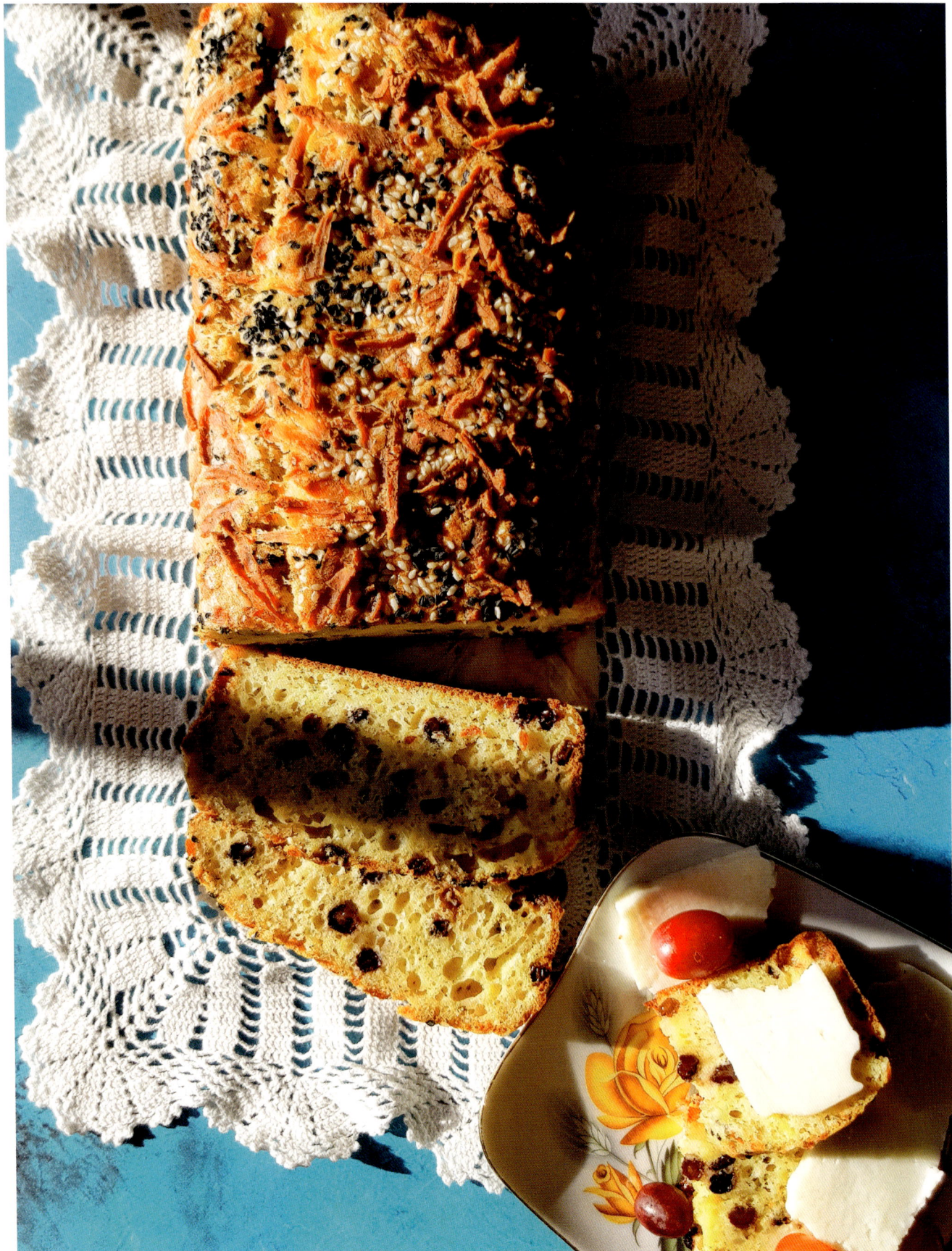

This is the first Cypriot recipe I have added to any of my books. I thought I'd dip my toes into at least one recipe from this region, seeing that I am adding "simply more" foods to this book. This bread has a combination of a few of my favorite flavors: mastic and mahlepi spices together with currants. The combination with the mellow halloumi cheese is so delicious. The texture of this bread is soft and slightly chewy. It can be eaten as is, served with jam for a somewhat sweet treat or topped with cheese for a more savory note.

Makes: 2 loaves · 1.5 hours

Preheat oven to 180° C/356° F.

In a large bowl, add the olive oil and egg yolks, whisking until well combined and a creamy consistency is achieved. Sift in the flour and baking powder. Add the milk and whisk to combine well.

In a separate bowl, whisk the egg whites until soft peaks are formed. Gently fold into the flour mixture in two additions. Now add the cheeses, dried mint, mastic, mahlepi, and currants. Fold gently until combined.

Pour mixture into two rectangular lined loaf tins (25x14 cm or 10x5.5 in.). Sprinkle white and black sesame seeds and additional grated halloumi cheese over the top.

Bake for 45–50 minutes or until a skewer inserted comes out clean. Set aside to cool on a rack. Can be eaten warm or at room temperature.

*Mastic and mahlepi spices can be purchased at European grocers.

Κυπριακή Φλαουνόπιτα
- CYPRIOT FLAOUNOPITA -

1 cup olive oil

5 whole eggs, separated

400 g (14 oz.) all-purpose flour

3 teaspoons baking powder

2 cups whole milk

200 g (7.0 oz.) halloumi cheese, grated, divided

1 cup Pecorino Romano or strong cheddar cheese

2 teaspoons dried mint

1 teaspoon powdered mastic*

3 teaspoons powdered mahlepi*

175 g (6.1 oz.) currants

TOPPING

1 tablespoon each of white and black sesame seeds

20 g (0.7 oz.) additional halloumi cheese, grated for topping

Τυροκούλουρα με γλυκάνισο

- FETA CHEESE AND FENNEL *KOULOURI* -

These feta cheese and fennel *koulouria* are next-level in terms of flavor. This filling is added to the soft-centered bread (the renowned street food of Thessaloniki) which has a crunchy and slightly sweetened exterior from grape must. The addition of fennel seeds adds a great balance to the savory feta cheese and sweet outer crust. They can be eaten for breakfast or as a snack throughout the day. If you prefer a less sweetened type, you can omit the dunking in grape must and instead just use water to allow the sesame to stick.

Makes: 8 pieces · 1.5 hours

- 225 ml (7.6 fl. oz.) lukewarm water, divided
- 3 teaspoons dried instant yeast
- 1½ tablespoons castor (superfine) sugar
- 2 tablespoons olive oil
- 100 ml (3.38 fl. oz.) whole milk, lukewarm
- 1 whole egg
- 1½ teaspoons salt
- 630 g (1.38 lb.) all-purpose flour

FILLING

- 300 g (10.5 oz.) feta cheese, crumbled
- 1 tablespoon fennel seeds, roughly ground

- ⅓ cup grape must syrup (*petimezi*), diluted in ¼ cup water*
- 2½ cups sesame seeds, toasted

Attach a dough hook to a stand mixer. In the bowl of the mixer, add the water, yeast, sugar, oil, milk, egg, and salt. Mix, and then, on medium speed, slowly add the flour (reserve the last 20 g or 0.7 oz. in case the flour mixture does not need it). Mix for approximately 5 minutes or until the mixture comes away from the bowl. It will be slightly sticky but also soft. Add a little more flour if it is too sticky and difficult to handle. Remove, knead for 2 minutes on a work surface, and form into a ball. Place covered in an oiled bowl and allow to rise for 40 minutes.

Combine the filling ingredients into a bowl and set aside.

In the meantime, take two bowls. In one bowl, place the grape must with water, mixing to incorporate. In the other bowl, place the toasted sesame.

Preheat the oven to 200º C/392º F. Line two baking trays with parchment paper.

Once the dough has risen, remove from the bowl and divide into 8 pieces (100 g. or 3.52 oz. each). Do not flour your workbench as you want the dough to stick slightly. Knead each piece slightly to deflate any air. Roll each piece into a rope approximately 35 cm (14 in.) long, and stretch them out to a 5 cm (2 in.) width with your fingers. Take about 2 tablespoons of the filling and place along the center of the koulouri. Gently bring the pastry together to enclose the filling. Bring the ends together into a ring shape and press to seal.

Dip each *koulouri* into the grape must and then immediately into the sesame. Coat well and place onto the baking tray. Wash and wipe hands after each *koulouri* as the sesame mixture sticks to your hands.

Bake for 20 minutes or until golden. These can be eaten warm or cold.

*Petimezi/grape must is available at Middle Eastern or Mediterranean delicatessens. *Petimezi* is a concentrated grape juice that resembles a thick, sweet syrup without any added sugars.

*To make an egg *koulouri*, crack open and egg and place into the hole of the bagel 10 minutes before the bagel is fully cooked. Continue to bake until the egg is cooked to your liking.

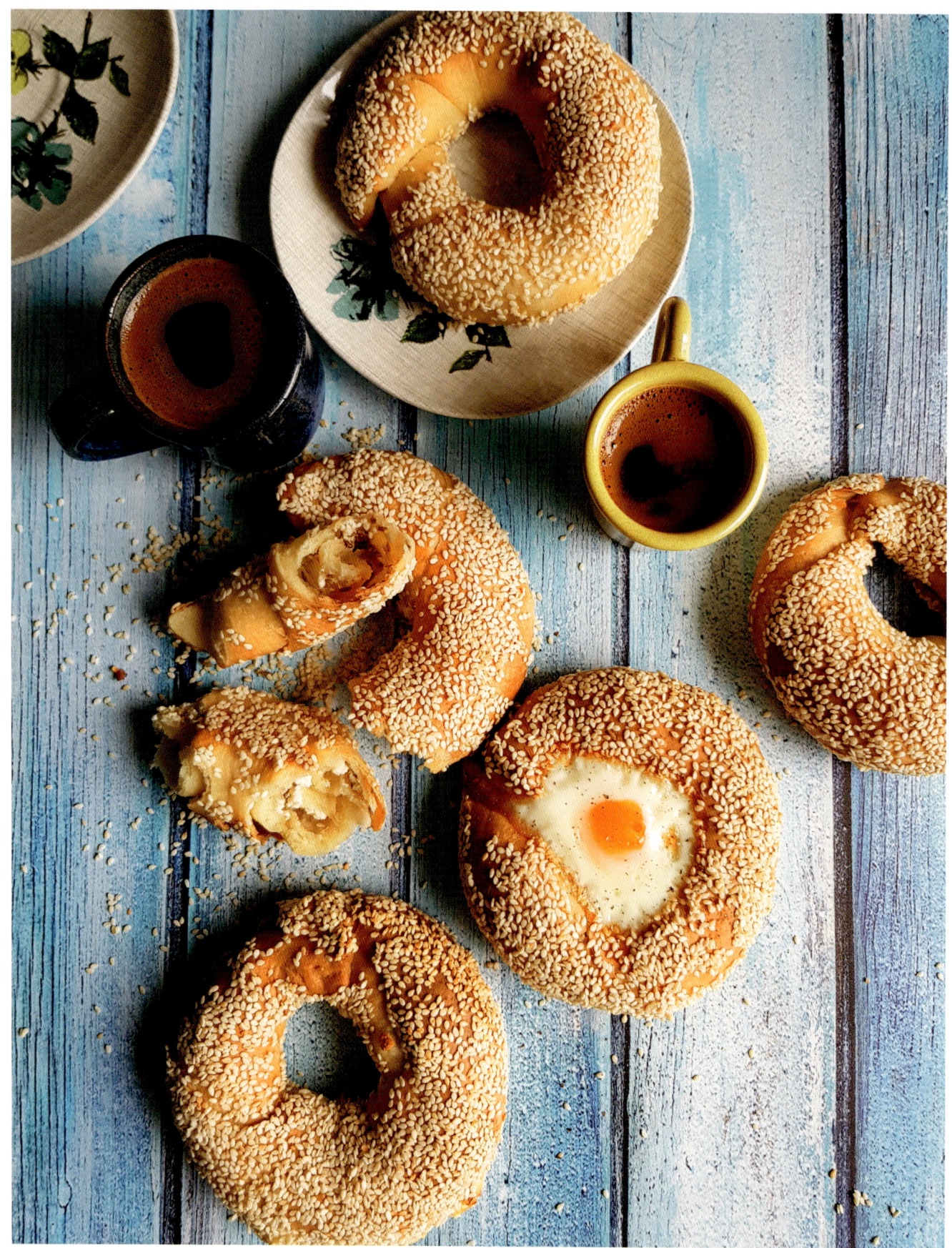

Feta Cheese and Fennel Koulouri, page 170-171.

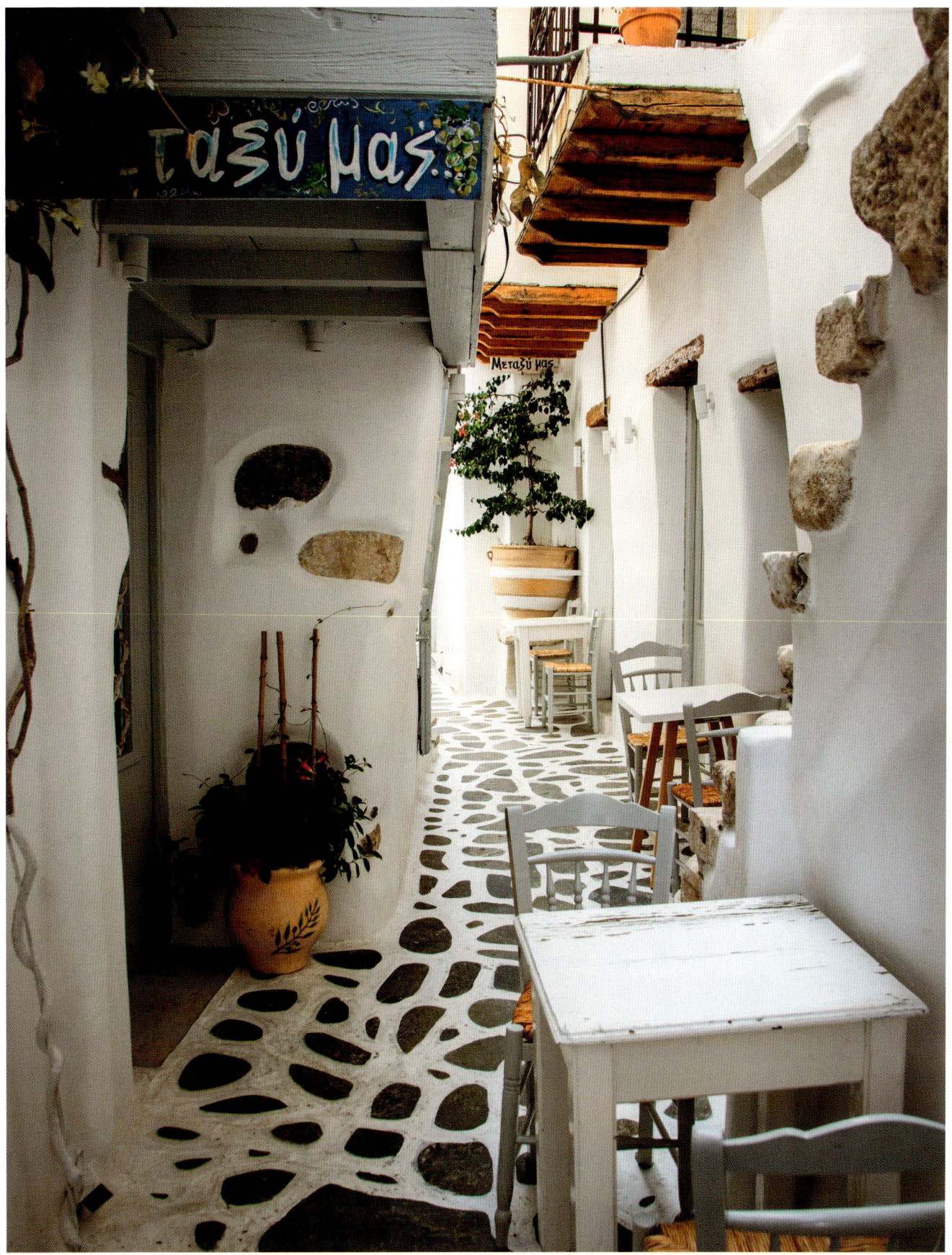

ΤΗΣ ΓΛΥΚΑΣ ΤΑ ΚΑΜΩΜΑΤΑ
THE SWEET BAKER

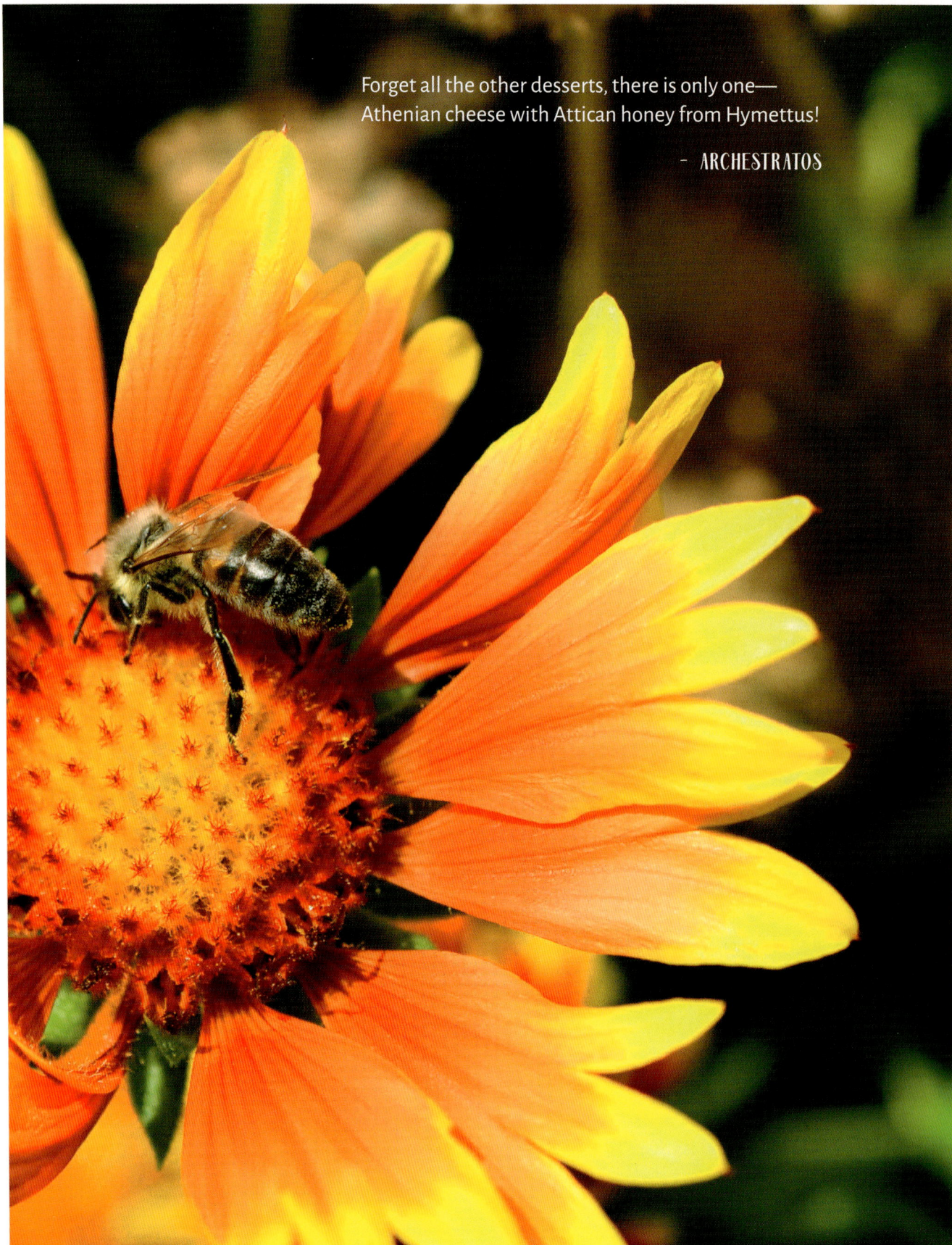

Forget all the other desserts, there is only one—
Athenian cheese with Attican honey from Hymettus!

– ARCHESTRATOS

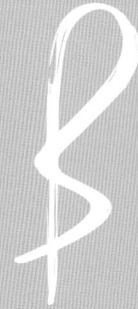

ΓΛΥΚΟ ΜΕ ΕΣΠΕΡΙΔΟΕΙΔΗ ΚΑΙ ΑΜΥΓΔΑΛΟ
178 CITRUS ALMOND CAKE (GF)

ΓΙΑΟΥΡΤΟΓΛΥΚΟ ΨΥΓΕΙΟΥ
180 YOGURT JELLY CAKE

ΓΑΛΑΤΟΠΙΤΑ - ΣΟΥΦΡΑ ΜΕ ΒΑΝΙΛΙΑ
182 RUFFLED VANILLA MILK PIE

ΡΥΖΟΓΑΛΟ ΓΛΥΚΟ
184 RICE PUDDING CAKE (GF)

ΜΗΛΟΠΙΤΑ ΜΕ ΕΛΑΙΟΛΑΔΟ ΚΑΙ ΟΥΙΣΚΙ
186 APPLE CAKE WITH OLIVE OIL AND WHISKEY

ΚΑΝΤΑΪΦΙ
188 PASTRY PARCELS WITH NUTS, SPICES, AND ORANGE SYRUP

ΡΟΞΑΚΙΑ
190 ROXAKIA—COCOA AND ORANGE WHEELS

ΦΟΙΝΙΚΙΑ ΑΠΟ ΙΚΑΡΙΑ
192 FINIKIA FROM IKARIA

ΡΟΖΕΔΕΣ ΚΥΘΗΡΩΝ
194 ALMOND SPICED KITHIRIAN COOKIES

ΚΕΡΚΥΡΑΪΚΗ ΦΟΓΑΤΣΑ
196 CORFIOT EASTER BREAD

ΜΠΑΚΛΑΒΑΔΑΚΙΑ
200 BITE-SIZE CASHEW AND ORANGE BAKLAVA

GF DENOTES GLUTEN-FREE RECIPES

Γλυκό με εσπεριδοειδή και αμύγδαλο
- CITRUS ALMOND CAKE -

Citrus trees are grown throughout Greece, and therefore myriads of cake recipes exist. Every region has its own version of orange and lemon pies. Some are with pastry, and some are without. I stumbled across a unique recipe many years ago. It combines three citrus fruits: oranges, mandarins, and lemons. This combination gives the cake a sweet and sour tone that balances very well. It is super light and fluffy. This cake keeps well in the refrigerator for a few days. The thickened cream and caramelized mandarins are a wonderful combination and topping to the cake.

Makes: 16–18 pieces • 2.5 hours • GLUTEN FREE

CANDIED MANDARINS*

3 whole mandarins

1 cup castor (superfine) sugar

¼ cup water

CAKE BATTER

2 medium oranges, whole

3 mandarins, whole, skin off

6 whole eggs

250 g (8.8 oz.) castor (superfine) sugar

Zest of one lemon

1 teaspoon baking powder

250 g (8.8 oz.) almond meal

50 g (1.7 oz.) slivered almonds

TO SERVE

300 ml thickened cream

Pistachios, to decorate

Line a (26x28 cm or 10x11 in.) springform tin with parchment paper. Set aside.

Prepare candied mandarins: Remove skins and separate mandarin segments. In a wide fry pan, place the sugar and ¼ cup water. Simmer on medium heat for 3–4 minutes or until sugar has dissolved. Add the mandarin slices and reduce heat to low. Cook for 8–10 minutes or until sugar syrup has thickened and starts to caramelize and turn light brown. Remove from heat and pour onto parchment paper to cool. Once cooled, break up into small pieces. Set aside.

Take two saucepans. Place the whole oranges in one pot and mandarins in the other. Cover both fruits with water. Simmer oranges on medium heat for 1½ hours and the mandarins for 20 minutes. Remove fruit and allow to cool. Cut the oranges in half, remove pips, and place into a blender together with the mandarins. Pulse until puréed. Pour into a large bowl. Set aside.

Preheat the oven to 160º C/320º F.

In a large bowl, beat eggs and sugar for 10 minutes or until white and fluffy. Stir in the puréed citrus. Add the zest, baking powder, and almond meal. Gently mix. Pour the batter into prepared tin and sprinkle the slivered almonds over the top.

Bake for 1 hour or until a skewer inserted comes out clean. Allow to cool completely, and then remove from the tin. Add whipped cream and top with candied mandarins and crushed pistachios.

*If you want a simpler version, dust with icing sugar instead of candied mandarins.

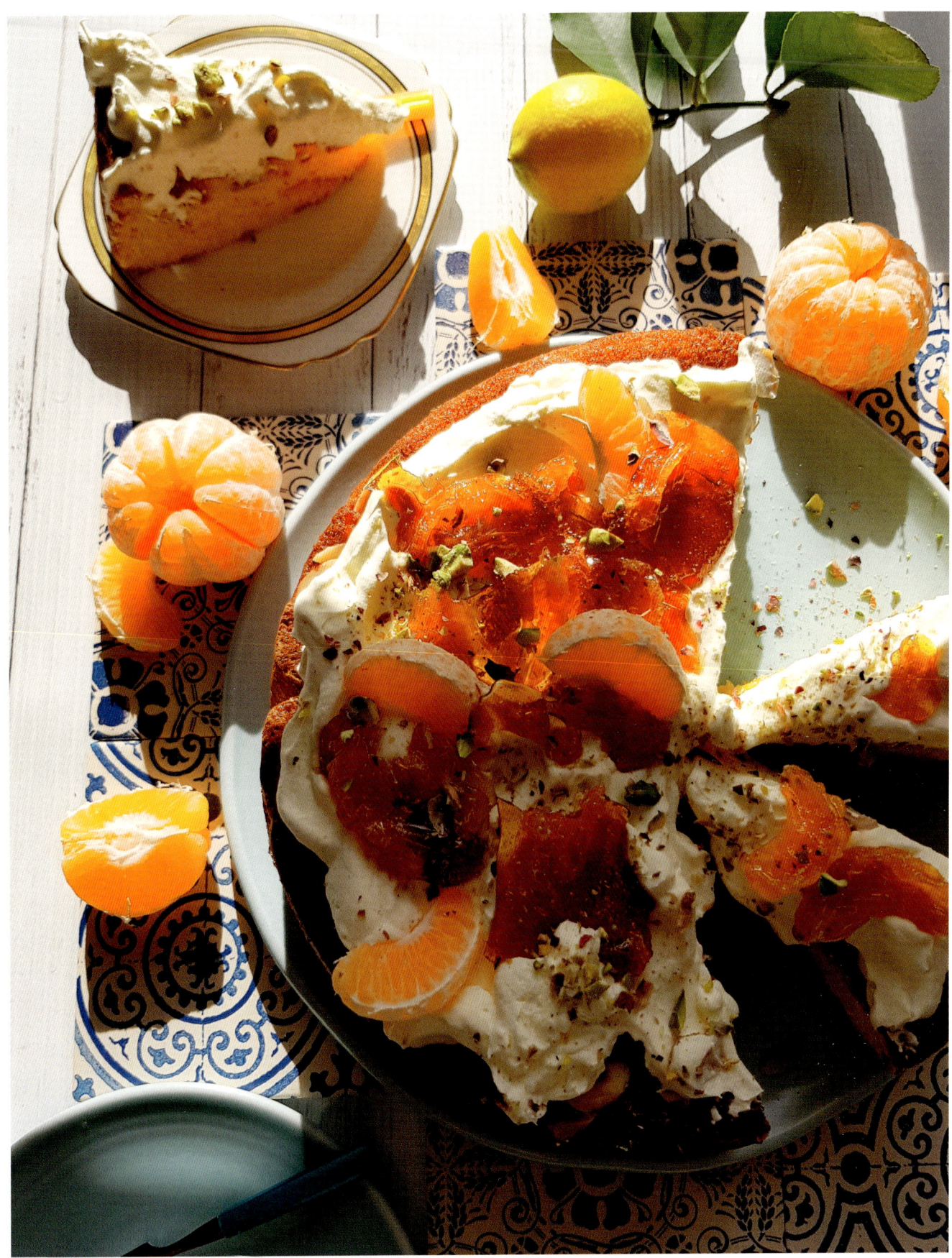

Γιαουρτόγλυκο ψυγείου
- YOGURT JELLY CAKE -

90 ml whole milk, warm

225 g (7.9 oz.) teddy bear or semi-sweet cookies (I use the Papadopoulou brand)*

2 packets (85 g each or 2.99 oz.) strawberry jelly

500 g (17.6 oz.) fresh strawberries, thinly sliced

1 kg (35.2 oz.) yogurt

Every Greek child has grown up eating this classic yogurt jelly cake. It is reminiscent of a trifle, but instead of custard and sponge cake, it has a biscuit base and a yogurt jelly center. Improvisations can be made depending on what fruit is in season, such as peaches or pineapple, though a strawberry version is most common in Greece in the summer months. This is simple to prepare. It has no added sugars other than what is in the jelly. It is best made a day before serving so that the jelly and yogurt mixture set well.

Serves: 20 · 15 minutes (plus overnight setting)

Use a 25x35 cm/10x14 in. dish.

Place the warm milk into a small bowl. Dip each cookie into the milk (just in and out, no need to soak), and then place one row on the bottom of the dish. Layer a second row of dipped cookies directly on top of the first. Layer a row of sliced strawberries over the top of the cookies. Set aside.

In another bowl, prepare one packet of the jelly as directed on the packet. Once the jelly has dissolved (with both hot and cold water), add the yogurt and whisk to incorporate it into the jelly mixture.

Gently pour this mixture over the cookie base, and then top with the remaining sliced strawberries.

Place in the fridge to set around 2–3 hours before adding the second box of jelly.

In a bowl, prepare the second box of jelly as directed on the packet. Pour over the set yogurt and return to the fridge to set overnight. Slice and serve cold.

*Papadopoulou cookies are available at European grocers.

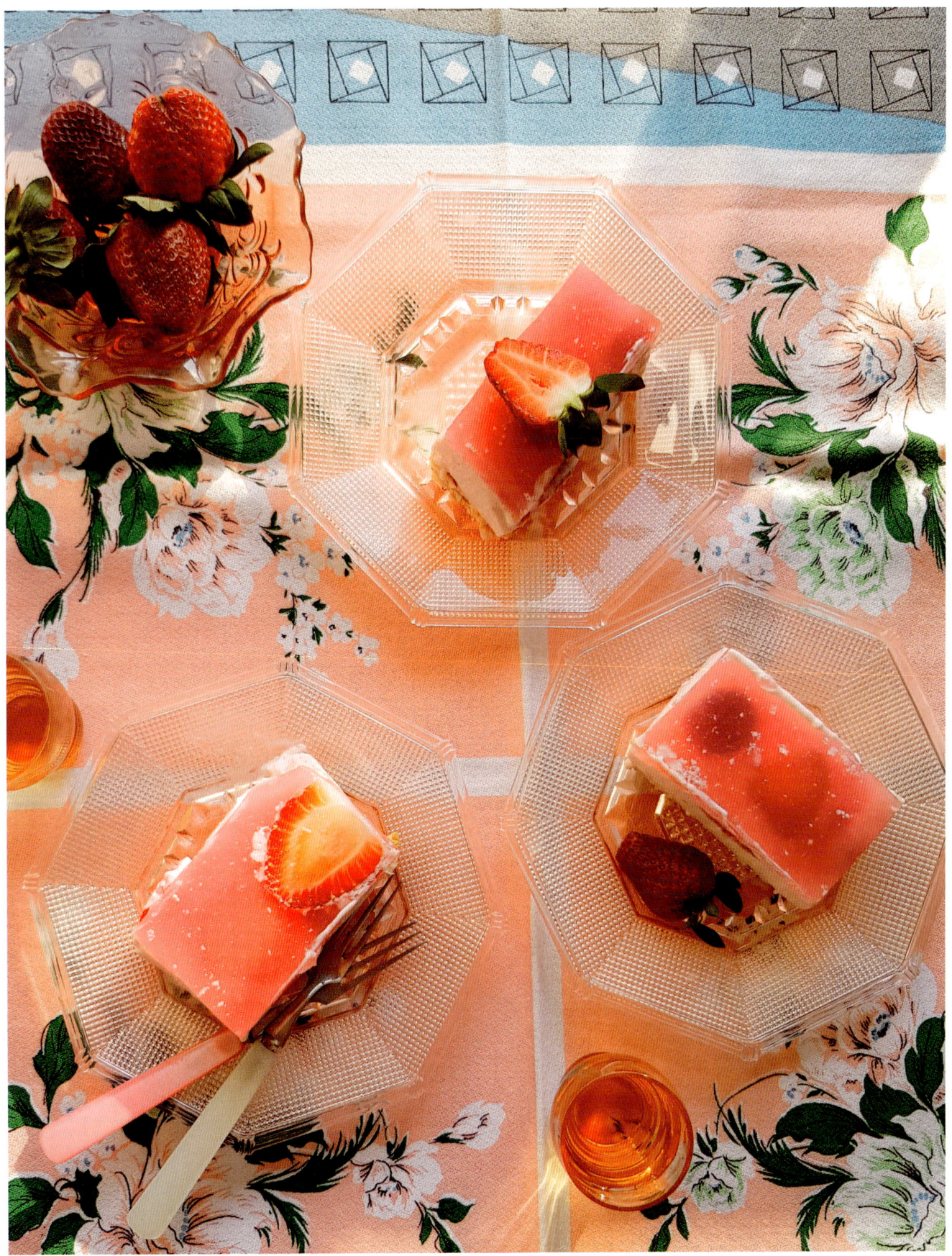

Γαλατόπιτα σούφρα με βανίλια
- RUFFLED VANILLA MILK PIE -

250 g (10 sheets) store-bought phyllo pastry

8–10 tablespoons olive oil or melted butter

1 teaspoon cinnamon powder

FILLING

3 whole eggs

2½ cups whole milk

Seeds of one vanilla bean

¾ cup castor (superfine) sugar

½ teaspoon baking powder

Zest of one orange

2–3 tablespoons dark brown (muscovado) sugar

TO SERVE

Cinnamon powder

Icing (confectioners) sugar

There are so many ways to make a Greek milk pie. Some recipes use homemade pastry, and some do not. Some only line pastry on the bottom of the pie, and some do not, and so on. This recipe, however, is a great take on using store-bought pastry. The pastry is scrunched up, which ensures you get a great crunch with the soft, milky mixture. This is a great recipe for a last-minute dessert or even a breakfast treat. It is best eaten warm. It is very quick to make and not overly sweet, so feel free to adjust sweetness if preferred. Lemon zest can also be added. It is Greek simplicity at its finest!

Makes: 10 pieces • 1 hour

Preheat oven to 200º C/390º F.

Oil a 29 cm (11 in.) round baking tray.

Lay one sheet of phyllo onto kitchen counter and brush with some oil or butter. Scrunch it lengthwise into a loose fan (do not worry if it breaks or tears), and then roll into a scroll. Place the rolled-up sheet into the center of the dish. Continue to fold the rest of the sheets like fans and wrap them around the first scroll in the dish. Continue to layer until the whole pan is full. Sprinkle cinnamon powder over the top.

Bake for 20 minutes or until the pastry is golden. The more golden, the better as this will give a good crunch to the texture of the overall pie. A lighter, slightly undercooked pastry will result in a soggy pie.

Remove from oven and prepare the filling.

Place the eggs, milk, vanilla, sugar, baking powder, and orange zest into a bowl. Whisk to combine, and then pour over the cooked pastry. Sprinkle dark brown sugar over the top.

Return to the oven and bake for another 20 minutes or until custard has set. Remove from oven and immediately dust with cinnamon powder.

Allow to cool slightly. Dust with icing sugar, slice, and serve warm.

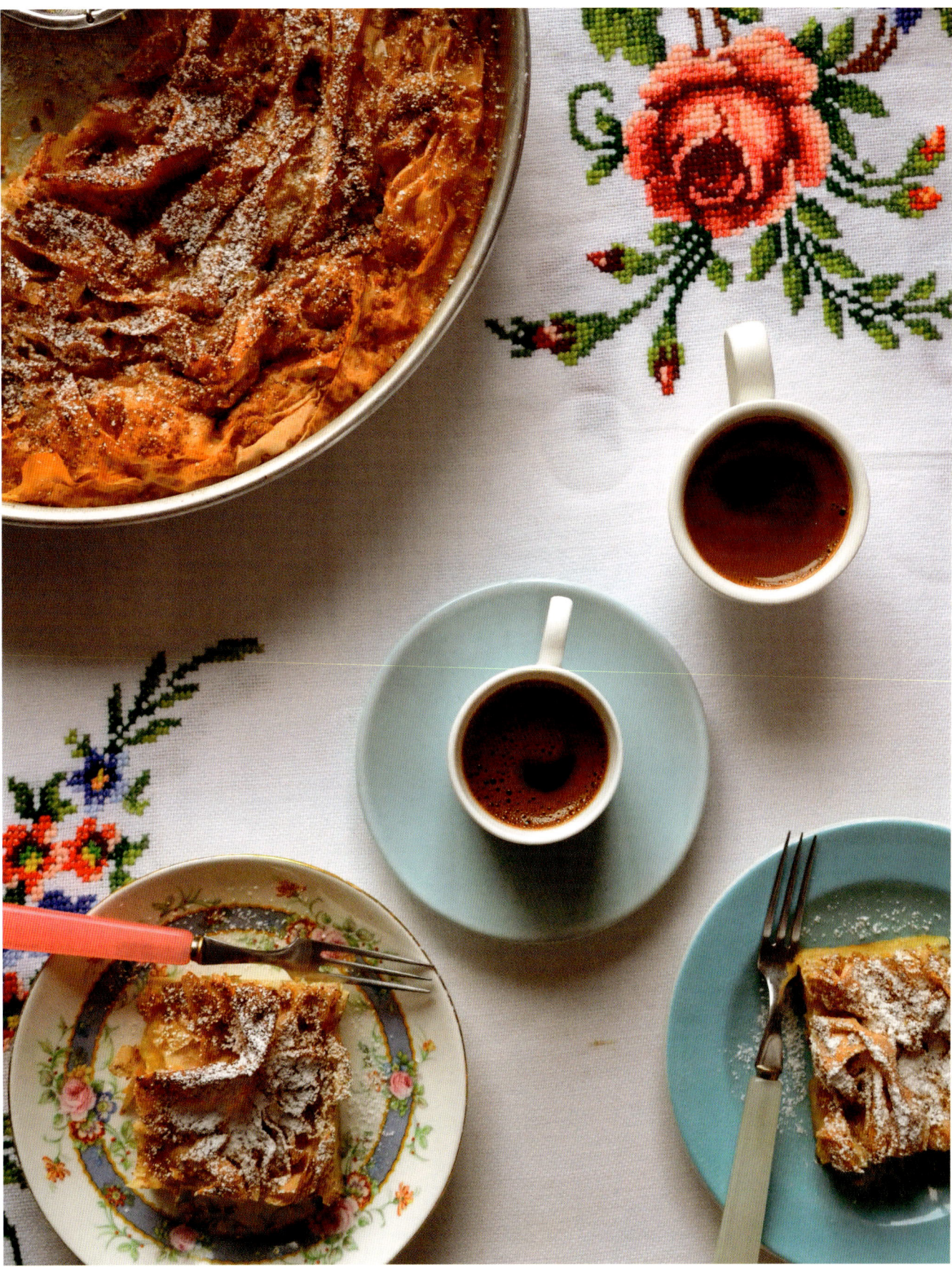

Ριζόγαλο γλυκό
- RICE PUDDING CAKE -

2 tablespoons orange liqueur

1 orange, zested

¼ cup raisins

3½ cups whole milk

1 vanilla pod, deseeded

1 cinnamon stick

1 piece of lemon rind (3 cm long)

¾ cup arborio rice

3 whole eggs, separated

2 tablespoons runny honey

TO SERVE

Icing (confectioners) sugar

This cake tastes like a cross between a brioche and traditional *rizogalo* (rice pudding). It is incredibly delicious and easy to make with very few ingredients. I first saw this when visiting Greece over two decades ago. *Rizogalo* is usually cooked on the stovetop and served in small individual plates. However, this recipe is baked and thickened by the addition of eggs and then baked in a tin and served as a large cake. It is light in texture and fragrant from the orange liquor and zest. It is not overly sweet, so feel free to drizzle additional honey or add some pieces of *loukoumi* (as pictured) when serving.

Makes: 16 pieces · 1.5 hours · GLUTEN FREE

Line a 20 cm/8 in. springform tin with parchment paper.

Place orange liqueur, orange zest, and raisins in a bowl. Set aside.

In a saucepan, combine milk, vanilla, cinnamon stick, lemon rind, and rice. Bring to a boil, whisking regularly so the rice does not stick. Lower heat and simmer a further 20 minutes or until the rice has fully cooked and the milk has mostly evaporated into a thick rice pudding consistency like that of a risotto. Every so often, whisk so that the rice does not stick.

Remove the rind and cinnamon stick and add the honey. Mix. Once the honey is added, it will liquidize slightly, so place the saucepan back on the stove and cook for a further few minutes until it has thickened again. Set aside to cool.

Preheat oven to 170° C/340° F.

Once cooled, mix in the egg yolks and sultana mixture.

With an electric mixer, beat egg whites until still peaks form. Fold gently into rice mixture. Pour into prepared tin and bake for 50 minutes or until a skewer inserted comes out clean. Cool in tin.

Remove and serve warm or cold with a dusting of icing sugar. Best eaten the day it is made.

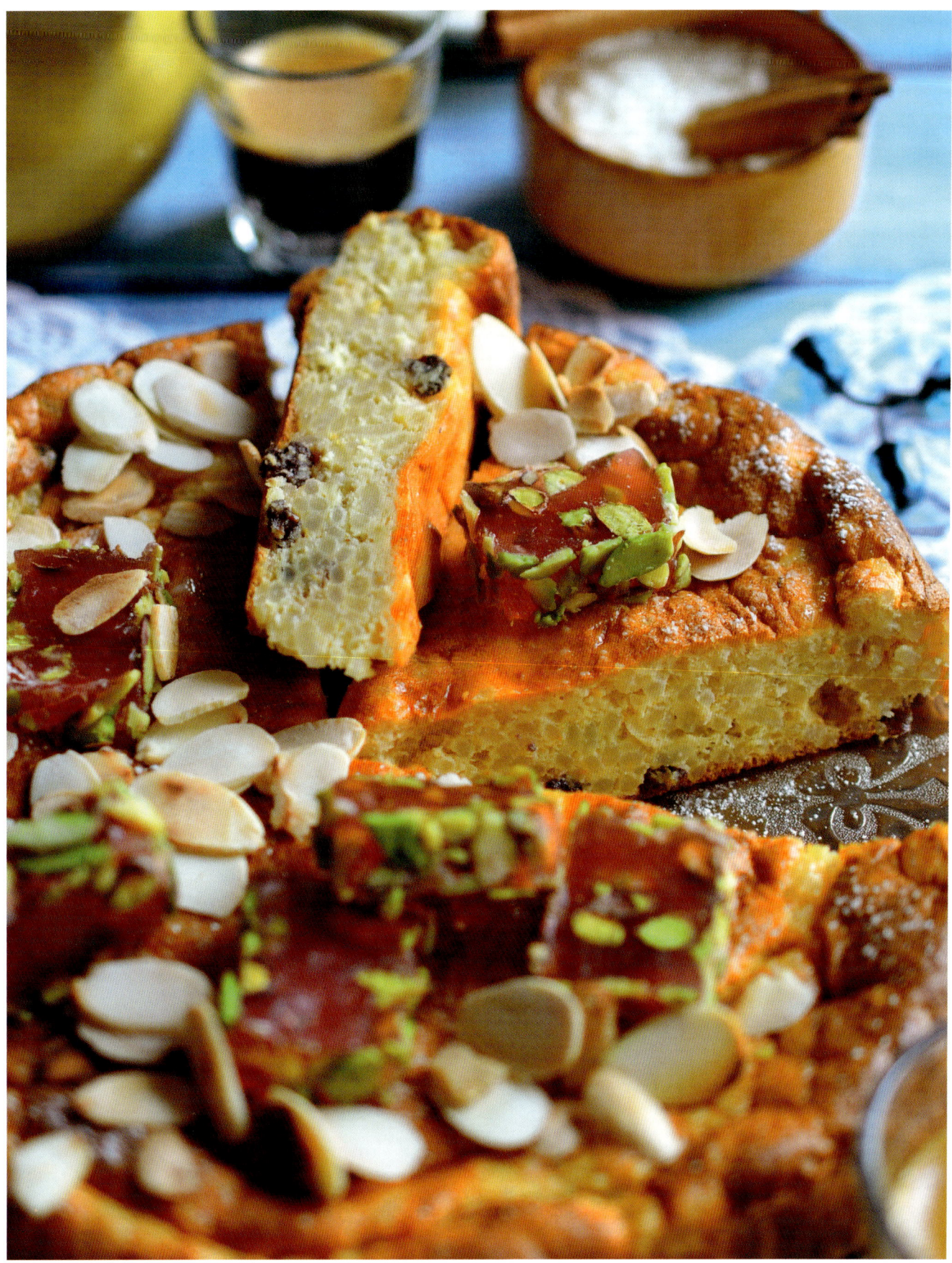

Μηλόπιτα με ελαιόλαδο και ουίσκι

- APPLE CAKE WITH OLIVE OIL AND WHISKEY -

7 large pink lady apples (1.2 kg) sliced with skins on into ¼ in. pieces

1 cup dark brown (muscovado) sugar, divided*

1½ tablespoons whiskey or rum

1 lemon, juiced

3 whole eggs, room temperature

1 teaspoon vanilla extract

¼ teaspoon salt

1½ teaspoons baking powder

1 cup all-purpose flour, sifted

¾ cup light olive oil

Milopita (*milo* for "apple," *pita* for "pie") is one of those cakes that is made all over Greece. Once again, the variations are many. Some use yogurt in the batter, spices, butter, a small number of apples, and so on. One thing for certain with this recipe is that the apples are the star ingredient. As you can see by the number of apples, it really is more about the fruit than cake itself. To intensify the apple flavor, the apples are cored, sliced thinly (skin on), and then baked to remove moisture. The apples are then added to the batter mixture. It is a simple technique that adds optimum taste.

Makes: 16 pieces • 2 hours

Preheat oven to 200° C/390° F.

Line a 23 cm/9 in. springform tin (base and sides) with parchment paper. Set aside.

In a large bowl, mix the sliced apples, 2 tablespoons of sugar, whiskey, and lemon juice. Line two flat baking trays with parchment paper and divide apples evenly onto both. Spread out evenly. Bake for 20–30 minutes, turning halfway through. The apples will shrink a little due to the moisture being drawn out.

Set aside to cool for 10 minutes.

In a large bowl, whisk the eggs for 2–3 minutes or until fluffy and pale. Then add the remaining sugar (set aside 3 tablespoons for the topping) and whisk to combine well. Add the vanilla, salt, baking powder, and half the flour, mixing well. Now add the olive oil and whisk to combine. Finish with the remaining flour. Whisk until you have no lumps and a smooth consistency.

Reduce oven temperature to 180° C/350° F. Reserve 20–25 of the baked apples for the top.

Using a large wooden spoon, fold the apples into the batter. Ensure that all the apples are coated well. Pour this batter into the prepared tin, pressing down evenly to distribute batter. Smooth into an even layer, and then arrange the reserved apples on the top, pressing in slightly. Sprinkle the remaining 3 tablespoons of sugar over the top and bake for 1 to 1½ hours or until a skewer inserted comes out clean. Serve hot or cold with custard or ice cream.

*Castor (superfine) sugar can be substituted with dark brown (muscovado) sugar.

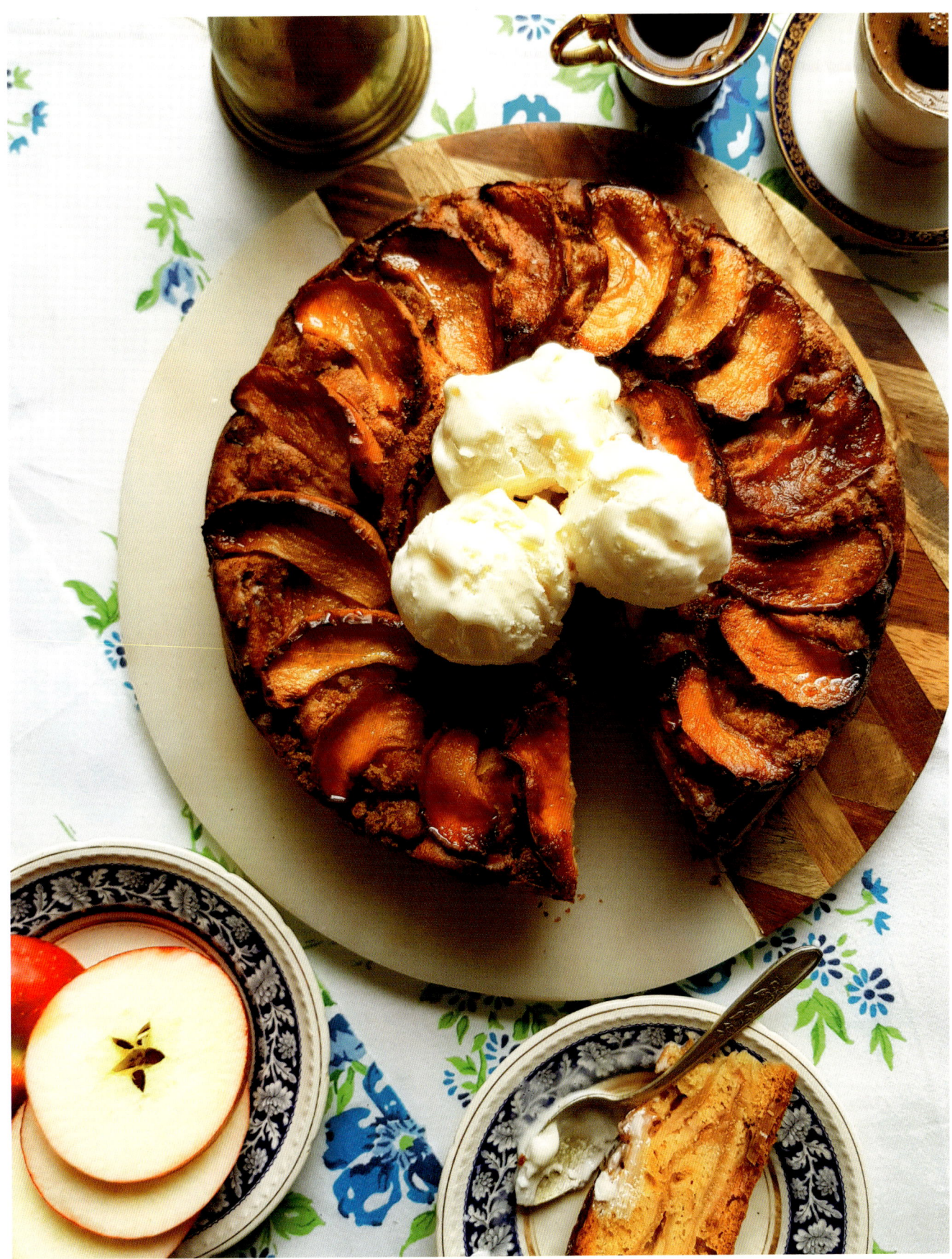

Κανταΐφι

- PASTRY PARCELS WITH NUTS, SPICES, AND ORANGE SYRUP -

Reminiscent of baklava, this dessert is made with nuts and spices, but rather than using phyllo pastry, it has shredded pastry. To finish the dessert, a sugar syrup is poured over the top. It is a quintessential Greek dessert that is always showcased front and center in sweet stores known in Greece as *zaharoplasteia*. There are two key points to a great *kataifi*. One, use an exceptionally good organic butter. Two, bake it low and slow to ensure the pastry cooks all the way through.

Makes: 14 pieces · 2.5 hours

SYRUP

- 2 cups castor (superfine) sugar
- 330 ml water
- 1 cinnamon stick
- Peel of 1 orange

FILLING

- 90 g (0.19 lb.) roasted almonds (½ ground, ½ roughly chopped)
- 90 g (0.19 lb.) roasted walnuts (½ ground, ½ roughly chopped)
- 2 teaspoons cinnamon powder
- ½ teaspoon clove powder
- 1 tablespoon castor (superfine) sugar
- Zest of 1 orange

- 350 g (0.77 lb.) butter, room temperature
- 1 packet (375 g or 13.2 oz.) *kataifi* pastry, room temperature

Preheat oven to 150° C/300° F.

Place the syrup ingredients into a saucepan and simmer on low heat until the sugar has completely dissolved. Set aside to cool.

Place filling ingredients into a bowl, mix, and set aside.

Remove *kataifi* pastry from the packet and gently pull apart the shreds with your hands (try not to tear), creating a fluffy heap of pastry. Divide the pastry into 19 piles. Take 14 piles and set aside covered with a damp cloth so they don't dry out. Wrap the extra 5 piles and refrigerate to use another time. This recipe and syrup are for 14 pieces.

Take one pile and spread lengthwise (do not make it too long—otherwise the filling will fall out). Place 1 tablespoon of filling on the end closest to you. On top of the filling, add 1 teaspoon of butter (or a small knob) and gently enclose, bringing in the sides and tightly rolling forward to create a roll.

Grease a baking tray with a little butter, and then place the rolls seam side down, placing each roll side by side. Once all the rolls have been done, melt the remaining butter and pour over the kataifi and bake for 1½ hours. Do not rush the baking time. You want the *kataifi* to cook right through (without the top burning).

Once the *kataifi* is slightly golden, remove from the oven and immediately pour the cold syrup over it.

Allow the *kataifi* to sit for 1 hour so that the syrup can be absorbed.

Keeps 1–2 days in the refrigerator.

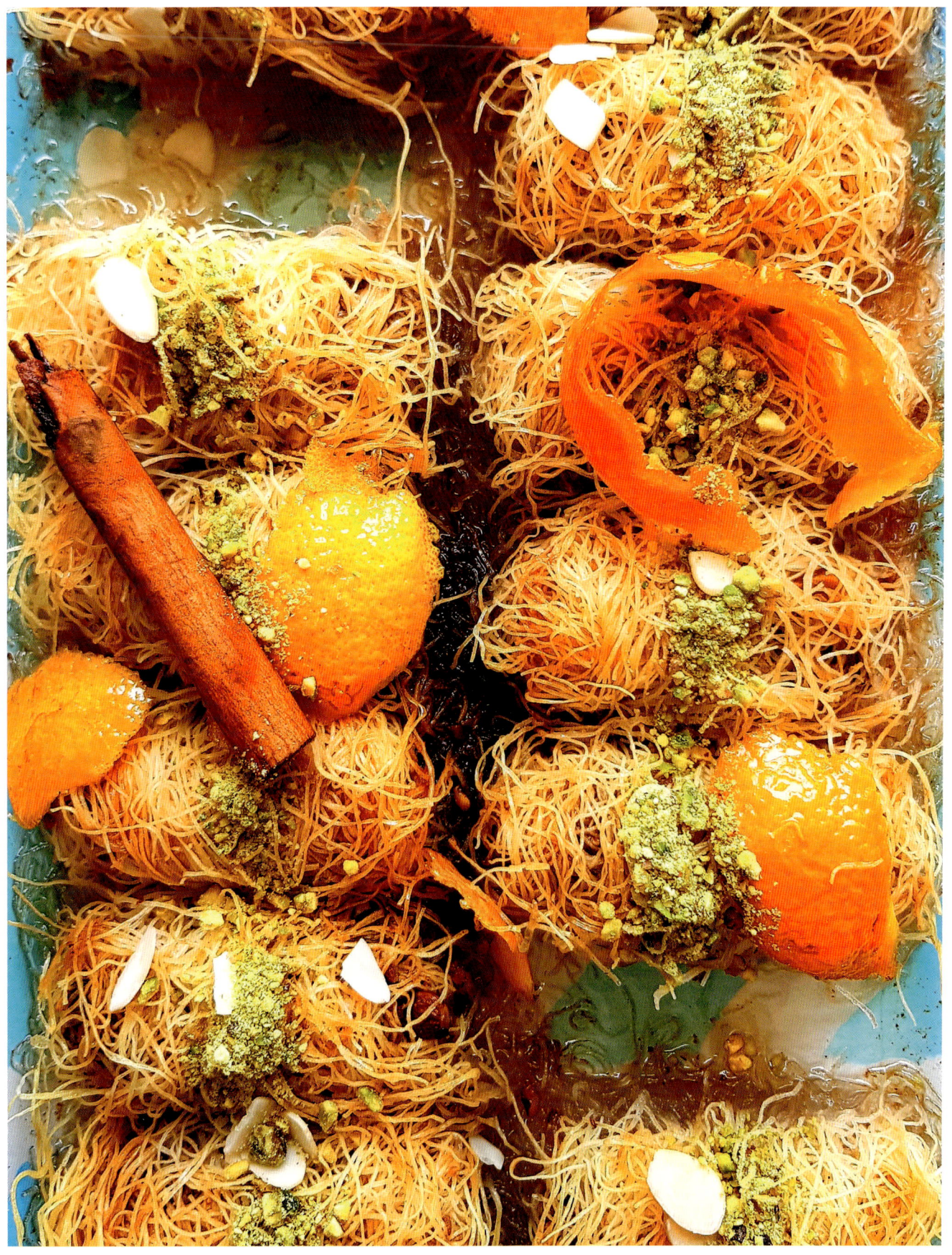

Ροξάκια
– ROXAKIA— COCOA & ORANGE WHEELS -

These biscuits are a winner for the syrup lover! If you have grown up in Greece, it was probably one of your childhood favorites. I know it is for my husband. He regularly talks about going to the local bakery and devouring them. It is an orange dough with a spiced cocoa center soaked in an orange syrup. The texture is spongy and super moist with a burst of intense flavor. I will say no more—you need to try these. Serve with a Greek coffee or a glass of milk.

Makes: 16–18 pieces · 45 minutes (plus soaking time)

DOUGH

- 2¼ teaspoons instant yeast
- 100 ml whole milk, warm
- 140 ml light olive oil
- 1 whole egg
- ½ teaspoon baking powder
- Zest of one orange
- 300 g (10.5 oz.) all-purpose flour

COCOA FILLING

- 1½ teaspoons cinnamon powder
- 2 tablespoons cocoa powder
- ½ teaspoon clove powder
- Zest of ½ orange
- 1–2 teaspoons olive oil (or as needed)

SYRUP

- 300 g (10.5 oz.) castor (superfine) sugar
- 400 ml water
- 1 slice of orange rind

Preheat oven to 180° C/350° F.

In a large bowl, place the yeast and warm milk. Mix and allow to sit for 10 minutes for the yeast to activate. Now add the oil, egg, baking powder, zest, and flour and mix with a wooden spoon until a dough is formed. It should come together easily. Knead the dough for 1–2 minutes until smooth. Place in a bowl covered with a tea towel to rest for 30 minutes.

Take ¾ of the dough and set aside. Place the remaining ¼ dough in a bowl together with the cocoa filling of cinnamon, cocoa, clove powder, orange zest, and 1 teaspoon oil. Using your hands, knead to combine well until the dough is dark brown in color. You may find one more teaspoon of oil is needed to help combine the ingredients. Roll this mixture into a long rope 30 cm (11 in.) long. Leave it to one side.

Now take the other dough and roll out into a rectangular shape 30x15 cm wide (11x6 in.). Place the cocoa dough on the edge closest to you and roll it up to enclose the cocoa filling like a sausage roll. Cut 1 cm (0.4 in.) pieces and place onto a lined baking tray. Press down slightly on each roll to flatten (but not too much).

Bake for 25 minutes or until slightly golden but not too dark—otherwise they will taste burned.

Remove from oven and allow to cool completely.

To make the syrup, place all the syrup ingredients into a saucepan and bring to a boil. Reduce heat and simmer for 6 minutes. Remove from heat and immediately pour the hot syrup over the cold *roxakia*. It will seem as though you have too much syrup; that's okay. Allow to sit for a minimum 2–3 hours in the syrup. Place onto a serving plate, scatter walnuts on top, and serve.

Discard any leftover syrup.

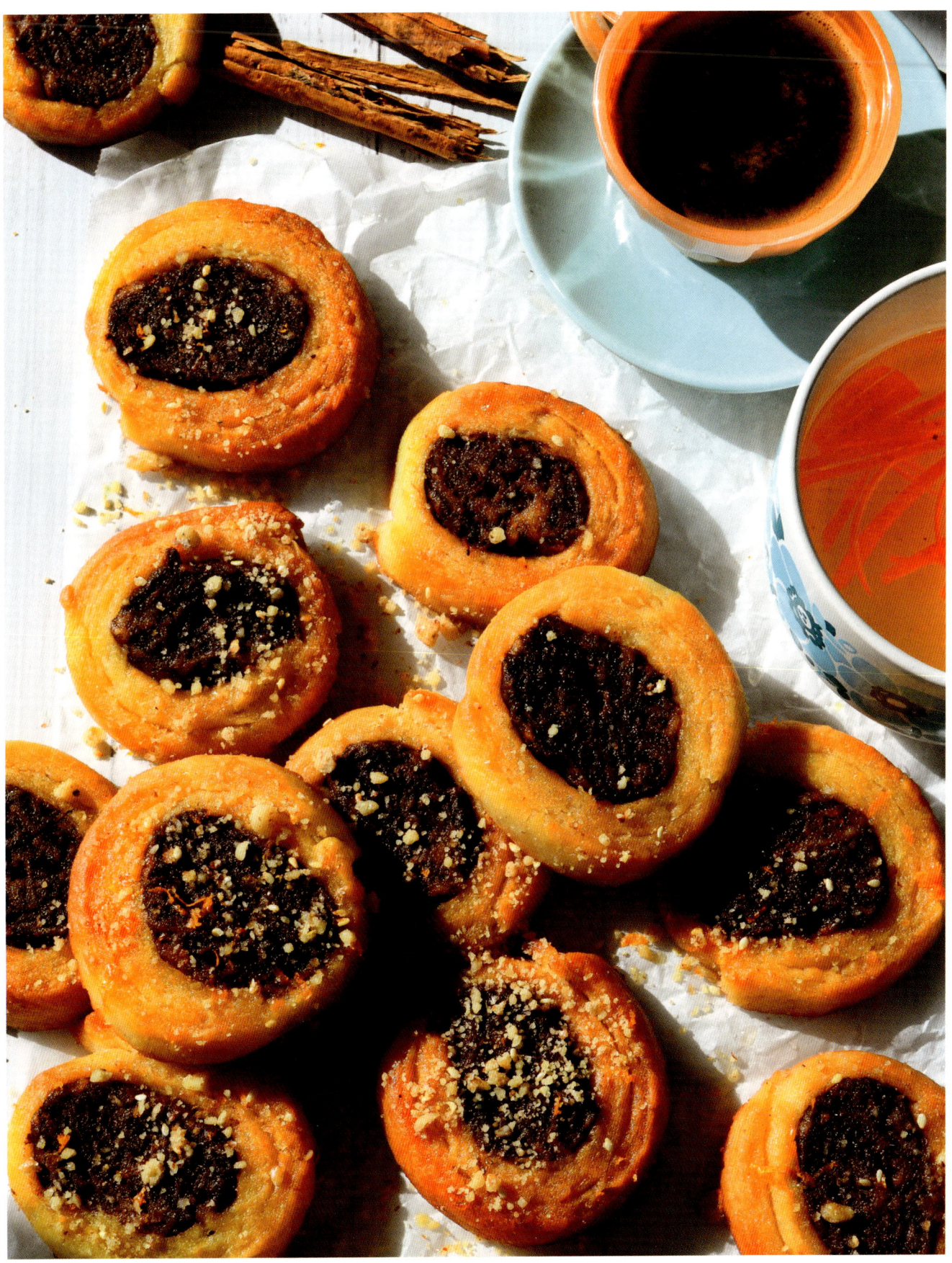

Φοινίκια από Ικαρία
- FINIKIA FROM IKARIA -

100 ml orange juice

1 teaspoon baking powder

½ teaspoon baking soda

¾ cup (180 ml) olive oil

½ cup castor (superfine) sugar

30 ml ouzo, mastic or metaxa liquor*

1½ teaspoons cinnamon powder

½ teaspoon clove powder

Zest of one orange

Zest of ½ lemon

400 g (2–3 cups) all-purpose flour

SYRUP

½ cup honey

1 cup water

3 slithers of orange peel

TOPPING

200 g chocolate, melted

Crushed pistachios, optional

Finikia are not to be mistaken for *melomakarona*, the honey-soaked cookie covered with walnuts (this recipe can be found in my cookbook *Hellenic Kanella: Memories Made in a Greek Kitchen*), though in many regions the same name is used. They have similar flavors but are made slightly differently. *Finikia* are also much smaller; they do not have any dairy or eggs and are primarily made with extra-virgin olive oil. They are quickly dipped in a honey syrup for an added sweetness. These little delicacies are super quick to make without needing a mixer. You just need a bowl and whisk. They are unbelievably delicious with a cup of coffee or even a glass of milk. I have topped these with melted chocolate, but they are most traditionally served with a dusting of cinnamon and/or sugar.

Makes: 45 pieces · 1.5 hours

Preheat oven to 170° C/340° F.

Place the orange juice, baking soda, and baking powder in a small bowl and mix. It will fizz. Set aside.

In a bowl, place the olive oil and sugar. Whisk to combine well. Add the orange mixture, ouzo, cinnamon powder, clove powder, and zest of the orange and lemon. Whisk to combine, and then, with a wooden spoon, gradually mix in the flour, adding spoonfuls at a time. The dough must be soft and not stick to your hands. Add a little more flour if needed, but do not overwork it.

Divide the dough into approximately 45 pieces, each piece weighing around 20 g/0.70 oz. Roll into a ball with your palms, and then shape it into a small oval. Place onto a lined baking pan and flatten it slightly with your hands. Bake for 20–30 minutes or until just golden on the bottom. Do not allow them to burn as they are small and will go hard.

While the cookies are baking, bring the syrup ingredients to a boil in a small saucepan. Reduce heat and simmer for 5 minutes. Keep warm (or reheat a few minutes before removing cookies from the oven as this must be hot). Immediately dip the hot cookies into the hot syrup, turning over once and then placing onto a platter. Do not let them soak too long. Allow to cool, and then drizzle melted chocolate over the top and sprinkle crushed pistachios. Alternatively, dust with some cinnamon powder.

Keep in a container in the refrigerator for up to 2 weeks.

*Liquors are usually available at European grocers. You can substitute with an orange liqueur.

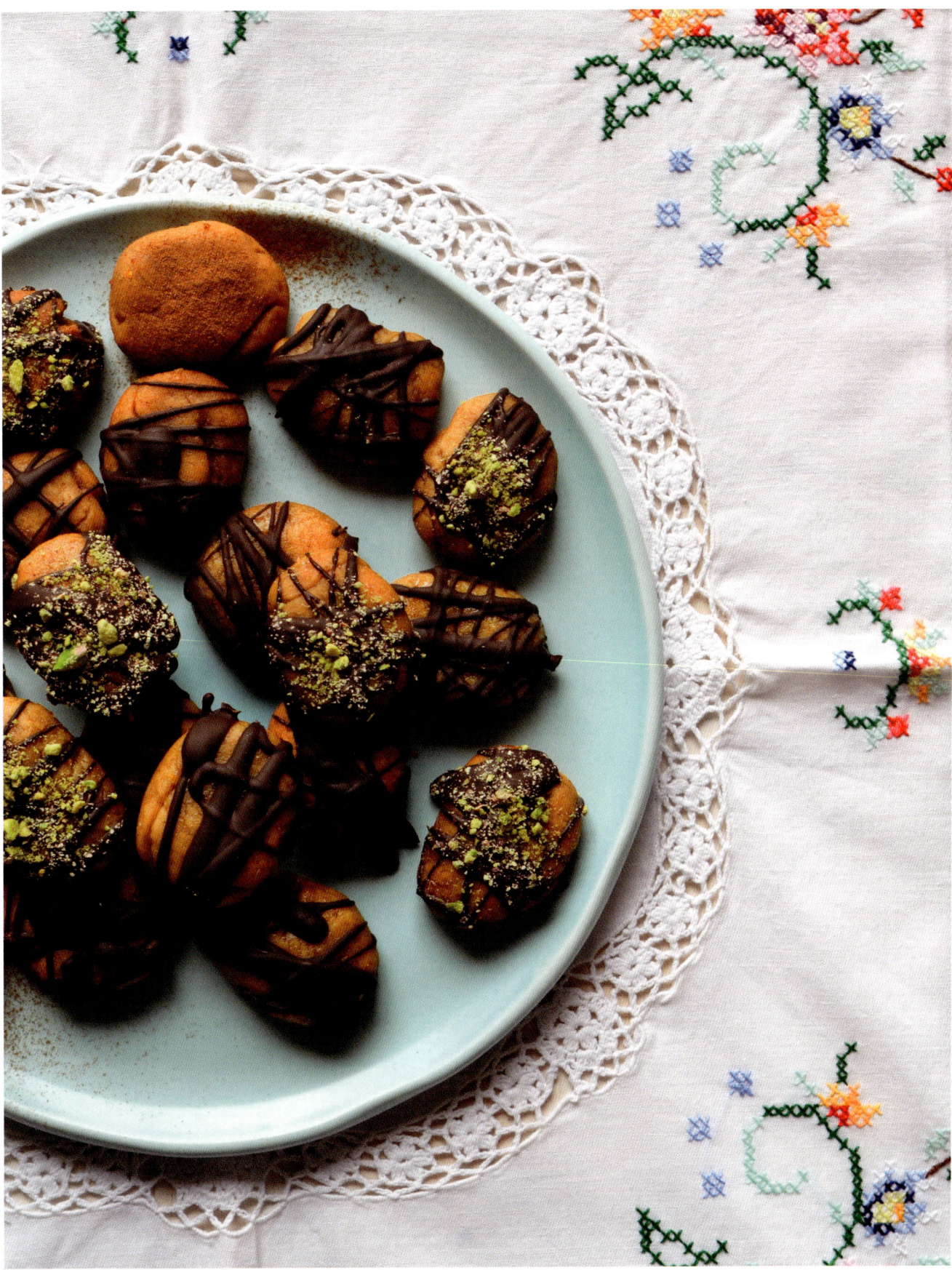

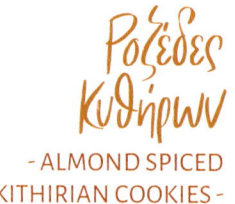

Ροζέδες Κυθήρων

- ALMOND SPICED KITHIRIAN COOKIES -

½ cup water

⅓ cup honey

2 cups raw almonds (skin on), ground, but not as fine as almond meal

½ cup roasted almonds (skin on) ground, but not as fine as almond meal

½ cup castor (super fine) sugar

¾ cup fine semolina

1½ teaspoon ground cloves

3 teaspoon cinnamon powder

1 cup rose water

1½ cups icing (confectioners) sugar

Rozedes are traditional almond cookies from Kithira, an island opposite the southeastern tip of the Peloponnese. They are nutty and beautifully spiced with cinnamon and clove and have a mellow sweetness from the honey. Once cooked and cooled, they are dipped into rose water and then liberally dusted with icing sugar to create a crust on the exterior. They are egg and dairy free and delightful with a cup of coffee. I enjoy the intensity of the added roasted almonds, but if you prefer a less nutty flavor, you can use raw almonds.

Makes: 40 pieces · 1 hour

Preheat oven to 160º C/320º F. Line a baking tray with baking paper.

Place water and honey into a small saucepan and heat on the stove to melt the honey. Add this to a bowl together with the almonds, sugar, semolina, round gcloves, and cinnamon powder. Using the back of a spoon, press down to dampen the nut mixture.

Using slightly wet hands, take a dessert spoon amount (no more than 18 g each) of mixture and gently squeeze in your palm to create a thin oval shape. The amount may seem small, but they will rise once baked. It will be sticky and a little tedious, but they should hold their shape. Keep wetting your hands to make it easier.

Place onto baking tray and bake for 25–30 minutes or until firm and slightly golden on the outside. Remove from oven and allow to cool on a rack for at least 15–20 minutes. They will seem a little hard but will soften once they get dipped in the rose water.

Take two bowls. Pour the rose water in one and put the icing sugar in the other.

Dip the cookies quickly in the rose water and immediately toss in the icing sugar. Place onto a plate. Once they are all done, repeat the icing for a second time to create a second crispy coating (the first gets absorbed by the rose water). Place onto a platter. Do not cover or store in a container as they will not retain their crispy exterior. Consume within 2–3 days.

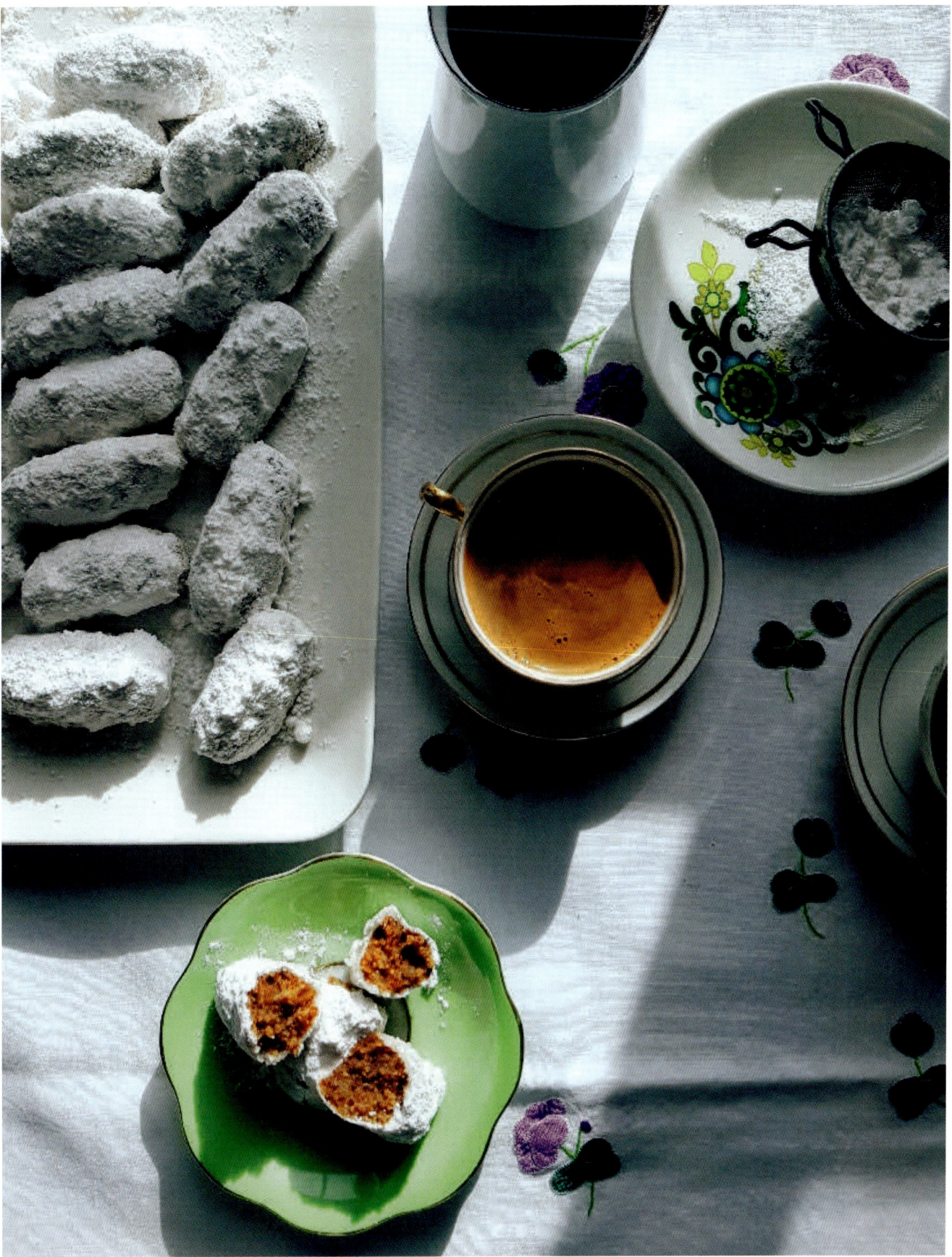

Κερκυραϊκή φογάτσα
- CORFIOT EASTER BREAD -

250 g (8.8 oz.) whole milk

250 g (8.8 oz.) castor (superfine) sugar

2 whole eggs, room temperature

1 additional whole egg (white and yolk separated)

Zest of 1½ oranges

Zest of 1 lemon

40 ml kumquat liqueur*

650 g (22.9 oz.) all-purpose flour

35 g (1.2 oz.) instant yeast

75 g (2.6 oz.) orange and lemon glacé fruits*

100 g (3.5 oz.) butter, room temperature (must be soft)

Whenever I visit a region in Greece, my curiosity to taste and learn about a produce is always at the forefront. Without a doubt, in Corfu, the kumquat fruit triggered my curiosity. Kumquats are grown extensively on this Ionian island. Hence some of the best kumquat treats such as jams, sweets, and liqueur are made there. I was so intrigued by the kumquat liquor that I even brought a bottle back with me to Australia. I knew I needed to add this traditional local recipe for Corfiot Easter bread to this chapter. This Easter bread is somewhat like the traditional tsoureki bread (recipe in my book *Hellenic Kanella: Memories Made in a Greek Kitchen*) known in all other regions of Greece except that it is flavored with kumquat, orange, and lemon rather than spices such as mastic and mahlepi. It is also made with the similar process of proving the dough twice, but it is baked as a loaf and not a braided bread. It is best enjoyed dunked into a glass of milk, coffee, or even with a shot of kumquat liqueur. You can substitute the kumquat liquor for a brandy or orange liqueur.

Makes: 16 pieces · 3.5 hours (including proving time)

Place the milk in a saucepan and heat slightly. Do not overheat. You should be able to place your finger in the milk. Remove from heat and immediately add the sugar, mixing to dissolve. Whisk together the 2 whole eggs plus one yolk, and then add this to the milk mixture. Mix. Now add the zests and liqueur, mixing well. Set aside.

Place the flour and yeast into the bowl of a mixer and mix with a spoon to distribute the yeast throughout the flour. Add the glacé fruits and pour in the milk mixture. With the paddle attachment, mix on low speed for 2–3 minutes or until all the flour has been incorporated and there is no flour around the bowl.

Now add the butter in small amounts with the mixer running on medium to high speed. Do not worry if it seems as though the dough is separating or becoming a little liquid. It will come together in the end. Once all the butter is incorporated, it will look quite stringy and chewy around the paddle. This is the texture you want to achieve. Do not add any additional flour. With buttered hands, remove the dough and gently bring together to form a ball. Place in an oiled bowl with the seam sides down so you have a perfect ball on top. Cover well with plastic wrap and set aside to rest in a warm area for a minimum of 2 hours.

Line a 20 cm/0.8 in. springform tin (base and sides) with parchment paper.

Oil your hands and gently punch the dough to deflate. Pick it up into your hands and create a ball shape again, placing the ball into the tin seam down. Press down slightly with your hands so it is even in the tin, and then set it aside in a warm place covered with a tea towel to rise for a second time. I like to heat my oven for 10 minutes on 100° C/210° F, turn it off, and place the tin in the oven (uncovered) and allow the heat to help the second rise. Leave for 1 hour and 30 minutes.

Remove from oven. Brush the egg yolk over it, and then snip the center (or use a knife) to create a cross in the center.

Preheat oven to 160° C/320° F.

Bake for 45 minutes or until a skewer inserted comes out clean and the top is golden. Allow it to cool in the tin, and then remove, slice, and enjoy with coffee.

Keeps for 3–4 days wrapped in aluminum foil or in a sealed cake tin at room temperature.

*Orange liqueur or brandy can be substituted.

*Glacé fruits can be purchased from Mediterranean grocers. Another lovely substitute is to add small chopped pieces of kumquat spoon sweet.

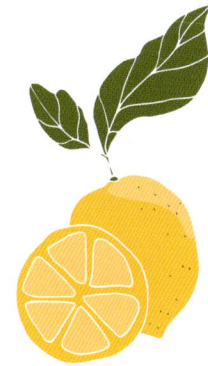

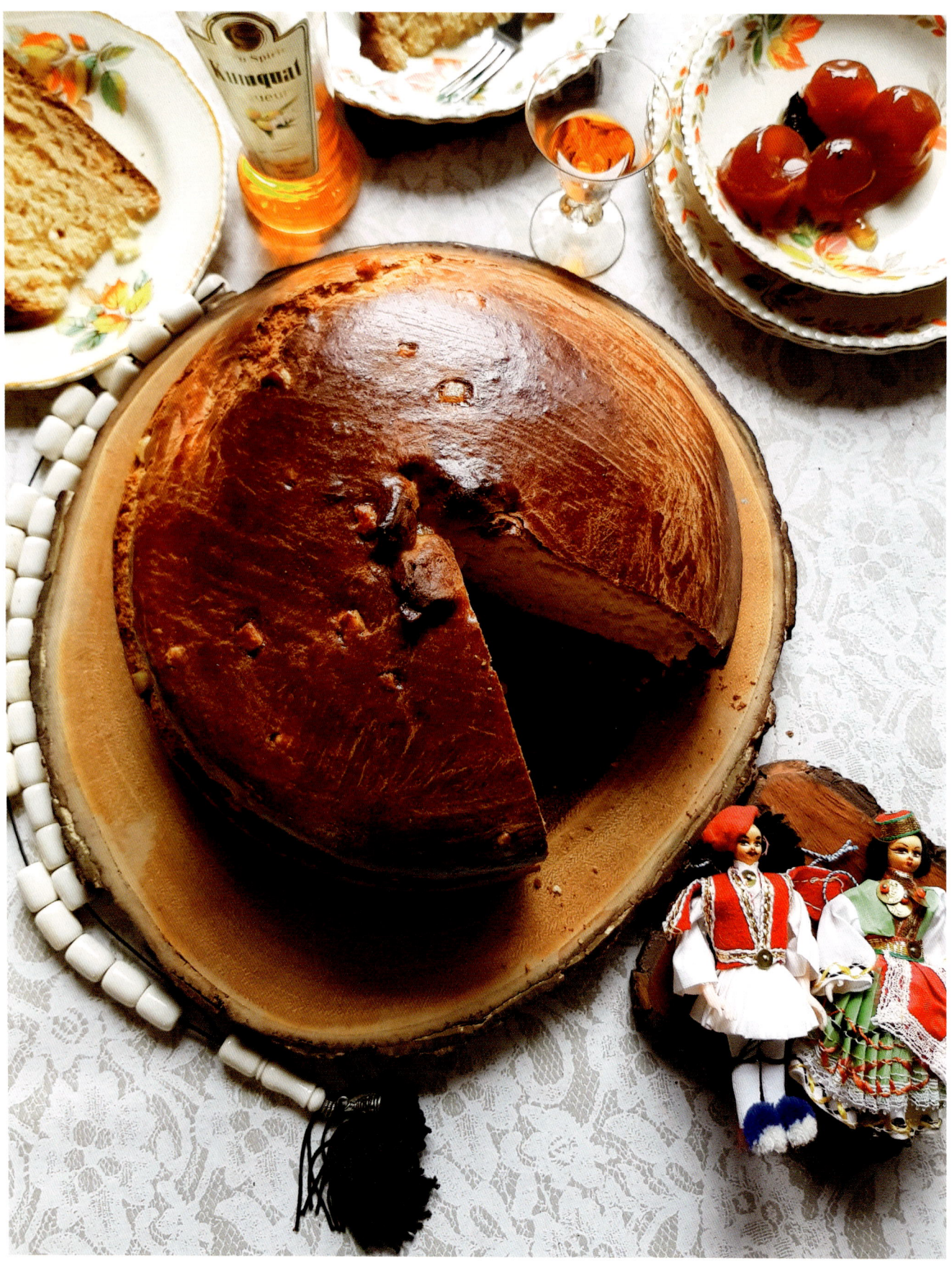

Corfiot Easter Bread, page 196-197.

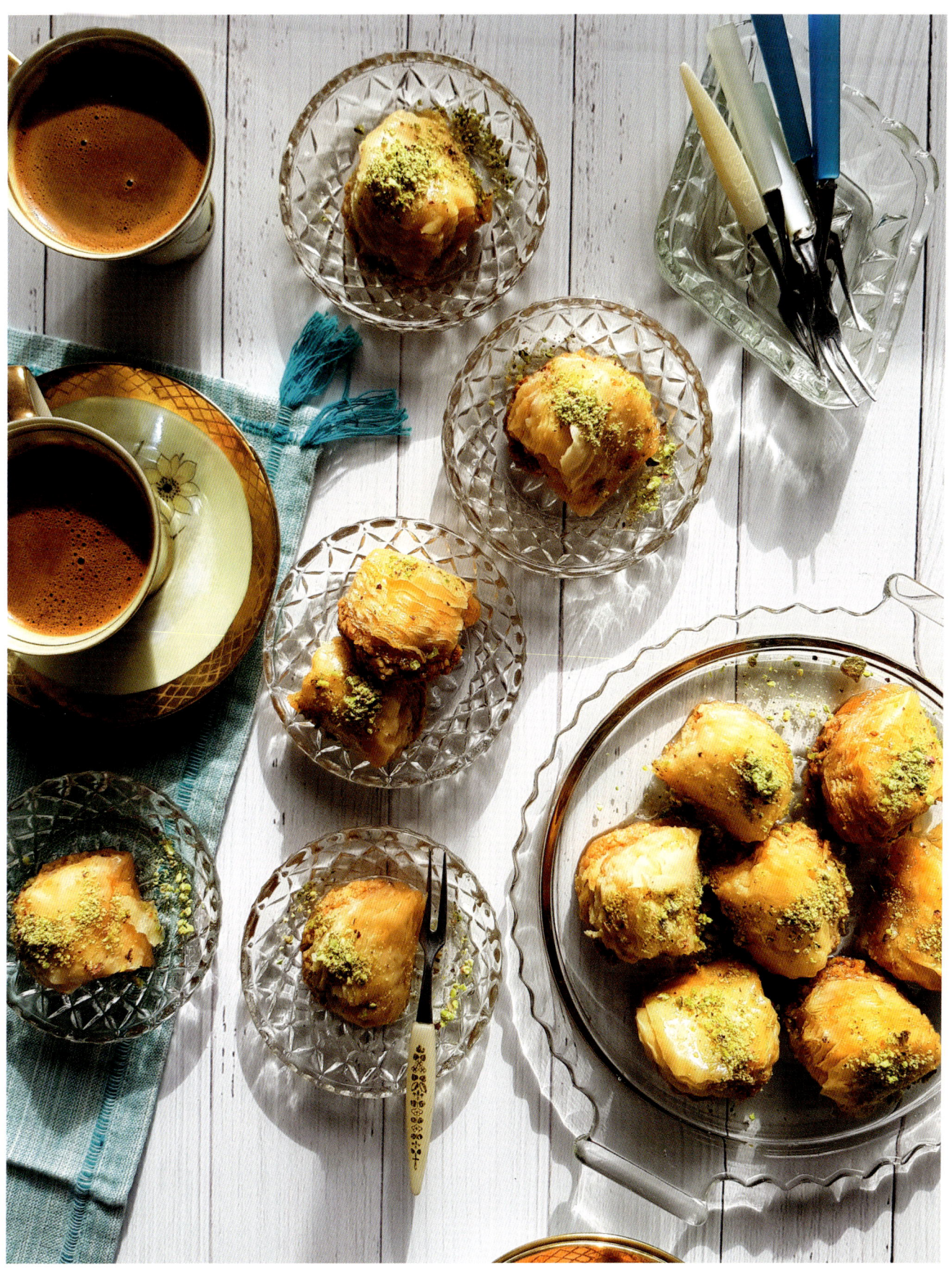

Bite-Size Cashew and Orange Baklava, page 200-201.

Μπακλαβαδάκια

- BITE-SIZE CASHEW AND ORANGE BAKLAVA -

SYRUP

2 cups castor (superfine) sugar

1 cup water

2 tablespoons lemon juice

FILLING

1½ cups crushed raw cashews

2 tablespoons castor (superfine) sugar

5 tablespoons orange blossom water*

---

18 sheets store-bought phyllo pastry, room temperature

250 g (1 cup) unsalted butter, melted

Baklava needs no specific introduction. Most people know this fabulous nutty, syrupy pastry-based dessert. Baklava comes in many shapes and sizes and is made with various nuts and spices. For this recipe, I have chosen cashews (although almonds and or walnuts can be used instead of cashews). They are bite-size and sufficiently rich to enjoy with a strong cup of Greek coffee.

Makes: 35 pieces · 1.5 hours

Preheat oven to 160° C/320° F.

Prepare the syrup first. Place the sugar and water into a saucepan. Bring to a boil, and then simmer over low heat for 8 minutes. Remove from heat and add the lemon juice. Set aside to cool completely.

Combine the cashews, sugar, and orange blossom water in a bowl. With the back of a spoon, press the mixture until evenly blended and the cashews seem damp.

Divide pastry into 3 piles of 6 sheets.

On a workbench, butter and layer 6 sheets of pastry, placing them lengthwise one at a time on top of the other. The longest length of the pastry should be facing you from left to right.

Lift the bottom left and right corners, folding it in half lengthwise. The seam should be closest to you. Brush the top with butter. Fold the phyllo in half again, keeping the seam toward you. Brush the top. Place 5–6 tablespoons of the cashew filling along the center of the phyllo. Use your fingers to bring the filling together and keep it along the middle of the pastry.

Now carefully fold the pastry in half again, tucking the filling inside. You should have a long thin pastry log filled with cashew filling. Brush the top with butter.

Use a 1½ inch cookie cutter to cut the individual *baklavadakia*. Start at one end of the pastry. Place the cookie cutter just below the upper edge where the two flaps meet. Press down and cut all the way through. By cutting just below the edges, you will be cutting through the phyllo creating the layers. The seam end should not be cut at all—otherwise they will fall apart. In essence, the bottom section of the cutter is not cutting anything. It should be placed just below the seam. Each log should cut around 10 *baklavadakia*.

Repeat with the other 2 piles of pastry.

Place *baklavadakia* onto a lined baking tray and bake for 40 minutes or until golden underneath. You do not want them too golden on the top. Remove from oven and place onto a dish.

Pour cooled syrup over the *baklavadakia* and allow to soak for a minimum of 3 hours.

Sprinkle crushed pistachios over the top and enjoy.

*Orange blossom water can be purchased from international grocers. It can be substituted with rose water.

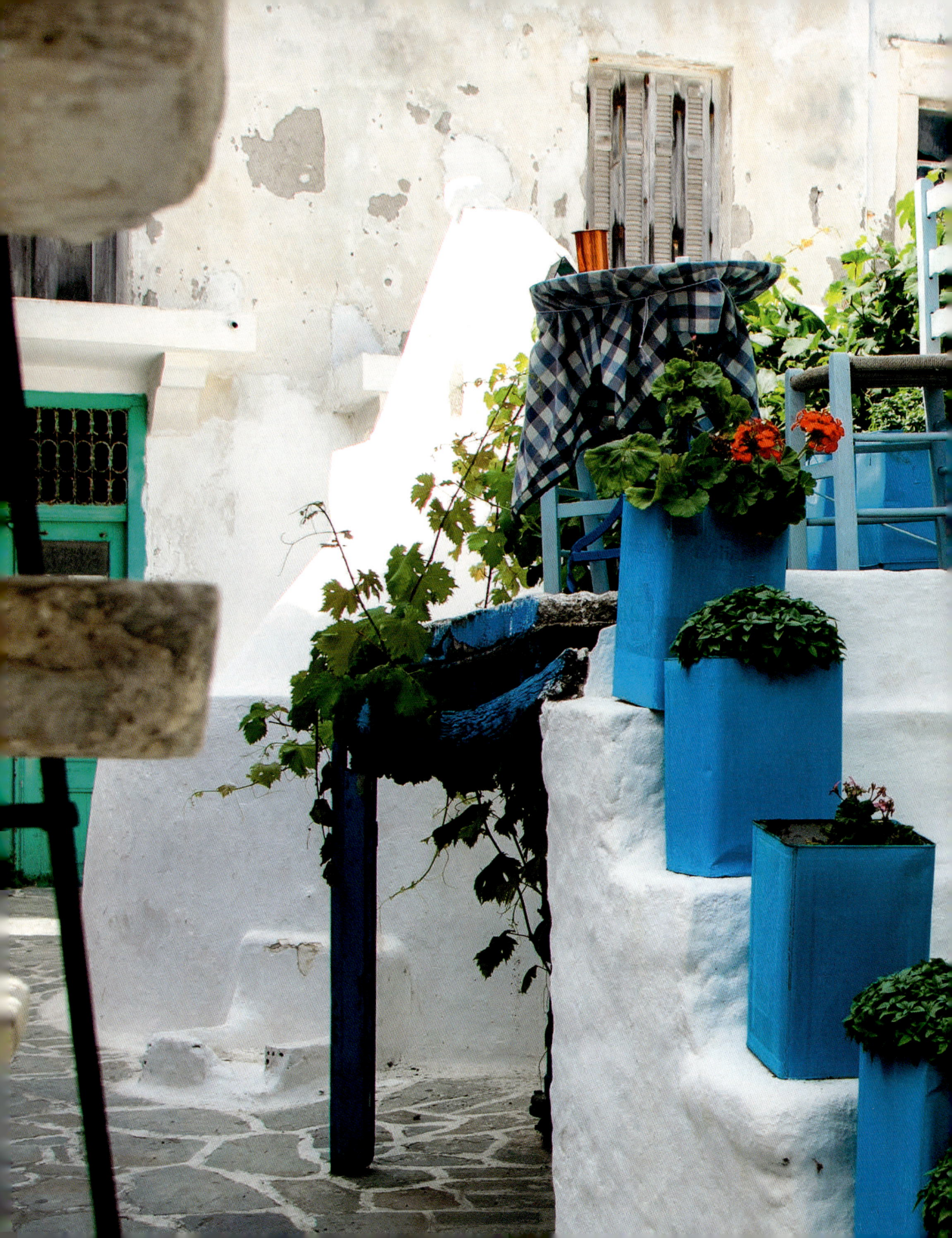

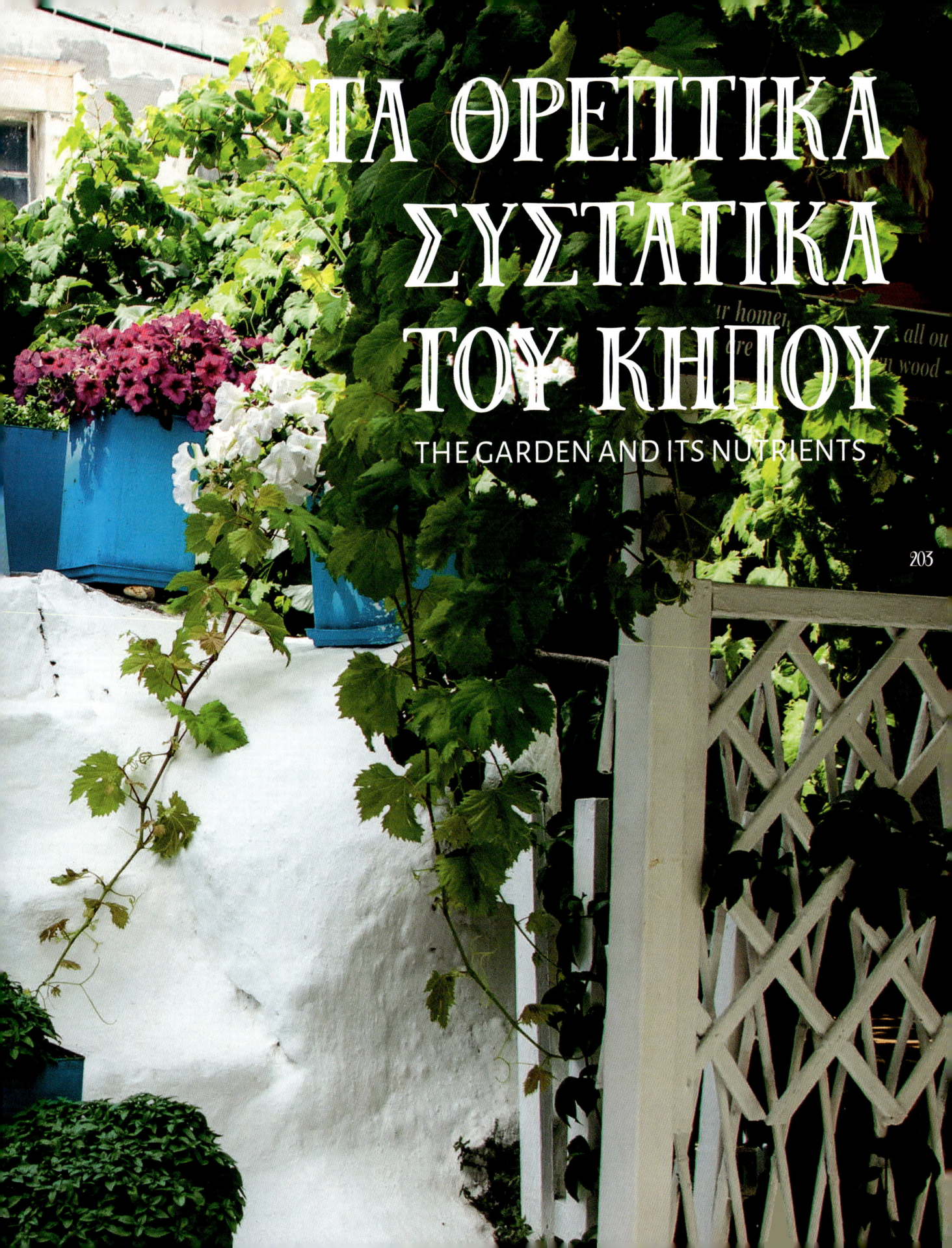

ΤΑ ΘΡΕΠΤΙΚΑ ΣΥΣΤΑΤΙΚΑ ΤΟΥ ΚΗΠΟΥ

THE GARDEN AND ITS NUTRIENTS

LICORICE
ΓΛΥΚΑΝΙΣΟΣ

DESCRIPTION:
The licorice plant is an herbaceous perennial legume native to Western Asia, North Africa, and Southern Europe. Licorice is a woody-stemmed perennial herb that grows to about 1–2 meters.

CULTURE:
You can grow licorice plants from seeds or from a broken-off rhizome. If planting from seeds, start seeds indoors in the fall and transplant in the spring. Rhizomes can be planted directly outdoors in the spring or summer.

BENEFITS:
Licorice root is said to have anti-inflammatory, antiviral, antibacterial, antifungal, and anti-allergic qualities.

IT MAY:
· relieve stomach ailments,
· prevent tooth decay,
· relieve rheumatoid arthritis,
· boost the immune system,
· and alleviate depression.

USES:
Used to flavor meats, fish dishes, breads, desserts, and liquors. Can also be made into tea.

BASIL
ΒΑΣΙΛΙΚΟΣ

DESCRIPTION:
Basil, also called great basil, is a culinary herb of the family Lamiaceae.

CULTURE:
Best grown from seeds and planted in summer.

BENEFITS:
Basil herb contains minerals such as potassium, manganese, copper, magnesium, iron, and vitamin K.

IT MAY:
· aid digestion,
· decrease inflammation,
· help lower cholesterol,
· and help prevent anemia.

USES:
Basil can be eaten raw in salads, in pesto, and is great in green smoothies. It pairs wonderfully with tomato dishes.

BELL PEPPERS
ΠΙΠΕΡΙΕΣ

DESCRIPTION:
Bell peppers are also called sweet pepper or capsicums. They are from the nightshade family (Solanaceae).

CULTURE:
Seeds or small plant. Best planted in the spring.

BENEFITS:
High in iron, vitamins C, B6, K1, E, potassium, and folate.

IT MAY:
· prevent hypertension,
· lower bad cholesterol,
· boost eye health,
· and boost immunity.

USES:
Can be eaten raw or cooked.

BEANS
ΦΑΣΟΛΑΚΙΑ

DESCRIPTION:
Green beans are an herbaceous plant that belongs to the legume family (Fabaceae).

CULTURE:
From seeds. Best planted in the spring.

BENEFITS:
Full of dietary fiber, loaded with vitamin C, A, K, iron, and folic acid.

THEY MAY:
· control blood sugar,
· lower high blood pressure,
· promote cardiovascular health,
· and help strengthen immunity.

USES:
Can be eaten cooked or raw.

Note: I am not a health professional.
Consult your physician for any further clarification.

DESCRIPTION:
Beets (Beta vulgaris) are biennial root vegetables grown for their edible root and leaves.

CULTURE:
Plant with either seeds or seedlings. Best to plant in the warmer (not wet) seasons.

BENEFITS:
High in iron, folate, and manganese. Also high in thiamine, riboflavin, vitamin B6, choline, phosphorus, potassium, zinc, selenium, magnesium, and pantothenic acid.

IT MAY:
· aid the immune system,
· aid nerve and muscle function,
· lower blood pressure,
· detoxify the liver,
· and boost energy.

USES:
It can be eaten raw or cooked

BEETS
ΠΑΤΖΑΡΙ

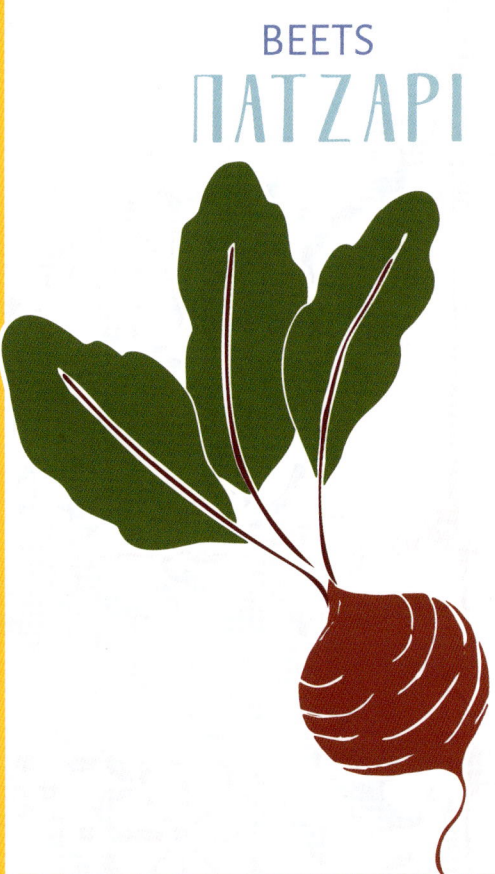

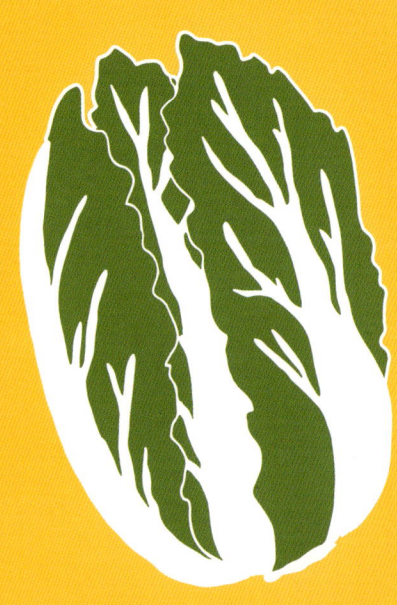

LETTUCE
ΜΑΡΟΥΛΙ

DESCRIPTION:
Lettuce (Lactuca sativa) is an annual leaf vegetable of the aster family (Asteraceae).

CULTURE:
Best grown from seeds and planted through the cooler months.

BENEFITS:
Lettuce is generally a rich source of vitamins K and A, though the nutritional quality varies depending on the variety.

IT MAY:
· aid with weight loss,
· fight inflammation,
· relieve constipation,
· help treat insomnia,
· and boost immunity.

USES:
Most lettuce varieties are eaten fresh and are commonly served as the base of green salads.

CUCUMBER
ΑΓΓΟΥΡΙ

DESCRIPTION:
Cucumber (Cucumis sativus) is a warm season annual plant grown for its edible fruit.

CULTURE:
Best grown from seeds and planted in the spring.

IT MAY:
· relieve arthritic pain,
· promote joint health,
· dissolve kidney and bladder stones,
· regulate body temperature,
· promote hair growth,
· hydrate (it is 98 percent water),
· and prevent headache.

BENEFITS:
High in nutrients, antioxidants, micronutrients, and promotes hydration.

USES:
Eaten raw, used in smoothies, or tossed in fresh salads.

EGGPLANT
ΜΕΛΙΤΖΑΝΑ

DESCRIPTION:
The eggplant, also known as aubergine, is a plant species in the nightshade family, Solanaceae. Typically used as a vegetable in cooking, it is a berry by botanical definition.

CULTURE:
Plant seeds in the spring.

BENEFITS:
Packed with fiber, vitamins B1, B3, B6, C, K, and phytonutrients.

IT MAY:
· improve blood flow,
· promote bone health,
· control cholesterol levels,
· and regulate blood pressure.

USES:
Eggplants in cooking can be mashed, roasted, grilled, and baked. Mostly used in savory cooking, eggplants can also be used in a dessert such as spoon sweet.

DILL
ΑΝΗΘΟΣ

DESCRIPTION:
Dill is an annual herb in the celery family, Apiaceae.

CULTURE:
Best grown from seeds. Plant in the spring or early summer.

BENEFITS:
Excellent source of antioxidants, vitamin C, and fiber.

IT MAY:
· help aid digestion and reduce gas,
· soothe menstrual disorders,
· boost the immune system,
· and protect against arthritis and other inflammatory diseases.

USES:
Used as a garnish in salads and stews. Pairs well with fish dishes.

GARLIC
ΣΚΟΡΔΟ

DESCRIPTION:
Because of the odor, garlic is sometimes known as the "stinking rose." Allium sativum is a perennial flowering plant grown from a bulb.

CULTURE:
Garlic cloves are planted in the ground. Garlic is an annual crop that is best planted in autumn.

BENEFITS:
Garlic is an excellent source of vitamin B6 (pyridoxine), manganese, selenium, antioxidants, and vitamin C. Garlic is a good source of other minerals, including phosphorous, calcium, potassium, iron, and copper.

It has antibacterial, antiviral, and antifungal properties and may
· aid in weight loss,
· boost immunity,
· aid in cold and flu prevention,
· and promote eye health.

USES:
Can be eaten raw or cooked in savory dishes.

MINT
ΔΥΟΣΜΟΣ

DESCRIPTION:
A very aromatic herb that comes from the Lamiaceae family.

CULTURE:
Recommended from cuttings. Best to plant spring or autumn.

BENEFITS:
Good source of protein, thiamine, niacin, phosphorus, fiber, vitamin A, C, B6, riboflavin, folate, calcium, iron, and magnesium.

IT MAY:
· promote digestion,
· improve oral health,
· help treat nausea and headaches,
· improve memory,
· relieve indigestion,
· and prevent allergies.

USES:
Best matched with vegetables, lamb, fruit, and sauces.

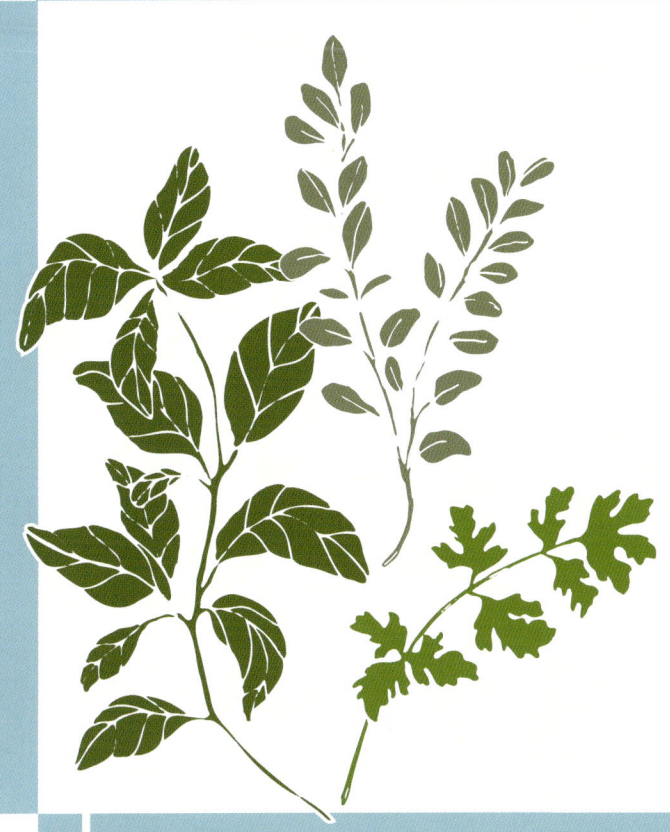

OREGANO
ΡΙΓΑΝΗ

DESCRIPTION:
Oregano is a plant derived from the mint family and is native to the Mediterranean region. The name is derived from the Greek word origanon, meaning "joy of the mountain" (oros, meaning "mountain," and the verb ganousthai, "delight in").

CULTURE:
Can be grown from seeds or cuttings. Best to plant late spring and early summer.

BENEFITS:
Oregano has folate, magnesium, vitamin A, and potassium, is rich in antioxidants and omega-3 fatty acids, and has antifungal and antibacterial properties.

IT MAY:
· boost the immune system,
· improve digestion,
· strengthen the bones,
· improve heart health,
· help aid against diabetes,
· and increase production of white blood cells, which aids in faster recovery from illness.

USES:
Best matched with meats, fish, vegetables, salads.

PARSLEY
ΜΑΪΝΤΑΝΟΣ

DESCRIPTION:
Parsley (Petroselinum crispum) is a hardy biennial herb of the family Apiaceae (or Umbelliferae) native to the Mediterranean.

CULTURE:
From seeds or cutting. Best planted in the spring.

BENEFITS:
Loaded with vitamins A, C, and K.

IT MAY:
· soothe indigestion,
· boost immunity,
· prevent bladder infection,
· reduce gas and constipation,
· decrease inflammation,
· and improve bone health.

USES:
Parsley can be used as garnish and in salads and be eaten fresh or cooked. Pairs well with fish and rice.

DESCRIPTION:
A robust woody herb native to the Mediterranean with a lemon-pine, slightly peppery flavor.

CULTURE:
Recommended from cuttings. Best to plant during spring in well-drained soil.

BENEFITS:
Fresh rosemary is a source of minerals like calcium, magnesium, iron, manganese, and copper. It also has high levels of vitamin C, A, B6 and antioxidants, and it has anti-inflammatory properties.

IT MAY:
· improve memory,
· stimulate brain function,
· stimulate hair growth,
· alleviate headaches,
· prevent high blood sugar,
· and improve digestion.

USES:
Best matched with meats, legumes, and vegetables.

ROSEMARY
ΔΕΝΤΡΟΛΙΒΑΝΟ

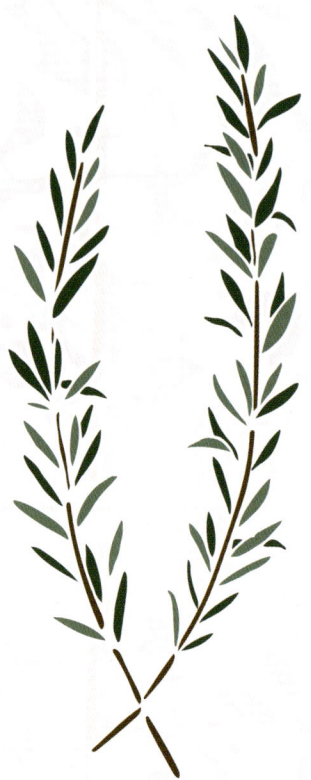

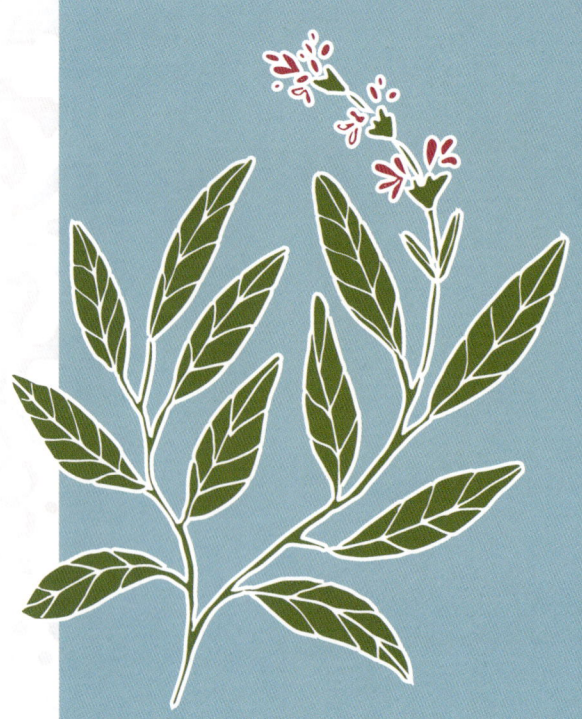

SAGE
ΦΑΣΚΟΜΗΛΟ

DESCRIPTION:
Sage, known as Salvia officinalis and also called common sage or garden sage, is an aromatic herb of the mint family (Lamiaceae). Sage is native to the Mediterranean region.

CULTURE:
The easiest and best way to grow sage is to plant a small cutting.

BENEFITS:
Sage is rich in vitamins K, A, C and antioxidants.

IT MAY:
· boost cognition,
· treat inflammation,
· strengthen immunity,
· improve bone health,
· and aid digestion.

USES:
Can be eaten fresh or dried. Pairs with poultry and pork and is used in stuffing sausages. Also consumed as a tea.

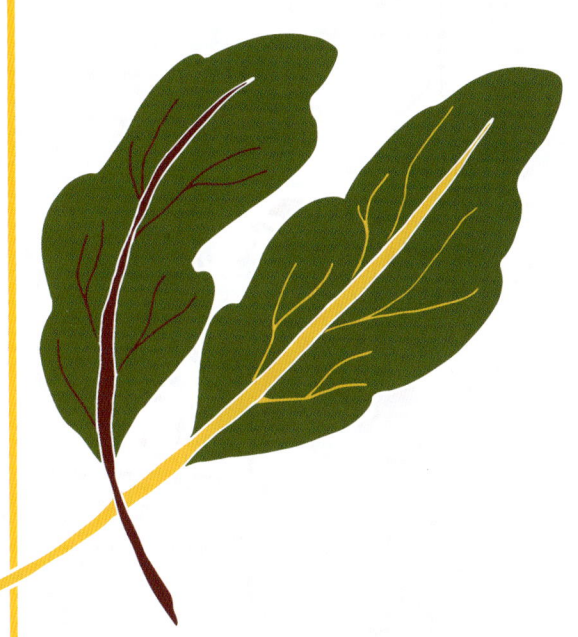

SILVERBEET
ΣΕΣΚΟΥΛΑ

DESCRIPTION:
Silverbeet is also known as Swiss chard. It is an annual or biennial vegetable with large leaves.

CULTURE:
Can be grown from a small plant or seeds generally all year round.

BENEFITS:
Good source of calcium, magnesium, and vitamin K, C, and A. It is rich in fiber and a great source of iron.

IT MAY:
· promote bone health,
· regulate blood sugar levels,
· help boost immunity,
· and promote brain health.

USES:
Eaten raw or cooked.

DESCRIPTION:
Spinach is an annual cool season green, leafy vegetable.

CULTURE:
Seeds are best. Plant through the colder months, autumn through winter.

BENEFITS:
Rich in vitamins K1, K2, C, folate, fiber, and antioxidants.

IT MAY:
· aid digestion,
· reduce inflammation,
· lower high blood pressure,
· strengthen bones,
· promote eye health,
· and strengthen the cardiovascular system.

USES:
Eaten raw or cooked.

SPINACH
ΣΠΑΝΑΚΙ

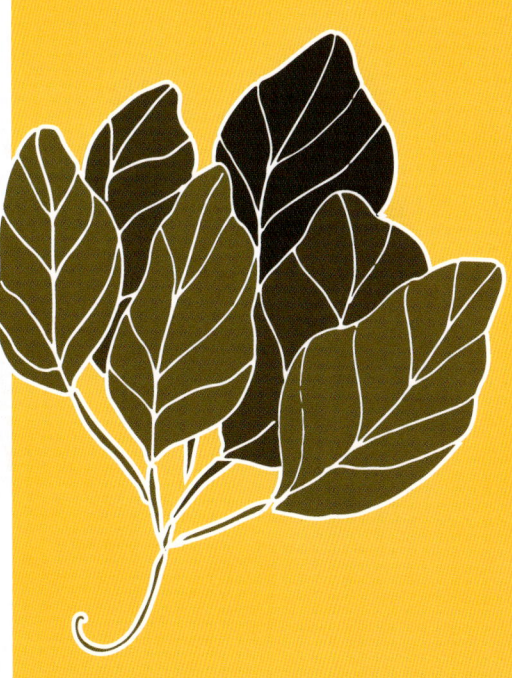

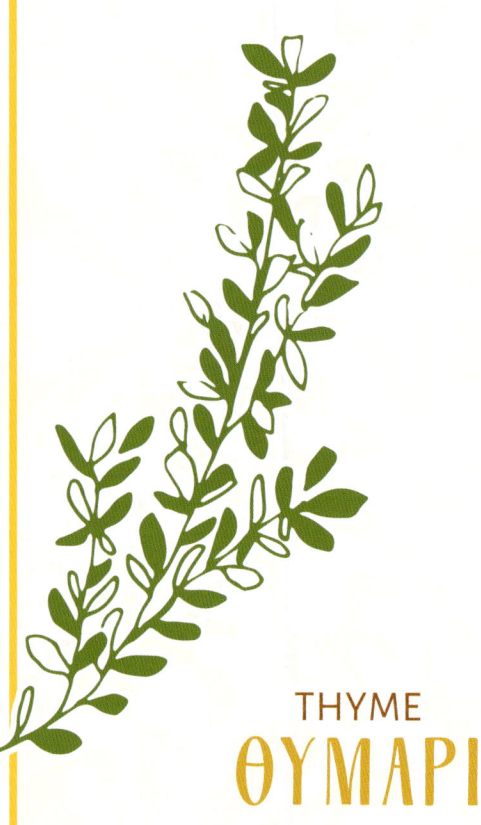

THYME
ΘΥΜΑΡΙ

DESCRIPTION:
Thyme, Thymus vulgaris, is a perennial evergreen shrub from the mint family (Lamiaceae). Stems are stiff and woody, and leaves are small. Flowers can be white to lilac and grow in small clusters. Thyme is highly aromatic and has a hint of clove and mint fragrance.

CULTURE:
Thyme can be grown from seeds, plant divisions, or seedlings. However, growing thyme from seeds can be difficult, so thyme cuttings are best. Best grown in the spring and harvested in the summer.

BENEFITS:
Thyme is packed with vitamin C, A, copper, iron, manganese, potassium, phosphorus, and antioxidants like thymol and carvacrol.

IT MAY:
· relieve sore throat,
· lower blood pressure and cholesterol,
· boost immunity,
· and aid in brain health.

USES:
Brewed and drunk as a tea. Thyme pairs with meat such as lamb or chicken, tomatoes, and beans. Also used to flavor stews and soups.

DESCRIPTION:
Spring onions, known as Allium cepa (Allium means "garlic" in Latin and fistulosum means "hollow stemmed"). They are young onion plants that have been harvested prematurely, belonging to the Amaryllidaceae family. Both the long, slender green tops and the small white bulb are edible.

CULTURE:
You can grow spring onions from a previous spring onion or seed. Best planted in the spring.

BENEFITS:
It is rich in antioxidants, vitamins K, C, and B, including folate (B9) and pyridoxine (B6), and it has traces of copper, magnesium, chromium, phosphorus, potassium, and sulfur. It also has antiviral and anti-inflammatory properties.

IT MAY:
prevent arthritis and reduce nasal congestion.

USES:
Can be eaten raw in salads or as garnish and cooked in savory dishes.

SPRING ONION
ΦΡΕΣΚΟ ΚΡΕΜΜΥΔΑΚΙ

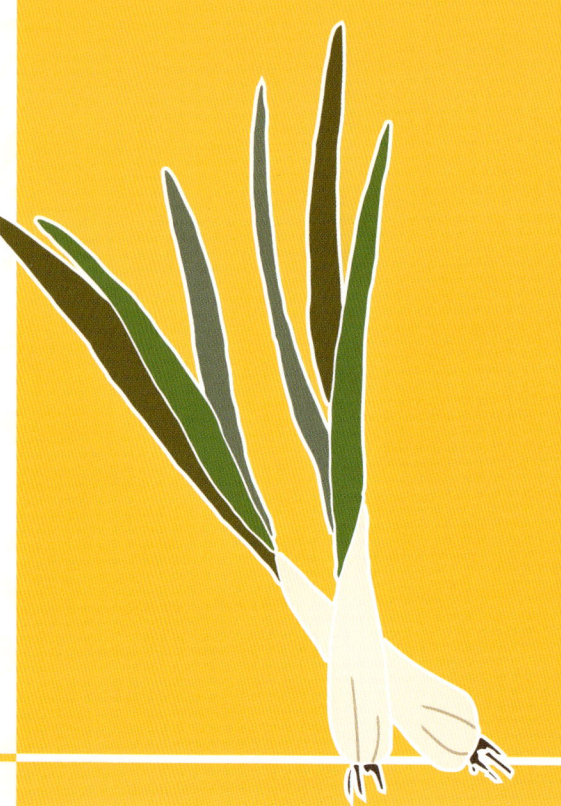

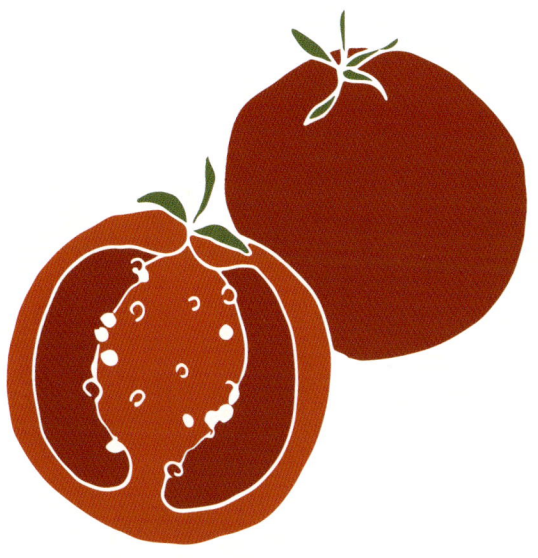

TOMATO
ΝΤΟΜΑΤΑ

DESCRIPTION:
Tomato (Solanum lycopersicum) is a flowering plant of the nightshade family cultivated extensively for its edible fruits.

CULTURE:
Best planted in the late spring.

BENEFITS:
High in vitamin A, E, C, potassium, and antioxidants.

IT MAY:
· reduce risk of heart disease,
· boost immunity,
· promote healthy skin,
· reduce migraines,
· improve vision,
· support healthy prostate,
· and lower hypertension.

USES:
Eaten raw and cooked.

DESCRIPTION:
Zucchini (Cucurbita pepo), also called a courgette, is a variety of summer squash grown for its edible fruits. Zucchini fruit grows quickly and is harvested within two to seven days of flowering.

CULTURE:
From seeds in the spring.

BENEFITS:
High in antioxidants, vitamin C, potassium, and is rich in water.

IT MAY:
· promote good digestion,
· help lower cholesterol,
· help lower blood pressure,
· fight inflammation,
· and prevent heart attacks and strokes.

USES:
Eaten raw in salads. It also can be baked, grilled, and fried.

ZUCCHINI
ΚΟΛΟΚΥΘΑΚΙ

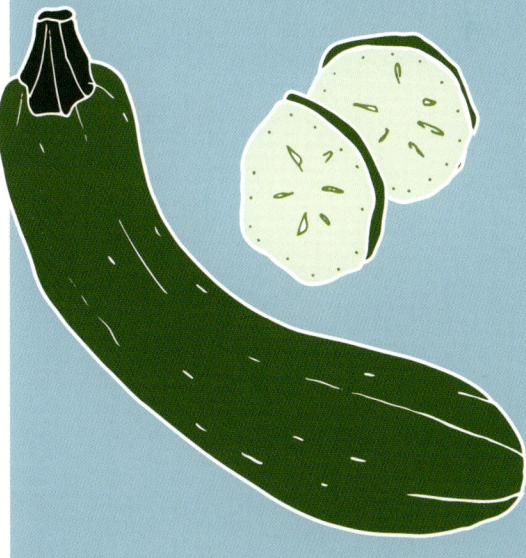

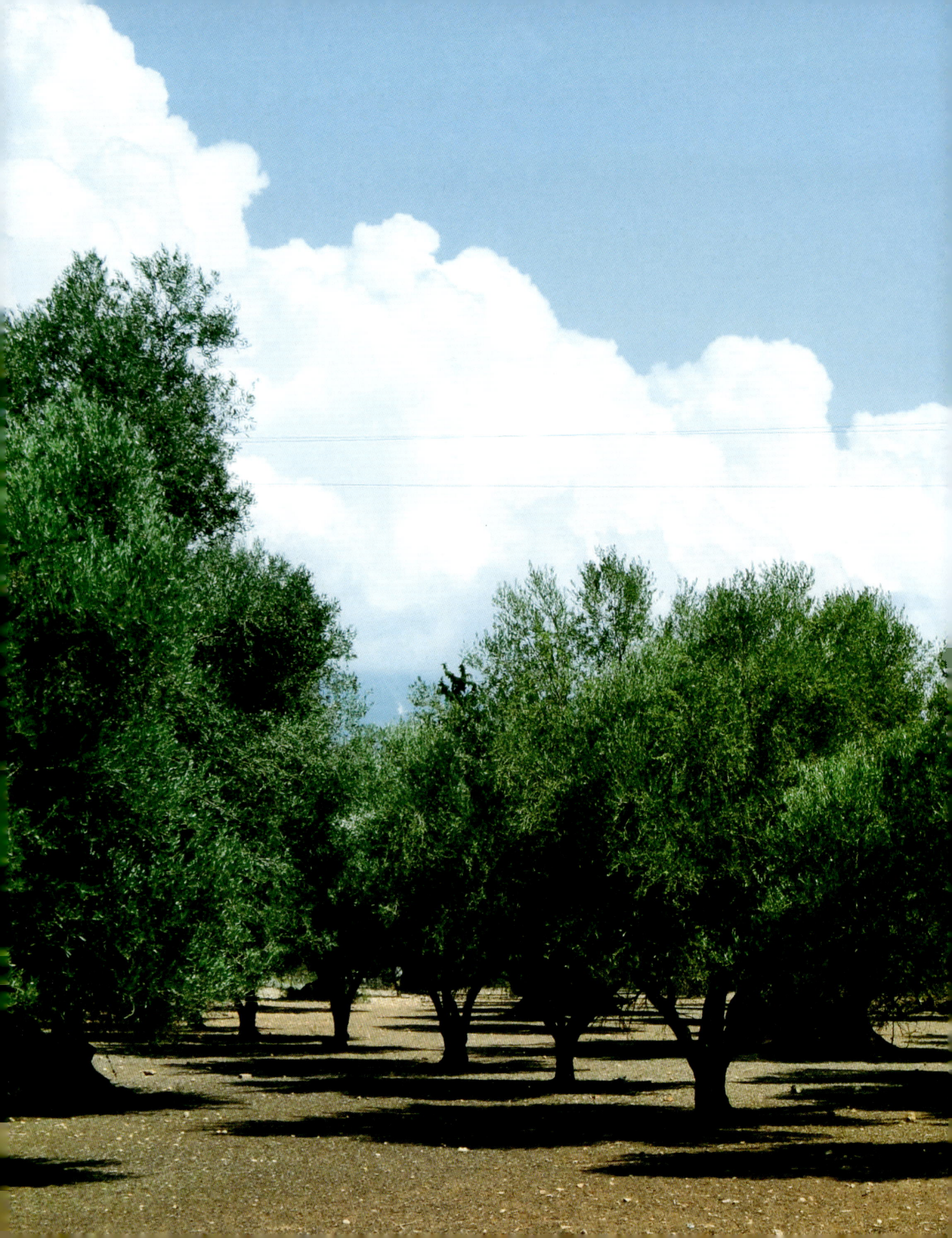

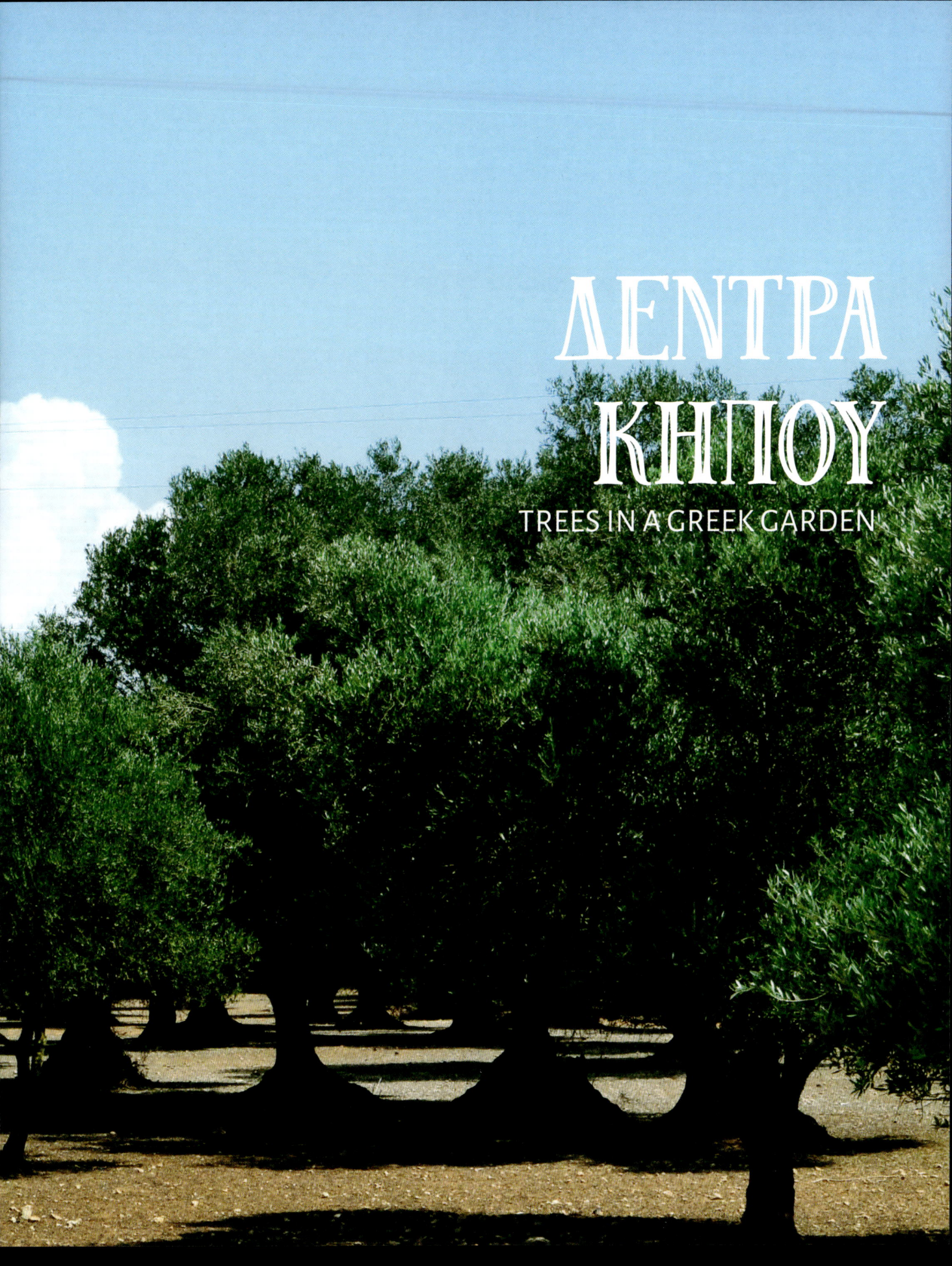

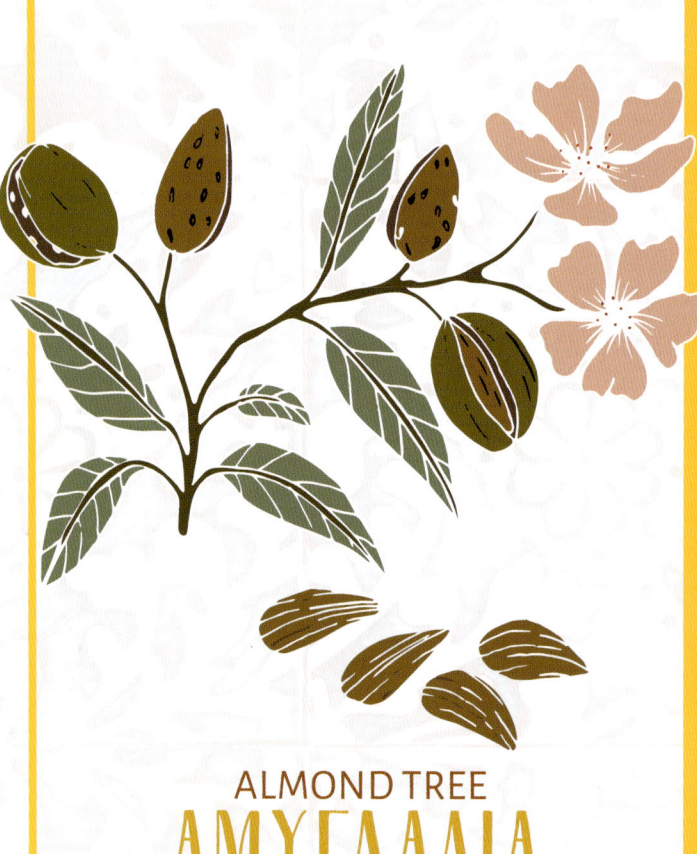

ALMOND TREE
ΑΜΥΓΔΑΛΙΑ

DESCRIPTION:
The almond belongs to the rose family (Rosaceae).

CULTURE:
Small plant. Best to plant in winter.

BENEFITS:
High levels of vitamin E and B12. Almonds are high in magnesium, phosphorus, and calcium.

IT MAY:
· help reduce LDL cholesterol,
· lower blood pressure,
· strengthen bones,
· prevent cardiovascular disease,
· and reduce inflammation.

USES:
Eaten raw as a snack, tossed in salads, and added to desserts.

DESCRIPTION:
Bay leaves, botanically classified as Laurus nobilis, are the foliage of the shrublike evergreen tree the bay laurel, which belongs to the avocado family.

CULTURE:
Spring is the best time to plant a bay tree.

BENEFITS:
Excellent source of vitamins B, C, niacin, and riboflavin. Bay leaves also have minerals such as copper, potassium, calcium, manganese, iron, selenium, zinc, and magnesium.

IT MAY:
· lower cholesterol,
· aid in managing diabetes,
· help lower stress hormones in body,
· and reduce inflammation of sore joints and arthritis.

USES:
Can be used fresh or dry. Leaves must be removed as you cannot eat them. They are used to flavor soups, stews, braises, and dessert syrups.

BAY TREE
ΔΑΦΝΗ

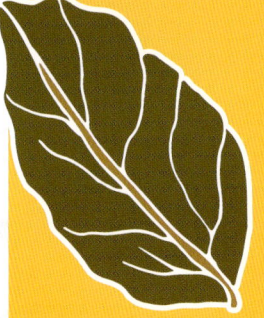
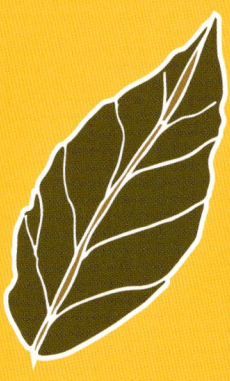

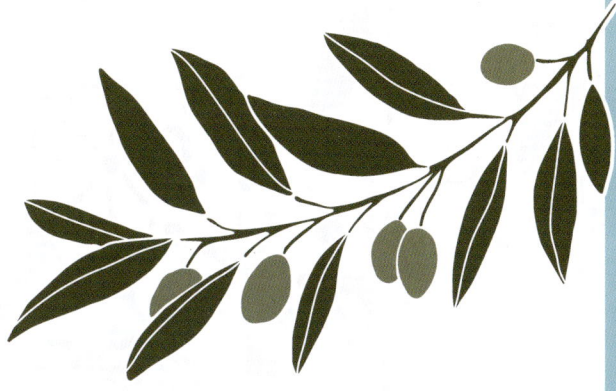

OLIVE TREE
ΕΛΙΑ

DESCRIPTION:
The olive tree, Olea europaea, is an evergreen tree or shrub native to Mediterranean Europe, Asia, and Africa.

CULTURE:
Small plant. Planted in autumn or spring.

BENEFITS:
Olives are rich in antioxidants, iron, calcium, fiber, copper, vitamin E and K, choline, sodium, phenolic compounds, and oleic acid.

IT MAY:
· help fight inflammation,
· aid in digestion,
· protect against colon and other cancers,
· help decrease inflammation,
· lower cholesterol,
· prevent osteoporosis,
· improve skin and hair,
· and protect against peptic ulcers.

USES:
Eaten as a snack, tossed through salads, incorporated in stews.

DESCRIPTION:
Oranges are a hybrid of the pomelo, or Chinese grapefruit (which is pale green or yellow), and the tangerine.

CULTURE:
From either seeds or plant. Best planted in the spring.

BENEFITS:
It is high in calcium, fiber, vitamin C, potassium, folate, and antioxidants. It also has antibacterial, anti-inflammatory, and antiaging properties.

IT MAY:
· promote good gut health,
· fight viral infections,
· regulate blood pressure,
· help manage diabetes,
· and prevent cardiovascular disease.

USES:
It can be used in desserts and salads, and it can be juiced or eaten raw.

ORANGE TREE
ΠΟΡΤΟΚΑΛΙΑ

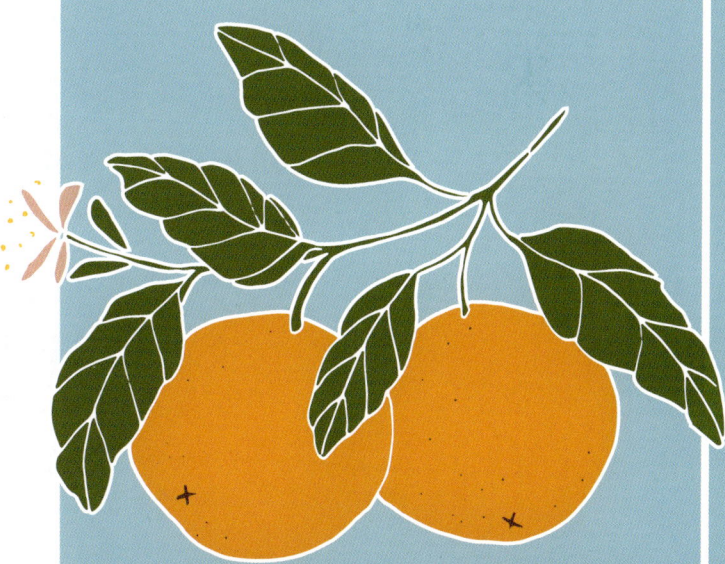

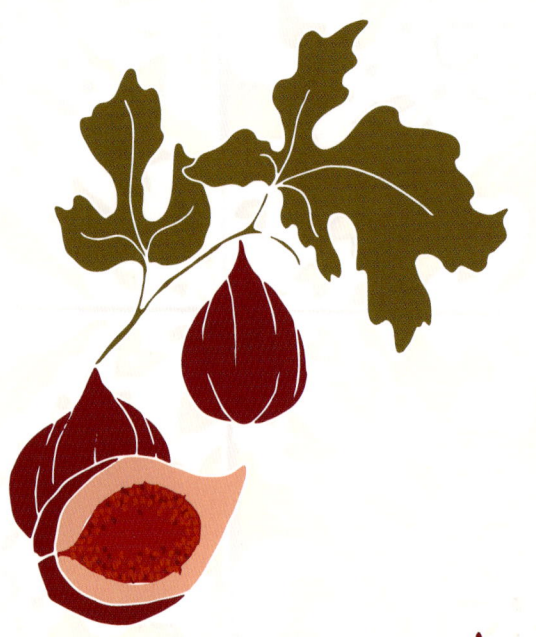

FIG TREE
ΣΥΚΙΑ

DESCRIPTION:
Figs are grown on the Ficus tree, which is a part of the mulberry family (Moraceae). Wild fig trees were first grown in West Asia, South Asia, Africa, and the Mediterranean Sea.

CULTURE:
A small fig tree is best planted from a cutting. Plant during the autumn and winter so the trees can establish themselves while it is cold.

BENEFITS:
Figs are an excellent source vitamins and minerals essential for bone health, including potassium, calcium, potassium, phosphorus, copper, iron, and vitamin A. They contain more dietary fiber than any other fresh or dried fruit and are rich in antimicrobial properties.

IT MAY:
· boost immunity,
· promote heart health,
· treat constipation,
· and help control blood sugar.

USES:
Figs can be eaten raw or cooked. Figs enhance meat dishes and can be tossed in salads, drizzled with honey and served with yogurt, served alongside wine and cheese, or even be made into jams.

GRAPEVINE
ΚΛΗΜΑΤΑΡΙΑ

DESCRIPTION:
The grapevine is a vining plant. It has no solid upright trunk.

CULTURE:
Late winter and early spring are the best times to plant a grapevine.

BENEFITS:
Grapes are a good source of vitamin K, A, B1, B2, B6, C. Vine leaves have omega-3 fatty acids, antioxidants, magnesium, and calcium.

GRAPES MAY:
· strengthen muscle and bones,
· prevent constipation,
· lower blood pressure,
· and increase good cholesterol.

VINE LEAVES MAY:
· help with pain,
· fight inflammation,
· and improve blood circulation.

USES:
Grapes can be eaten raw. Vine leaves can be baked or fried, but they are always consumed cooked.

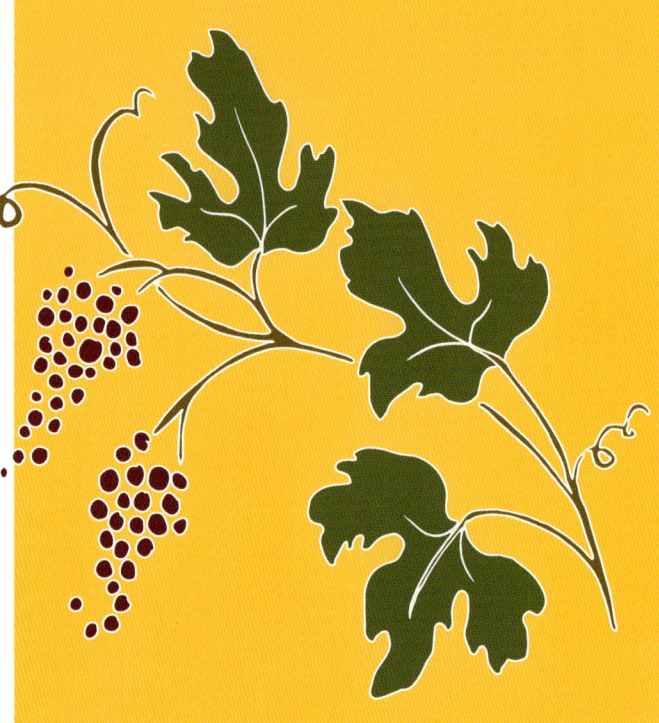

DESCRIPTION:
The lemon (Citrus limon) is a species of small evergreen tree in the flowering plant family Rutaceae.

CULTURE:
Plant trees any time of year, though preferably in warmer climates.

BENEFITS:
It is loaded with vitamin C and antioxidants.

IT MAY:
· boost immunity,
· purify liver, kidney, and blood,
· reduce fever,
· increase concentration,
· lower stress and anxiety,
· improve digestion,
· lower blood pressure,
· and improve cholesterol.

USES:
Lemons are used for culinary and nonculinary purposes, primarily for their juice, which has uses for both cooking and cleaning. Can be used raw or in cooking.

LEMON TREE
ΛΕΜΟΝΙΑ

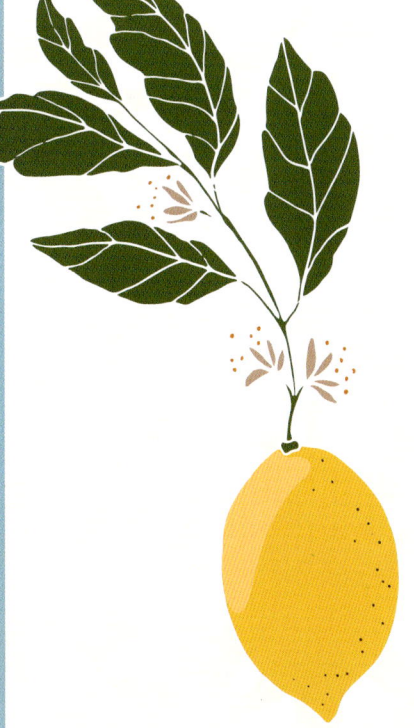

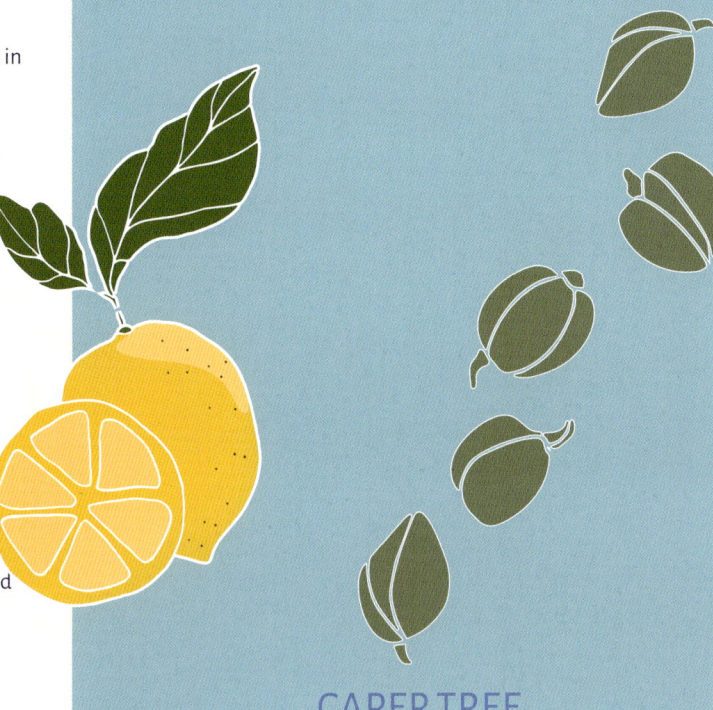

CAPER TREE
ΚΑΠΠΑΡΗ

DESCRIPTION:
The caper plant (Capparis spinosa) grows wild in hot climates on dry, rocky soil. It is a deciduous perennial low shrub utilized for its edible buds and berries. The caper is the bud before it flowers. The caper berry is the fruit after it flowers.

CULTURE:
Best grown from seeds. Must be planted in a dry, hot climate. Humidity kills the plant. Best to plant at the beginning of summer.

BENEFITS:
It is loaded with antioxidants and is high in fiber, sodium, vitamin K, and polyphenols.

IT MAY:
· boost bone health,
· help with blood clotting,
· and reduce inflammation.

USES:
Can be used in salads and dips.

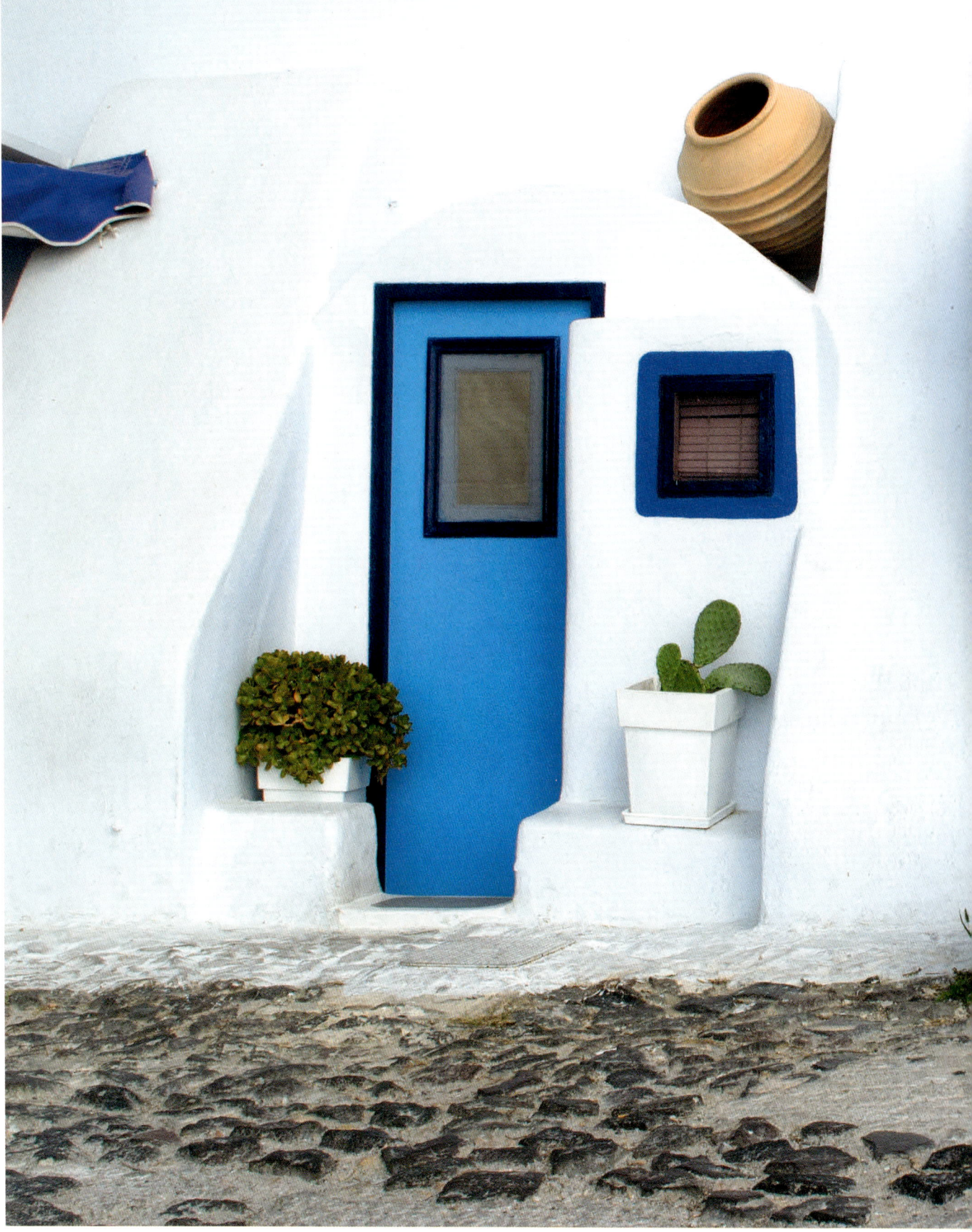

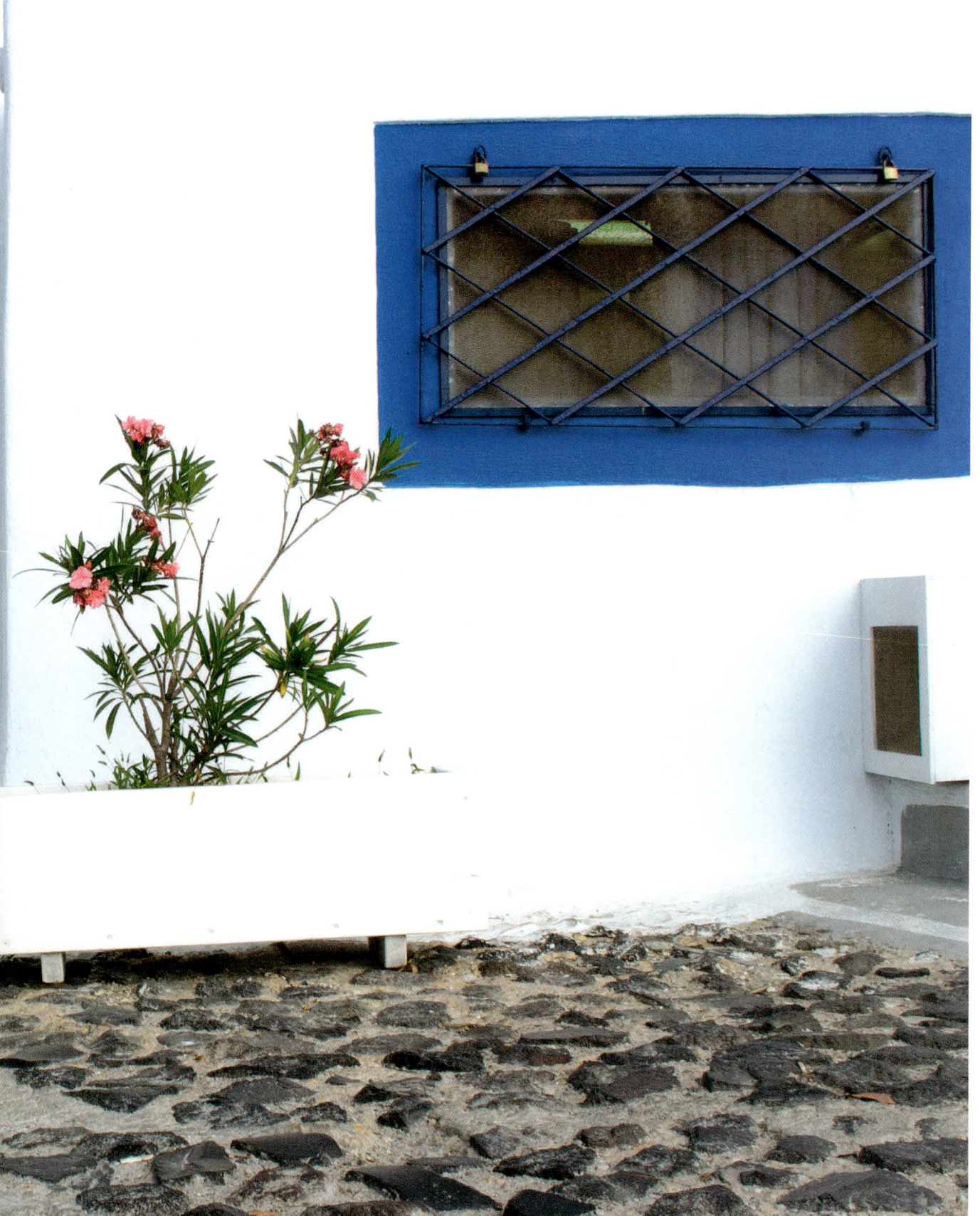

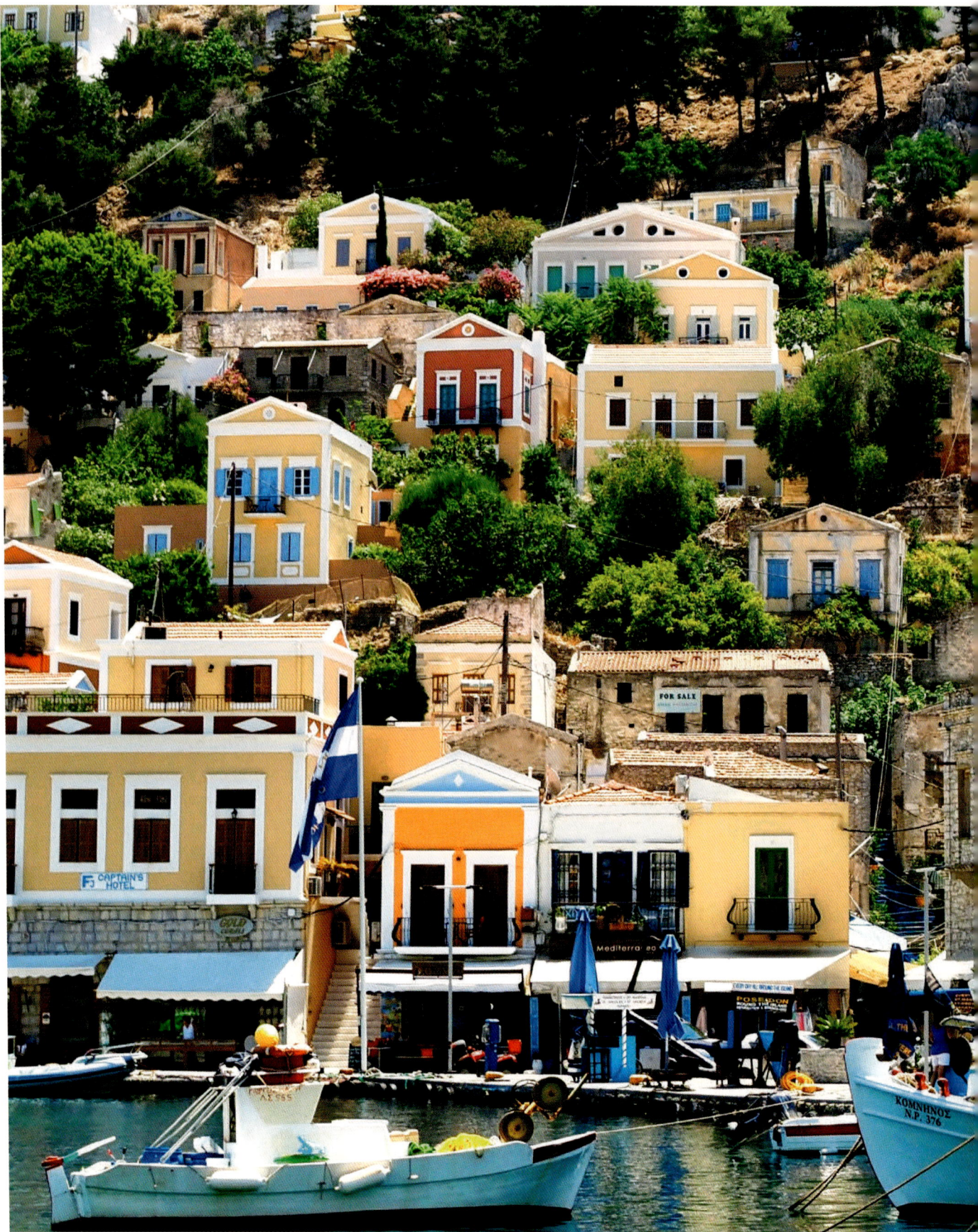

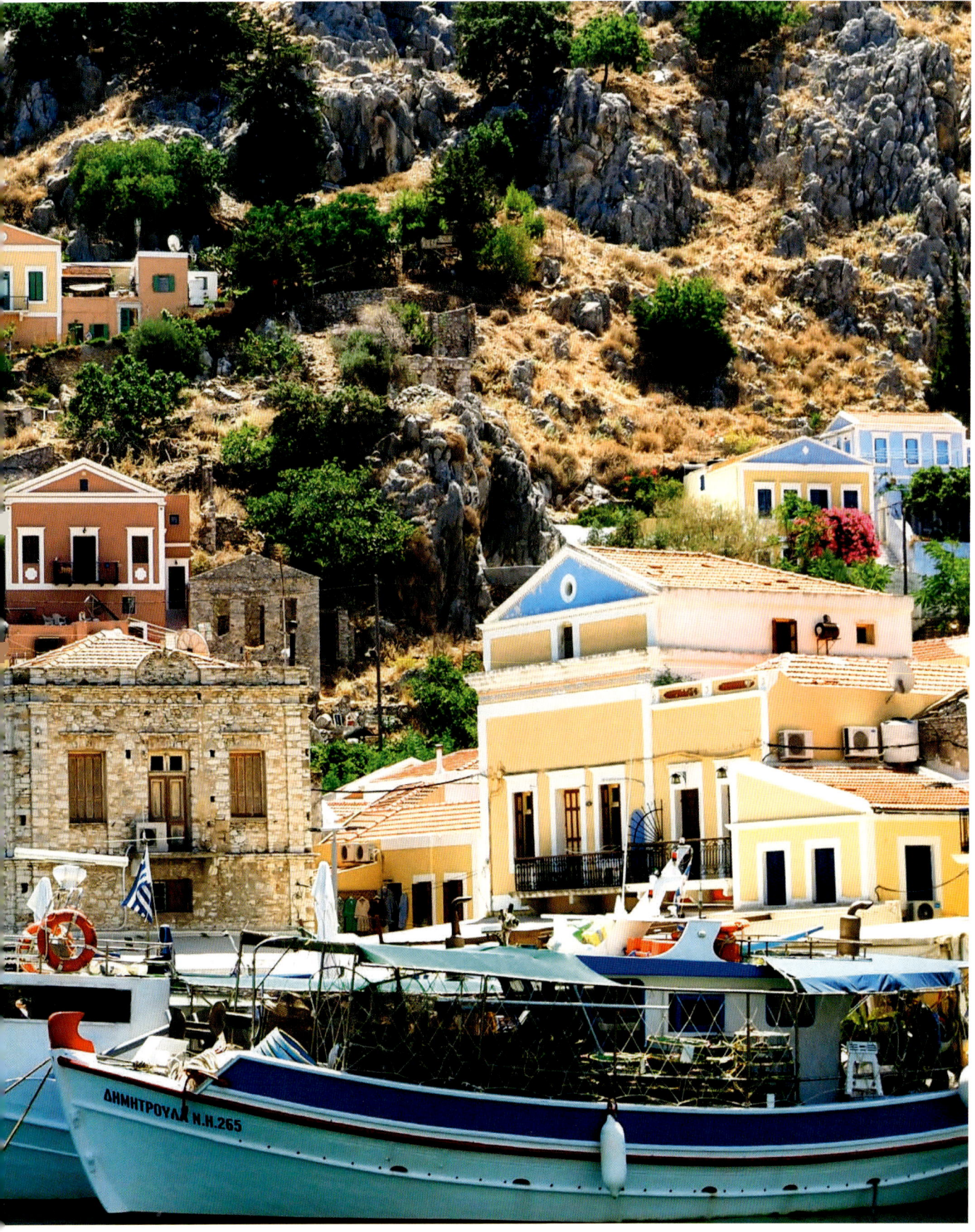

INDEX

A

ALMONDS
- Almond Spiced Kithirian Cookies, 194
- Citrus Almond Cake, 178
- Pastry Parcels with Nuts, Spices, and Orange Syrup, 188

APPLES
- Apple Cake with Olive Oil and Whiskey, 186

ARUGULA
- Arugula. See rocket

ASPARAGUS
- Wild Asparagus with Eggs, 85

B

- Baked Cod with Fried Potato, Zucchini, and Raisin Salsa, 116
- Baked Fish with Okra, 114
- Baked Silverbeet Rolls, 62
- Baklava, Bite-Size Cashew and Orange, 200–01

BEANS
- Black-Eyed Bean Salad, 37

BEETROOT
- Beetroot and Feta Dip, 77
- Roasted Beetroot and Parsley Salad with Honey Dressing, 39

BREAD
- Corfiot Easter Bread, 196–97
- Cypriot Flaounopita, 169
- Feta Cheese and Fennel Koulouri, 170–71
- No-Knead Olive Ciabatta, 165
- Peinirli, 167

C

CAKE
- Apple Cake with Olive Oil and Whiskey, 186
- Citrus Almond Cake, 178
- Rice Pudding Cake, 184
- Yogurt Jelly Cake, 180

CAPERS
- Caper Mash from Syros, 78
- Parsley Dip, 79

CAPSICUMS
- Black-Eyed Bean Salad, 37
- Capsicum and Cheese Pie with Village Pastry, 143
- Chickpea Salad with Marinated Capsicum and Sun-Dried Tomato, 31
- Cod Stew with Capsicums, 106
- Greek Salad, 40
- Lima Beans with Honey and Orange Octopus, 102

CASHEWS
- Bite-Size Cashew and Orange Baklava, 200–01

CAULIFLOWER
- Cauliflower Stew with Spices and Raisins, 87

CHEESE
- Beetroot and Feta Dip, 77
- Capsicum and Cheese Pie with Village Pastry, 143
- Cheese Pie in a Flash with Store-Bought Pastry, 157
- Cheese Pie Made with Yogurt and Milk Pastry, 145

Cheese-Stuffed Eggplants in a Spicy Tomato Sauce, 46

Chickpea Salad with Marinated Capsicum and Sun-Dried Tomato, 31

Cypriot Flaounopita, 169

Feta Cheese and Fennel Koulouri, 170–71

Florina Peppers with Cheese and Zucchini, 44

Greek Salad, 40

Greens with Eggs and Feta Cheese, 81

Kaseropita with Village Pastry, 158

Leek Pie with "Sunray" Phyllo Pastry, 146–47

Lima Beans with Spinach, 54

Mushroom Pastitsio, 66–67

Peinirli, 167

Potato, Olive, and Rosemary Pie with Village Pastry, 150–51

Prawn Saganaki with Lemon, Fennel, and Feta Cheese, 118

Pumpkin Cheese Pies with Village Pastry in Oil, 159

Spaghetti with Fried Cheese and Egg, 60

Spinach, Cheese, and Tomato Open Pie, 155

Stove Top Fried Cheese Pies with Village Pastry, 153

Zucchini Fritters, 88

CHESTNUTS

Chickpeas with Chestnuts, 75

CHICKPEAS

Chickpea Salad with Marinated Capsicum and Sun-Dried Tomato, 31

Chickpea Stew with Honey, 48

Chickpeas with Chestnuts, 75

CHOCOLATE

Finikia from Ikaria, 192

Roxakia (Cocoa and Orange Wheels), 190

Ciabatta, No-Knead Olive, 165

Citrus Almond Cake, 178

COD

Baked Cod with Fried Potato, Zucchini, and Raisin Salsa, 116

Cod Stew with Capsicums, 106

COOKIES

Almond Spiced Kithirian Cookies, 194

Finikia from Ikaria, 192

Yogurt Jelly Cake, 180

Corfiot Easter Bread, 196–97

Crispy Baked Sardine Rolls, 110

CUCUMBERS

Greek Salad, 40

CURRANTS

Cypriot Flaounopita, 169

Vine Leaves Stuffed with Rice, Currants, and Pine Nuts, 82

Cypriot Flaounopita, 169

D

Desserts. See sweets

DILL

Mung Bean and Dill Salad, 32

DIPS

Beetroot and Feta Dip, 77

Parsley Dip, 79

E

Easter Bread, Corfiot, 196–97

EGGPLANT

Cheese-Stuffed Eggplants in a Spicy Tomato Sauce, 46

EGGS

Greens with Eggs and Feta Cheese, 81

Spaghetti with Fried Cheese and Egg, 60

Wild Asparagus with Eggs, 85

F

FENNEL SEEDS

Feta Cheese and Fennel Koulouri, 170–71

Prawn Saganaki with Lemon, Fennel, and Feta Cheese, 118

FETA CHEESE

Beetroot and Feta Dip, 77

Capsicum and Cheese Pie with Village Pastry, 143

Cheese Pie in a Flash with Store-Bought Pastry, 157

Cheese Pie Made with Yogurt and Milk Pastry, 145

Chickpea Salad with Marinated Capsicum and Sun-Dried Tomato, 31

Feta Cheese and Fennel Koulouri, 170–71

Florina Peppers with Cheese and Zucchini, 44

Greek Salad, 40

Greens with Eggs and Feta Cheese, 81

Kaseropita with Village Pastry, 158

Leek Pie with "Sunray" Phyllo Pastry, 146–47

Lima Beans with Spinach, 54

Peinirli, 167

Potato, Olive, and Rosemary Pie with Village Pastry, 150–51

Prawn Saganaki with Lemon, Fennel, and Feta Cheese, 118

Pumpkin Cheese Pies with Village Pastry in Oil, 159

Spinach, Cheese, and Tomato Open Pie, 155

Stove Top Fried Cheese Pies with Village Pastry, 153

Zucchini Fritters, 88

Finikia from Ikaria, 192

FISH AND SEAFOOD

Baked Cod with Fried Potato, Zucchini, and Raisin Salsa, 116

Baked Fish with Okra, 114

Cod Stew with Capsicums, 106

Crispy Baked Sardine Rolls, 110

Lima Beans with Honey and Orange Octopus, 102

Married Sardines, 108

Octopus Stifado, 112

Prawn Saganaki with Lemon, Fennel, and Feta Cheese, 118

Roasted Garlic Mash and Honey Octopus, 122

Savoro (Sweet and Sour Whiting), 104

Stuffed Sardines Wrapped in Vine Leaves, 120

Flaounopita, Cypriot, 169

Florina Peppers with Cheese and Zucchini, 44

Fragrant Rice-Stuffed Onions with Pine Nuts, 58

Fritters, Zucchini, 88

#

GARLIC

Roasted Garlic Mash and Honey Octopus, 122

GLACE FRUITS

Corfiot Easter Bread, 196–97

Greek Salad, 40

GREENS

Baked Silverbeet Rolls, 62

Green Salad with Strawberries and Honey Dressing, 35

Greens with Eggs and Feta Cheese, 81

Leek Pie with "Sunray" Phyllo Pastry, 146–47

Lima Beans with Spinach, 54

Spinach, Cheese, and Tomato Open Pie, 155

Green Salad with Strawberries and Honey Dressing, 35

H

HALLOUMI CHEESE

Cypriot Flaounopita, 169

HONEY

Chickpea Stew with Honey, 48

Green Salad with Strawberries and Honey Dressing, 35

Lima Beans with Honey and Orange Octopus, 102

Roasted Beetroot and Parsley Salad with Honey Dressing, 39

Roasted Garlic Mash and Honey Octopus, 122

J

JELLY

Yogurt Jelly Cake, 180

K

KALAMATA OLIVES

Greek Salad, 40

Ladenia from Kimolos, 163

No-Knead Olive Ciabatta, 165

Potato, Olive, and Rosemary Pie with Village Pastry, 150–51

Kaseropita with Village Pastry, 158

KASSERI CHEESE

Kaseropita with Village Pastry, 158

Peinirli, 167

KATAIFI PASTRY

Pastry Parcels with Nuts, Spices, and Orange Syrup, 188

KEFALOGRAVIERA CHEESE

Cheese-Stuffed Eggplants in a Spicy Tomato Sauce, 46

Florina Peppers with Cheese and Zucchini, 44

Kaseropita with Village Pastry, 158

Mushroom Pastitsio, 66–67

Potato, Olive, and Rosemary Pie with Village Pastry, 150–51

Spinach, Cheese, and Tomato Open Pie, 155

Koulouri, Feta Cheese and Fennel, 170–71

KUMQUAT LIQUEUR

Corfiot Easter Bread, 196–97

L

Ladenia from Kimolos, 163

LEEKS

Leek Pie with "Sunray" Phyllo Pastry, 146–47

Leek with Prunes and White Wine, 83

LEGUMES

Black-Eyed Bean Salad, 37

Chickpea Salad with Marinated Capsicum and Sun-Dried Tomato, 31

Chickpeas with Chestnuts, 75

Lima Beans with Honey and Orange Octopus, 102

Lima Beans with Spinach, 54

Mung Bean and Dill Salad, 32

LEMONS

Prawn Saganaki with Lemon, Fennel, and Feta Cheese, 118

Citrus Almond Cake, 178

LIMA BEANS

Lima Beans with Honey and Orange Octopus, 102

Lima Beans with Spinach, 54

M

MANDARINS

Citrus Almond Cake, 178

Married Sardines, 108

MIZITHRA CHEESE

Spaghetti with Fried Cheese and Egg, 60

Mung Bean and Dill Salad, 32

MUSHROOMS

wild mushrooms, 64

Mushroom and Onion Stew, 68

Mushroom Pastitsio, 66–67

Peinirli, 167

N

No-Knead Olive Ciabatta, 165

NUTS

Almond Spiced Kithirian Cookies, 194

Bite-Size Cashew and Orange Baklava, 200–01

Chickpeas with Chestnuts, 75

Citrus Almond Cake, 178

Fragrant Rice-Stuffed Onions with Pine Nuts, 58

Pastry Parcels with Nuts, Spices, and Orange Syrup, 188

Vine Leaves Stuffed with Rice, Currants, and Pine Nuts, 82

O

OCTOPUS

Lima Beans with Honey and Orange Octopus, 102

Octopus Stifado, 112

Roasted Garlic Mash and Honey Octopus, 122

OKRA

Baked Fish with Okra, 114

OLIVE OIL

Apple Cake with Olive Oil and Whiskey, 186

Olive-Oil Fried Potatoes, 89

Pumpkin Cheese Pies with Village Pastry in Oil, 159

ONIONS

Fragrant Rice-Stuffed Onions with Pine Nuts, 58

Mushroom and Onion Stew, 68

Octopus Stifado, 112

ORANGE BLOSSOM WATER

Bite-Size Cashew and Orange Baklava, 200–01

ORANGES

Citrus Almond Cake, 178

Corfiot Easter Bread, 196–97

Finikia from Ikaria, 192

Lima Beans with Honey and Orange Octopus, 102

Pastry Parcels with Nuts, Spices, and Orange Syrup, 188

Roxakia (Cocoa and Orange Wheels), 190

OUZO

Finikia from Ikaria, 192

P

PAPRIKA

Tomato and Pasta Soup with Sweet Paprika, 56

PARMESAN CHEESE

Cheese Pie in a Flash with Store-Bought Pastry, 157

PARSLEY

Parsley Dip, 79

Roasted Beetroot and Parsley Salad with Honey Dressing, 39

PASTA

Mushroom Pastitsio, 66–67

Spaghetti with Fried Cheese and Egg, 60

Tomato and Pasta Soup with Sweet Paprika, 56

Pastitsio, Mushroom, 66–67

PASTRY, SAVOURY

Capsicum and Cheese Pie with Village Pastry, 143

Cheese Pie in a Flash with Store-Bought Pastry, 157

Cheese Pie Made with Yogurt and Milk Pastry, 145

Cypriot Flaounopita, 169

Feta Cheese and Fennel Koulouri, 170–71

Kaseropita with Village Pastry, 158

Ladenia from Kimolos, 163

Leek Pie with "Sunray" Phyllo Pastry, 146–47

No-Knead Olive Ciabatta, 165

Peinirli, 167

Potato, Olive, and Rosemary Pie with Village Pastry, 150–51

Pumpkin Cheese Pies with Village Pastry in Oil, 159

Spinach, Cheese, and Tomato Open Pie, 155

Stove Top Fried Cheese Pies with Village Pastry, 153

Patates Giahni Me Trahana, 50

PECORINO ROMANO CHEESE

Cypriot Flaounopita, 169

Peinirli, 167

PEPPERS

peppers, bell. See capsicums

peppers, Florina

Florina Peppers with Cheese and Zucchini, 44

PETIMEZI

Cauliflower Stew with Spices and Raisins, 87

Feta Cheese and Fennel Koulouri, 170–71

Savoro (Sweet and Sour Whiting), 104

PHYLLO PASTRY

Bite-Size Cashew and Orange Baklava, 200–01

Cheese Pie in a Flash with Store-Bought Pastry, 157

Leek Pie with "Sunray" Phyllo Pastry, 146–47

Ruffled Vanilla Milk Pie, 182

Pie, Ruffled Vanilla Milk, 182

PINE NUTS

Fragrant Rice-Stuffed Onions with Pine Nuts, 58

Vine Leaves Stuffed with Rice, Currants, and Pine Nuts, 82

POTATOES

Baked Cod with Fried Potato, Zucchini, and Raisin Salsa, 116

Caper Mash from Syros, 78

Leek with Prunes and White Wine, 83

Olive-Oil Fried Potatoes, 89

Parsley Dip, 79

Patates Giahni Me Trahana, 50

Peinirli, 167

Potato, Olive, and Rosemary Pie with Village Pastry, 150–51

Roasted Garlic Mash and Honey Octopus, 122

Spicy (Not Hot) Baked Potatoes, 52

Stuffed Potatoes and Tomatoes, 70

PRAWNS

Prawn Saganaki with Lemon, Fennel, and Feta Cheese, 118

PRUNES

Leek with Prunes and White Wine, 83

PUMPKIN

Pumpkin Cheese Pies with Village Pastry in Oil, 159

R

RAISINS

Baked Cod with Fried Potato, Zucchini, and Raisin Salsa, 116

Cauliflower Stew with Spices and Raisins, 87

Savoro (Sweet and Sour Whiting), 104

RICE

Baked Silverbeet Rolls, 62

Fragrant Rice-Stuffed Onions with Pine Nuts, 58

Rice Pudding Cake, 184

Stuffed Potatoes and Tomatoes, 70

Vine Leaves Stuffed with Rice, Currants, and Pine Nuts, 82

RICOTTA CHEESE

Cheese Pie Made with Yogurt and Milk Pastry, 145

Cheese-Stuffed Eggplants in a Spicy Tomato Sauce, 46

Florina Peppers with Cheese and Zucchini, 44

Roasted Beetroot and Parsley Salad with Honey Dressing, 39

Roasted Garlic Mash and Honey Octopus, 122

rocket

Athenian Rocket Salad with Tomato, Lemon Juice, and Rock Salt, 33

rosemary

Potato, Olive, and Rosemary Pie with Village Pastry, 150–51

rose water

Almond Spiced Kithirian Cookies, 194

Roxakia (Cocoa and Orange Wheels), 190

Ruffled Vanilla Milk Pie, 182

S

SALADS

Athenian Rocket Salad with Tomato, Lemon Juice, and Rock Salt, 33

Black-Eyed Bean Salad, 37

Chickpea Salad with Marinated Capsicum and Sun-Dried Tomato, 31

Greek Salad, 40

Green Salad with Strawberries and Honey Dressing, 35

Mung Bean and Dill Salad, 32

Roasted Beetroot and Parsley Salad with Honey Dressing, 39

SARDINES

Crispy Baked Sardine Rolls, 110

Married Sardines, 108

Stuffed Sardines Wrapped in Vine Leaves, 120

Savoro (Sweet and Sour Whiting), 104

SEAFOOD. *See fish and seafood*

SESAME SEEDS

Feta Cheese and Fennel Koulouri, 170–71

Silverbeet Rolls, Baked, 62

SNAPPER

Baked Fish with Okra, 114

Spaghetti with Fried Cheese and Egg, 60

Spicy (Not Hot) Baked Potatoes, 52

SPINACH

Leek Pie with "Sunray" Phyllo Pastry, 146–47

Lima Beans with Spinach, 54

Spinach, Cheese, and Tomato Open Pie, 155

STEW

    Cauliflower Stew with Spices and Raisins, 87

    Chickpea Stew with Honey, 48

    Cod Stew with Capsicums, 106

    Mushroom and Onion Stew, 68

Stove Top Fried Cheese Pies with Village Pastry, 153

STRAWBERRIES

    Green Salad with Strawberries and Honey Dressing, 35

    Yogurt Jelly Cake, 180

Stuffed Potatoes and Tomatoes, 70

Stuffed Sardines Wrapped in Vine Leaves, 120

SWEETS

    Almond Spiced Kithirian Cookies, 194

    Apple Cake with Olive Oil and Whiskey, 186

    Bite-Size Cashew and Orange Baklava, 200–01

    Citrus Almond Cake, 178

    Corfiot Easter Bread, 196–97

    Finikia from Ikaria, 192

    Pastry Parcels with Nuts, Spices, and Orange Syrup, 188

    Rice Pudding Cake, 184

    Roxakia (Cocoa and Orange Wheels), 190

    Ruffled Vanilla Milk Pie, 182

    Yogurt Jelly Cake, 180

T

TOMATOES

    Athenian Rocket Salad with Tomato, Lemon Juice, and Rock Salt, 33

    Greek Salad, 40

    Kaseropita with Village Pastry, 158

    Ladenia from Kimolos, 163

    Spinach, Cheese, and Tomato Open Pie, 155

    Stuffed Potatoes and Tomatoes, 70

TOMATOES, CANNED OR PUREED

    Baked Silverbeet Rolls, 62

    Cheese-Stuffed Eggplants in a Spicy Tomato Sauce, 46

    Chickpea Stew with Honey, 48

    Fragrant Rice-Stuffed Onions with Pine Nuts, 58

    Mushroom and Onion Stew, 68

    Tomato and Pasta Soup with Sweet Paprika, 56

TOMATOES, SUN-DRIED

    Chickpea Salad with Marinated Capsicum and Sun-Dried Tomato, 31

TRAHANA

    Patates Giahni Me Trahana, 50

V

    Vanilla Milk Pie, Ruffled, 182

    VILLAGE PASTRY

    Capsicum and Cheese Pie with Village Pastry, 143

    Kaseropita with Village Pastry, 158

    Potato, Olive, and Rosemary Pie with Village Pastry, 150–51

    Pumpkin Cheese Pies with Village Pastry in Oil, 159

    Stove Top Fried Cheese Pies with Village Pastry, 153

VINE LEAVES

    Stuffed Sardines Wrapped in Vine Leaves, 120

    Vine Leaves Stuffed with Rice, Currants, and Pine Nuts, 82

W

WALNUTS

Pastry Parcels with Nuts, Spices, and Orange Syrup, 188

WHISKEY

Apple Cake with Olive Oil and Whiskey, 186

WHITE WINE

Leek with Prunes and White Wine, 83

WHITING

Savoro (Sweet and Sour Whiting), 104

Wild Asparagus with Eggs, 85

Y

YOGURT

Cheese Pie Made with Yogurt and Milk Pastry, 145

Yogurt Jelly Cake, 180

Z

ZUCCHINI

Baked Cod with Fried Potato, Zucchini, and Raisin Salsa, 116

Florina Peppers with Cheese and Zucchini, 44

Zucchini Fritters, 88

COOK'S NOTES

Have kitchen scales handy when cooking from my book. I like to weigh things for accuracy.

All measurements in this book use American cup measurements, which are slightly smaller than a metric cup.

1 cup = 240 ml or 8.44 oz.

½ cup = 118 ml or 4.15 oz.

¼ cup = 59 ml or 2.0 oz.

⅓ cup = 79 ml or 2.7 oz.

1 tablespoon = 15 ml

1 teaspoon = 5 ml

UNLESS OTHERWISE STATED:

Oil is always extra-virgin olive oil

Onions are brown onions

Salt is sea salt

Capsicums are bell peppers

Eggs are organic

Yogurt is always Greek yogurt

Corn flour is corn starch

Parsely is always flat leaf variety

Kanella Productions P/L

ruth.bardis@gmail.com

Text copyright © 2021 by Ruth Bardis

Photographs copyright © 2021 by Ruth Bardis

Photography: Ruth Bardis

Unsplash images (page 12, 18, 34, 74, 113, 221) used with permission

Styling: Ruth Bardis

Graphic design: Kim Ellis

Digital art (page 33, 67, 78, 83, 88, 101, 116, 139, 197, 231, 204-217): Kim Ellis (kitellis.creates@gmail.com)

Digital art (page 21-23): Brydee Pilarinos

All rights reserved. No part of this work may be reproduced or utilized in any form or by any means, electronic or mechanical, including photocopying, recording or by any information storage and retrieval system, without the prior written permission of the publisher.

ISBN: 978-0-646-85431-1

Printed in China

ACKNOWLEDGMENTS

I always find it hard to list the amount of people who contribute to making my book dream a reality. Sometimes it needs to be as simple as this:

To all who have previously bought either of my other publications. As books get sold, the more I'm driven to keep writing about Greek food. You remind me of how much people love to eat Greek. The support I have received is humbling! Thank you for giving me an excuse to cook my heart out, write, and share this with the world.

To my big, fat Greek family! Jenny, Tony, Peter, James, Stephania, Anita, Abigail, Bill, Olga, Paula, Damian, JJ, Anna, Peter, Noah, Paulina, Matty, Brydee, Dominic, Emilyia, Gianni, Chistian, Hannah and Savvas-each one of you have, in some way or another (known to you or not), encouraged me to want to keep doing what I love to do. May my books inspire you to know more of your family roots and cook Greek for many generations to come.

To my inlaws for sharing with me, many more Greek foods.

Mum, my love for cooking Greek starts with you. What an amazing role model you are in hospitality. Thank you for teaching me how to appreciate and love cooking.

Dad, your business mind is in my genes. Thank you for always challenging me to keep reaching for the stars! As you have said, I may not reach them, but the journey there is exhilarating. Thank you for showing me the importance of working hard, being true to my strengths, and being loyal in my endeavors.

Kim Ellis, thank you for your hard work, time, and joy in working to bring my vision to book form. You are the best!

Tony, thank you for your Greek grammar expertise and the excitement you share in my food adventures. Brydee, thank you for your artwork in the folk medicine section. You depicted my hubby and I so well, I love your creativity and passion for art. Abigail, your painting on page 41 was such a cute addition to my book, your attention to detail is amazing.

Athanasios, my husband, how can I express enough appreciation to you, the person who knows my struggles, my achievements, my true journey in arriving here? Thank you for embracing my creativity in writing books. You know what you mean to me. I could easily write a book solely on you, but here I will say a humble thank you. I love you!

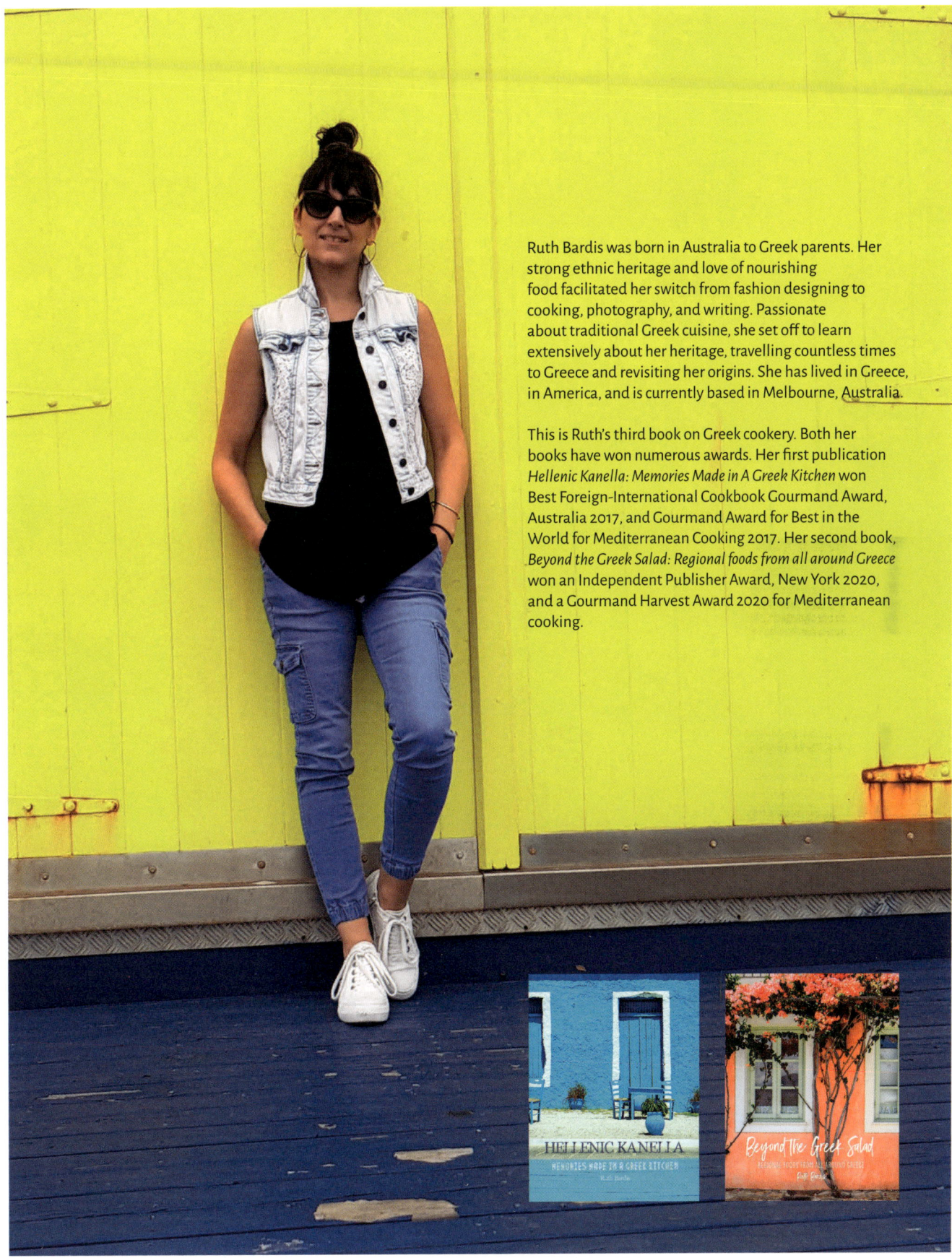

Ruth Bardis was born in Australia to Greek parents. Her strong ethnic heritage and love of nourishing food facilitated her switch from fashion designing to cooking, photography, and writing. Passionate about traditional Greek cuisine, she set off to learn extensively about her heritage, travelling countless times to Greece and revisiting her origins. She has lived in Greece, in America, and is currently based in Melbourne, Australia.

This is Ruth's third book on Greek cookery. Both her books have won numerous awards. Her first publication *Hellenic Kanella: Memories Made in A Greek Kitchen* won Best Foreign-International Cookbook Gourmand Award, Australia 2017, and Gourmand Award for Best in the World for Mediterranean Cooking 2017. Her second book, *Beyond the Greek Salad: Regional foods from all around Greece* won an Independent Publisher Award, New York 2020, and a Gourmand Harvest Award 2020 for Mediterranean cooking.

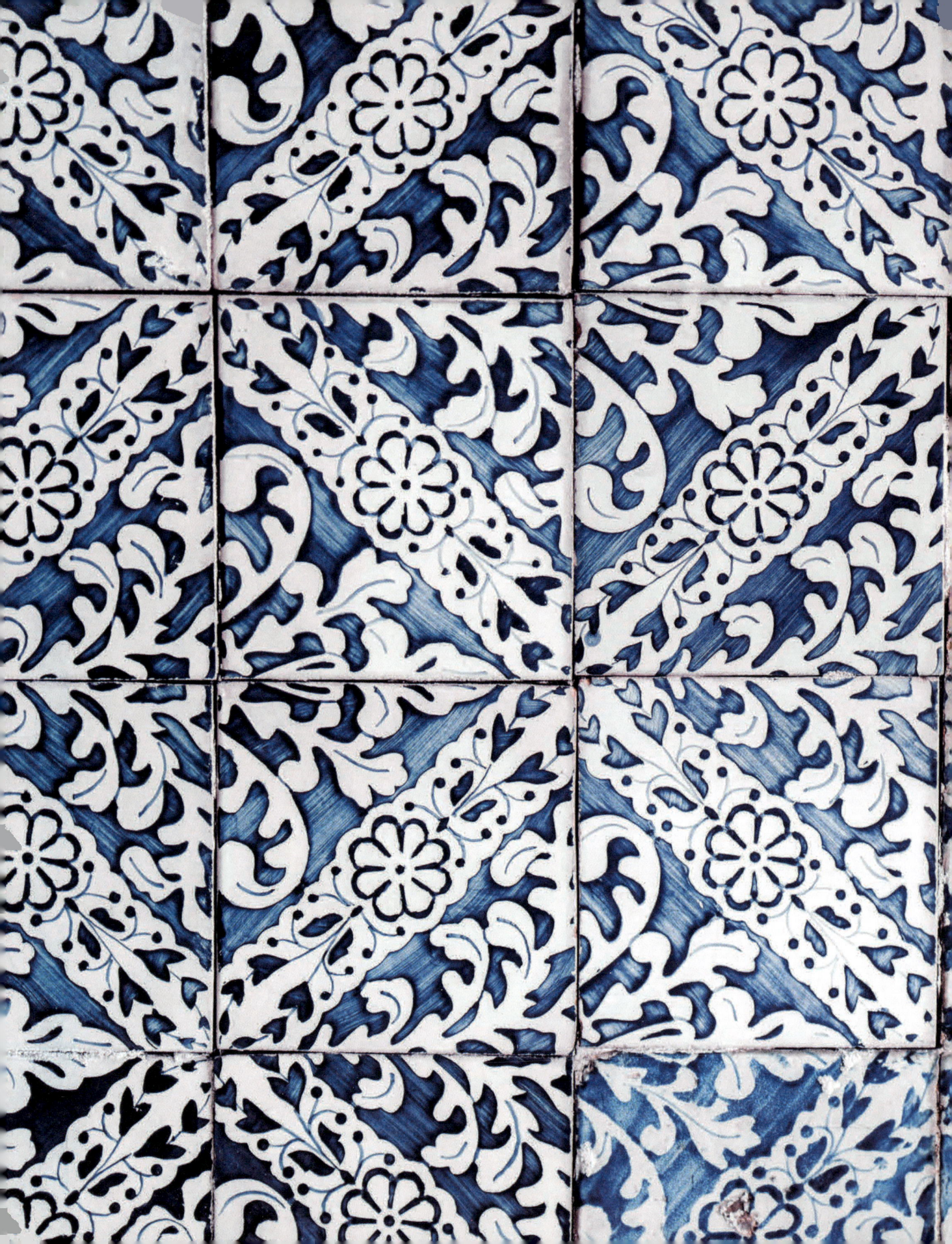